Epidermolysis Bullosa: Part II – Diagnosis and Management

Guest Editor

DÉDÉE F. MURRELL, MA, BMBCh, FAAD, MD

DERMATOLOGIC CLINICS

www.derm.theclinics.com

Consulting Editor

BRUCE H. THIERS, MD

April 2010 • Volume 28 • Number 2

SAUNDERS an imprint of ELSEVIER, Inc.

W.B. SAUNDERS COMPANY
A Division of Elsevier Inc.

1600 John F. Kennedy Boulevard ● Suite 1800 ● Philadelphia, PA 19103-2899

http://www.theclinics.com

DERMATOLOGIC CLINICS Volume 28, Number 2
April 2010 ISSN 0733-8635, ISBN-13: 978-1-4377-1813-3

Editor: Carla Holloway

Dermatologic Clinics (ISSN 0733-8635) is published quarterly by Elsevier Inc., 360 Park Avenue South, New York, NY 10010-1710. Months of publication are January, April, July, and October. Business and editorial offices: 1600 John F. Kennedy Blvd., Suite 1800, Philadelphia, PA 19103-2899. Customer service office: 11830 Westline Drive, St. Louis, MO 63146. Periodicals postage paid at New York, NY, and additional mailing offices. Subscription prices are USD 296.00 per year for US individuals, USD 431.00 per year for US institutions, USD 347.00 per year for Canadian individuals, USD 516.00 per year for Canadian institutions, USD 406.00 per year for international individuals, USD 516.00 per year for international institutions, USD 141.00 per year for US students/residents, and USD 204.00 per year for Canadian and international students/residents. International air speed delivery is included in all *Clinics* subscription prices. All prices are subject to change without notice. **POSTMASTER:** Send address changes to *Dermatologic Clinics*, Elsevier Health Sciences Division, Subscription Customer Service, 3251 Riverport Lane, Maryland Heights, MO 63043. **Customer Service: 1-800-654-2452 (U.S. and Canada); 314-447-8871 (outside U.S. and Canada). Fax: 314-447-8029. E-mail: journalscustomerservice-usa@elsevier.com (for print support); journalsonlinesupport-usa@elsevier.com (for online support).**

Reprints. For copies of 100 or more, of articles in this publication, please contact the Commercial Reprints Department, Elsevier Inc., 360 Park Avenue South, New York, New York 10010-1710. Tel.: (212) 633-3813; Fax: (212) 462-1935; Email: reprints@elsevier.com.

The *Dermatologic Clinics* is covered in *MEDLINE/PubMed (Index Medicus), Current Contents/Clinical Medicine, Excerpta Medica, Chemical Abstracts,* and *ISI/BIOMED.*

Contributors

CONSULTING EDITOR

BRUCE H. THIERS, MD
Professor and Chairman, Department
of Dermatology and Dermatologic Surgery,
Medical University of South Carolina,
Charleston, South Carolina

GUEST EDITOR

DÉDÉE F. MURRELL, MA, BMBCh, FAAD, MD
Professor and Head, Department of Dermatology,
St George Hospital, University of New South
Wales, Kogarah, Sydney, New South Wales,
Australia

AUTHORS

JEREMY ALLGROVE, MA, MD, FRCP, FRCPCH
Department of Paediatric Endocrinology, Barts
and the London NHS Trust, Royal London
Hospital, Whitechapel; Great Ormond Street
Hospital for Children NHS Trust, London, United
Kingdom

NOOR ALMAANI, MRCP
St John's Institute of Dermatology, Guy's and St
Thomas' NHS Foundation Trust, St Thomas'
Hospital, London, United Kingdom

H. ALAN ARBUCKLE, MD, FAAP, FAAD
Director, Epidermolysis Bullosa Center for
Excellence; Director, Wound Care Clinic, The
Children's Hospital, Aurora; Assistant Chief,
Dermatologic Services VA Medical Center,
Denver; Assistant Professor of Pediatrics and
Dermatology, University of Colorado School of
Medicine, Colorado

RICHARD G. AZIZKHAN, MD, PhD, FACS, FAAP
Surgeon-in-Chief, Lester Martin Chair of Pediatric
Surgery, Professor of Surgery and Pediatrics,
Division of Pediatric and Thoracic Surgery,
Epidermolysis Bullosa Treatment Center,
Cincinnati Children's Hospital Medical Center,
University of Cincinnati College of Medicine,
Cincinnati, Ohio

CATINA BERNARDIS, MBBS, BSc, FRCS (Plast)
Consultant Plastic Surgeon, Department of Plastic
Surgery, St Thomas' Hospital, London, United
Kingdom

CHRISTINE BODEMER, MD, PhD
Team Leader of the National Reference Center for
Genodermatosis MAGEC (*Maladies Génétiques à
Expression Cutanée*); Department of Dermatology,
Necker Enfants Malades Hospital, APHP Paris;
University René Descartes; Institut National
de la Santé et de la Recherche Médicale,
Paris, France

RACHEL BOX, BSc (Occupational Therapy)
Hand Therapist, Department of Hand Therapy,
St Thomas' Hospital, London,
United Kingdom

**CAROLINE BRAIN, MB, BS, MD, MRCP,
FRCPCH,**
Consultant Paediatric Endocrinologist,
Department of Paediatric Endocrinology, Great
Ormond Street Hospital for Children NHS Trust,
London, United Kingdom

LEENA BRUCKNER-TUDERMAN, MD
Department of Dermatology, University Medical
Center Freiburg, Freiburg, Germany

MITCHELL S. CAIRO, MD
Professor, Departments of Pediatrics,
Pathology, and Medicine, Morgan Stanley
Children's Hospital of New York-Presbyterian
Hospital, Columbia University, New York,
New York

DANIELE CASTIGLIA, PhD
Team Leader, Laboratory of Molecular and Cell
Biology, IDI-IRCCS, Rome, Italy

RODRIGO CEPEDA-VALDES, MD
DebRA MEXICO AC, Monterrey, Nuevo León,
Mexico

A. CHARLESWORTH, MSc
INSERM U634, Faculty of Medicine, Nice, France

C. CHIAVÉRINI, MD, PhD
French Reference Center of Hereditary
Epidermolysis Bullosa; Department of
Dermatology, Archet Hospital, Nice, France

ANGELA M. CHRISTIANO, PhD
Professor, Departments of Dermatology and
Genetics and Development, Columbia University,
New York, New York

JACQUELINE E. DENYER, RGN, RSCN, RHV
Clinical Nurse Specialist, Department of
Dermatology, Great Ormond Street Hospital,
London; DebRA UK, Crowthorne, United Kingdom

PATRICIA J.C. DOPPING-HEPENSTAL, BSc
Laboratory Head, National Diagnostic
Epidermolysis Bullosa Laboratory, GSTS
Pathology, St John's Institute of Dermatology,
St Thomas' Hospital, London, United Kingdom

JOSÉ C. DUIPMANS, MScN, RN
Specialist EB-nurse, Center for Blistering
Diseases, Department of Dermatology, University
Medical Center Groningen, University of
Groningen, Groningen, The Netherlands

ROBIN A.J. EADY, DSc, FRCP
Emeritus Professor, St John's Institute of
Dermatology, St Thomas' Hospital, London,
United Kingdom

HIVA FASSIHI, MD, MRCP (UK)
Specialist Registrar in Dermatology, Division of
Genetics and Molecular Medicine, Guy's Hospital,
St John's Institute of Dermatology, King's
College London (Guy's Campus), London,
United Kingdom

KENNETH R. GOLDSCHNEIDER, MD
Associate Professor of Clinical Anesthesiology
and Pediatrics, University of Cincinnati College
of Medicine; Director, Division of Pain
Management, Department of Anesthesiology,
Cincinnati Children's Hospital Medical Center,
Cincinnati, Ohio

LESLEY HAYNES, RD
Dietetic Department, Great Ormond Street
Hospital for Children NHS Trust, London,
United Kingdom

HELMUT HINTNER, MD
Professor of Dermatology, Head of the
Department of Dermatology and the EB House
Austria, Department of Dermatology, Paracelsus
Medical University, Salzburg, Austria

ALAIN HOVNANIAN, MD, PhD
Institut National de la santé et de la recherche
médicale; Department of Genetics and
Dermatology, Necker Hospital for Sick Children,
Paris; University René Descartes, Paris, France

**RICHARD HOWARD, BSc, MB, ChB, FRCA,
FFPMRCA**
Consultant in Anesthesia and Pain Medicine,
Department of Anaesthesia, Great Ormond Street
Hospital for Children, London, United Kingdom

LIZBETH RUTH A. INTONG, MD
Fellow, Department of Dermatology, St George
Hospital, Kogarah, Sydney, New South Wales,
Australia

MUNENARI ITOH, MD, PhD
Postdoctoral Fellow, Department of Dermatology,
Columbia University, New York, New York

MARCEL F. JONKMAN, MD, PhD
Professor and Chair, Center for Blistering
Diseases, Department of Dermatology, University
Medical Center Groningen, University of
Groningen, Groningen, The Netherlands

SAROLTA KÁRPÁTI, MD, PhD, DSc
Chair, Department of Dermato-Venereology and
Dermatooncology, Semmelweis University; Head,
Dermatology Division of the Molecular Medicine
Research Group, Hungarian Academy of
Sciences, Budapest, Hungary

**M. TARIQ KHAN, PhD, BSc (Hons),
BSc (Pod Med), DFHom (Pod)**
Director and Consulting Podiatrist, Marigold
Clinic, Royal London Homeopathic Hospital, NHS
Foundation Trust; Consultant Podiatrist, EB
Department, Great Ormond Street Hospital for
Sick Children, London, United Kingdom

MAIJA KIURU, MD, PhD
Postdoctoral Fellow, Department of Dermatology,
Columbia University, New York, New York

SUSANNE M. KRÄMER, DDS, MSc SND
Honorary Lecturer, Department of Oral Medicine
and Special Needs Dentistry, UCL Eastman Dental
Institute, London, United Kingdom; Lecturer,
Division of Pediatric Dentistry, School of Dentistry,
University of Chile, Independencia; DebRA Chile,
Las Condes, Santiago, Chile

J.P. LACOUR, MD
French Reference Center of Hereditary
Epidermolysis Bullosa; Department of
Dermatology, Archet Hospital, INSERM U634,
Faculty of Medicine, Nice, France

IRENE LARA-CORRALES, MD, MSc
The Hospital for Sick Children, Toronto, Ontario,
Canada

CARMEN LIY-WONG, MD
Department of Dermatology, Hospital Universitario
"Dr Jose E. Gonzalez" UANL, Monterrey, Nuevo
León, Mexico

ANNE W. LUCKY, MD
Volunteer Professor of Dermatology and
Pediatrics, University of Cincinnati College of
Medicine; Co-Director, Cincinnati Children's
Epidermolysis Bullosa Center; Division of Pediatric
Dermatology, Cincinnati Children's Hospital
Medical Center, Cincinnati, Ohio

MAGEC-NECKER TEAM
Department of Dermatology, Necker Enfants
Malades Hospital, APHP Paris, France

ANNA E. MARTINEZ, MBBS, MRCP, MRCPCH
Consultant Paediatrician, Department of
Paediatric Dermatology, Great Ormond Street
Hospital for Children NHS Trust, London,
United Kingdom

JOHN A. MCGRATH, MD, FRCP
Professor of Molecular Dermatology, Division
of Genetics and Molecular Medicine,
Guy's Hospital, St John's Institute of Dermatology,
King's College London (Guy's Campus),
London, United Kingdom

MÁRTA MEDVECZ, MD, PhD
Assistant Lecturer, Department of Dermato-
Venereology and Dermatooncology, Semmelweis
University; Researcher, Molecular Medicine
Research Group, Hungarian Academy of
Sciences, Budapest, Hungary

JEMIMA E. MELLERIO, BSc, MD, FRCP
Consultant Dermatologist, St John's Institute
of Dermatology, Guy's and St Thomas' NHS
Foundation Trust, St Thomas' Hospital;
Department of Paediatric Dermatology, Great
Ormond Street Hospital for Children NHS Trust,
London, United Kingdom

G. MENEGUZZI, PhD
INSERM U634, Faculty of Medicine, Nice, France

ALAN E. MORTELL, FRCSI, MD
Division of Pediatric and Thoracic Surgery,
Epidermolysis Bullosa Treatment Center,
Cincinnati Children's Hospital Medical Center,
University of Cincinnati College of Medicine,
Cincinnati, Ohio

DÉDÉE F. MURRELL, MA, BMBCh, FAAD, MD
Professor and Head, Department of Dermatology,
St George Hospital, University of New South
Wales, Kogarah, Sydney, New South Wales,
Australia

REEMA NANDI, MD, FRCA
Consultant in Anesthesia and Pain Medicine,
Department of Anaesthesia, Great Ormond Street
Hospital for Children, London, United Kingdom

KEN NATSUGA, MD
Department of Dermatology, Hokkaido University
Graduate School of Medicine, Sapporo,
Japan

WATARU NISHIE, MD, PhD
Department of Dermatology, Hokkaido University
Graduate School of Medicine, Sapporo, Japan

J.P. ORTONNE, MD, PhD
French Reference Center for Hereditary
Epidermolysis Bullosa; Department of
Dermatology, Archet Hospital, Nice, France

VALÉRIE PENDARIES, PhD
Institut National de la santé et de la recherche
médicale; University Paul-Sabatier, Toulouse,
France

GABRIELA POHLA-GUBO, PhD
Head of the Laboratory for Immunology,
Allergology and Molecular Diagnostics and the EB
Academy at the EB House Austria, Department of
Dermatology, Paracelsus Medical University,
Salzburg, Austria

ELENA POPE, MD, MSc
Associate Professor, University of Toronto; Head,
Section of Dermatology, The Hospital for Sick
Children, Toronto, Ontario, Canada

JULIO CESAR SALAS-ALANIS, MD
DebRA MEXICO AC, Monterrey, Nuevo León,
Mexico

HIROSHI SHIMIZU, MD, PhD
Professor and Chairman, Department of
Dermatology, Hokkaido University Graduate
School of Medicine, Sapporo, Japan

SATORU SHINKUMA, MD
Department of Dermatology, Hokkaido University
Graduate School of Medicine, Sapporo, Japan

ELI SPRECHER, MD, PhD
Tel Aviv Sourasky Medical Center, Department of
Dermatology, Tel Aviv, Israel

VIRGINIA P. SYBERT, MD
Clinical Professor of Medicine, Division
of Medical Genetics, University of Washington
School of Medicine; Pediatric Dermatologist,
Group Health Permanente, Seattle,
Washington

KAISA TASANEN, MD, PhD
Associate Professor, Department of
Dermatology, Clinical Research Center,
Oulu University Hospital, University of Oulu,
Oulu, Finland

MATTHIAS TITEUX, PhD
Institut National de la santé et de la recherche
médicale; University Paul-Sabatier, Toulouse,
France

ANDERS VAHLQUIST, MD, PhD
Professor, Department of Medical Sciences,
Uppsala University, University Hospital, Uppsala,
Sweden

SUPRIYA S. VENUGOPAL, BSc, MBBS, MMed
Department of Dermatology, St George Hospital,
University of New South Wales, Kogarah, Sydney,
New South Wales, Australia

ROSEMARIE WATSON, MD, FRCPI, FACP
Director, National EB Service, St James' Hospital;
Our Lady's Children's Hospital Crumlin;
Consultant Dermatologist, Senior Lecturer, Trinity
College, Dublin, Ireland

W.F. YAN, MBBS, MSc
Department of Dermatology, St George Hospital,
Kogarah; University of New South Wales, Sydney,
New South Wales, Australia

GIOVANNA ZAMBRUNO, MD
Director, Laboratory of Molecular and Cell Biology,
IDI-IRCCS, Rome, Italy

Contents

The definitive diagnosis of inherited epidermolysis bullosa is best made with positive immunofluorescence antigenic mapping, transmission electron microscopy, and epidermolysis bullosa–related monoclonal antibody studies. However, immunofluorescence microscopy is faster and easier as compared with electron microscopy for subtyping epidermolysis bullosa. The severity of the disease varies with the structural protein involved. A proper diagnosis should be made as soon as possible, and skin biopsies help with diagnosis. This article describes the technique of skin biopsy.

Immunofluorescence mapping is based on the detection of structural proteins of keratinocytes or of the dermo-epidermal junction using specific poly- or monoclonal antibodies. Through this method, the level of split formation can be determined by investigating the location of a given antigen in a natural or induced blister. This method also allows testing for the normal expression, reduction or absence of various structural proteins depending on the antibodies used. It has widely replaced transmission electron microscopy and is used as the initial laboratory test to prove the clinical diagnosis of epidermolysis bullosa.

Transmission electron microscopy (TEM) has long been the best available method for the diagnosis of epidermolysis bullosa. Today, TEM is largely superseded by immunofluorescence microscopy mapping, which is generally more available. This article discusses its continuing role in confirming or refining results obtained by other methods, or in establishing the diagnosis where other techniques have been unsuitable or have failed. It covers key steps for optimizing tissue preparation, features of analysis, recently classified epidermolysis bullosa disorders, and strengths and weaknesses of TEM.

The development of DNA technology and improved knowledge of the structure and function of the human genome have led to the identification of the causative genes responsible for the different forms of epidermolysis bullosa (EB) and provided the opportunity to determine the precise location and type of mutations present in EB patients, allowing diagnosis of this disease at the level of the defective gene itself. The large genetic heterogeneity of EB, however, precludes the direct use of molecular testing for EB diagnosis. In addition, only a few diagnostic or research laboratories in the world are equipped to perform mutational screening, which is still labor intensive and associated with considerable costs, because most mutations are unique to one or a few families. This article reviews the most popular methods used in EB molecular analysis.

One of the most significant benefits of translational research in dermatology has been the development of prenatal diagnosis for couples at risk of recurrence of severe inherited skin diseases. Indeed, over the last 30 years a greater understanding of the molecular basis of epidermolysis bullosa (EB), as well as technical refinements in laboratory procedures, has facilitated the development of several different approaches for prenatal diagnosis. Initial tests were based on fetal skin biopsy sampling, but these have largely been superseded by DNA based analyses, mostly using fetal DNA derived from chorionic villus sampling taken at around 10–12 weeks' gestation. Further advances, however, have led to the introduction of licensed preimplantation genetic screening for some forms of EB, an approach that defines a disease-associated genotype before implantation into the uterus. Pioneering research also continues to try to develop less invasive approaches with the prospects of maternal blood sampling early during the first trimester as a feasible objective. The availability of several different options for prenatal diagnostic testing therefore has led to an increased choice for families at risk of recurrence of EB.

This article contains the author's views on genetic counseling in cases concerning the epidermolysis bullosa syndromes. The provision of genetic counseling entails absolutes such as diagnosis, natural history, treatment, mode of inheritance, recurrence risks/prenatal diagnosis and referral. The genetic counselor needs to be informed and informative and answer all the needs of the patients and their families reliably both at the initial consultation and subsequently as needed over the course of the patient's life.

Epidermolysis bullosa simplex (EBS) is an inherited skin disorder characterized by separation of the epidermis from the underlying dermis, with the cleavage plane lying within the basal-cell layer of the epithelium. The major clinical subtypes of EBS have a dominant inheritance and have been associated with genetic defects in specific domains of keratins K5 and K14 that result in abnormal organization of the keratin network and cell disruption. Autosomal recessive forms of EBS associated with extracutaneous manifestations, such as muscular dystrophy (MIM 226670) or pyloric atresia (MIM 612138), have been linked to genetic mutations in the gene for plectin (*PLEC*). *PLEC* mutations have also been found in 2 families with the rare dominant Ogna form of EBS. This article reviews current knowledge on EBS.

MANAGEMENT

Skin and wound care in epidermolysis bullosa (EB) is specific both to the type of EB and to individual wounds within each child. Availability of dressings and personal preference are also paramount in the selection of materials. The ideal dressing is yet to be developed, although there are now a variety of suitable dressings available. This article discusses current techniques of wound and dressing management for EB simplex, junctional EB, and dystrophic EB. Factors adversely affecting healing include anemia, malnutrition, infection, and pruritus.

Bathing is very difficult for individuals with epidermolysis bullosa (EB), although anecdotally preferred to showering. This article reviews the as yet small body of research literature that documents or quantifies the impact of bathing on EB patients.

In all forms of epidermolysis bullosa (EB), skin fragility may result in bacterial colonization or infection, particularly in the more severe forms where wounds may be multiple and long-standing. A balance exists between a wound's bacterial load and the host defenses, such that there is a spectrum from simple contamination, through colonization, critical colonization, to overt infection. The increased bioburden in critically colonized or infected wounds impairs healing and therefore recognition of these situations, and appropriate measures to promote a healing environment, are fundamental to the care of EB wounds.

Tests to monitor in patients with severe types of epidermolysis bullosa are presented.

Pain is an unfortunate constant in the lives of most patients with epidermolysis bullosa (EB), especially for those with the more severe types of EB. Patients with EB have a broad spectrum of need for pain treatment, varying with the type of EB, the severity within that type, and the particular physical, emotional, and psychological milieu of each individual. Prevention of situations that precipitate trauma to the skin or exacerbate other pain-inducing complications of this multifaceted disorder is the primary goal of the treating physician. The approach to pain management is different in daily life, during intermittent exacerbations or injuries, or when hospitalizations or operative procedures occur.

Squamous cell carcinomas (SCCs) are highly aggressive in patients with epidermolysis bullosa (EB). Non–ultraviolet-related SCCs are the leading cause of death in patients with recessive dystrophic EB, particularly recessive dystrophic EB-generalized severe subtype (RDEB-GS). The mechanism of SCC development in patients with RDEB continues to be investigated and several theories have been reported in the literature.

Optimization of resistance to infection, growth, sexual maturation, wound healing, and provision of the best possible overall quality of life are important management goals in children with epidermolysis bullosa. However, all these goals rely on the maintenance of optimal nutritional status, and achieving this is extremely challenging in the severe types of the disease. Strategies to improve nutritional status have the best chance of success when the dietitian or nutritionist works as an integral member of the multidisciplinary team and is well informed of patients' situations, family dynamics, and prognoses. Even the best-coordinated dietetic interventions may exert only limited impact.

Dental treatment is an important part of the multidisciplinary care of patients with epidermolysis bullosa (EB). Routine dental treatment can be difficult to provide in patients with severe tissue fragility caused by mucosal sloughing, microstomia, ankyloglossia, and scarring. This article provides a review of dental practices, exploring different areas of oral management and highlighting the importance of early referral, preventive programs, and close follow-up to maintain oral health. It also discusses treatment modifications and precautions needed for each of the 4 mayor types of EB.

Epidermolysis bullosa (EB) is a spectrum of rare, inherited, blistering skin disorders, primarily affecting the skin and pharyngoesophageal mucosa. EB affects approximately 2 to 4 per 100,000 children each year. Blistering and scarring occur in response to even the most minor trauma. In this article, the authors outline the potential management options for patients with EB complicated by feeding difficulties secondary to esophageal strictures as well as those with nutritional deficiencies requiring a gastrostomy tube for supplemental feeding.

Patients with epidermolysis bullosa (EB) may present for anesthesia with an unrelated surgical condition or, more commonly, for diagnostic or therapeutic procedures. Children in particular may require frequent anesthetics. Safe and effective management of anesthesia presents a significant challenge and although there is little rigorous evidence available to aid decision-making, in this article the elements of current good anesthesia care in EB are summarized.

Epidermolysis bullosa (EB) results from genetic defects of molecules in the skin concerned with adhesion. Some of the most common problems seen with EB sufferers are blisters, vesicles, and bullas. Maintaining foot cleanliness, exercising, and wearing shoes are all good preventative measures and important in EB foot care.

Surgery of the Hand in Recessive Dystrophic Epidermolysis Bullosa   335

Catina Bernardis and Rachel Box

The underlying genetic abnormalities of epidermolysis bullosa (EB) cause destabilization at the dermo-epidermal junction. Patients with EB characteristically are subject to blistering following relatively minor trauma (the Nikolsky sign), and suffer from ulcers and erosions in all areas subject to persistent or repeated friction, such as the hand. Hand deformities occur in most patients with dystrophic EB (DEB), and include adduction contractures of the first web space, pseudosyndactyly, and flexion contractures of the interphalangeal, metacarpophalangeal, and wrist joints. All structures in the hand may be involved. The severity of the deformity worsens with age, and surgical correction becomes increasingly difficult. Recurrent deformity occurs within 2 to 5 years. Meticulous skin care and the use of well-fitted splints supervised within a multidisciplinary team setting are essential. To date there is no strong evidence base on which to plan surgical treatment of the hand in DEB.

Genitourinary Tract Involvement in Epidermolysis Bullosa   343

Noor Almaani and Jemima E. Mellerio

Involvement of the genitourinary tract has been described in many different types of epidermolysis bullosa (EB). Pathology may be broadly divided into problems resulting in obstruction, that may in turn lead to hydroureter or hydronephrosis, or disease primarily affecting the renal parenchyma. Left unrecognized and untreated, renal tract disease may lead to chronic renal failure, and consequent problems associated with providing renal replacement therapy. Management of the urogenital tract in EB should therefore focus on detecting symptoms suggestive of obstruction and regular monitoring to detect problems as early as possible.

Dilated Cardiomyopathy in Epidermolysis Bullosa   347

Irene Lara-Corrales and Elena Pope

Dilated cardiomyopathy (DC) is a rare but potentially fatal complication of epidermolysis bullosa. No clear cause for it has been identified, but iron overload, low carnitine, low selenium, concomitant viral illness, chronic anemia, and medications have been proposed as possible contributors to the development of DC in reported cases. Early detection allows for medical treatment that delays clinical progression and prolongs survival.

Osteopenia and Osteoporosis in Epidermolysis Bullosa   353

Anna E. Martinez and Jemima E. Mellerio

Patients with the more severe forms of epidermolysis bullosa (EB) are at risk of developing osteopenia, osteoporosis and fractures. The cause is likely to be multifactorial and includes reduced mobility, a generally proinflammatory state, poor nutrition and hormonal factors. Monitoring this group with dual energy X-ray absorptiometry (DEXA) scans and plain radiographs is necessary to detect these changes. Data are lacking about the optimal approach to managing poor bone health in EB, although it seems that encouraging mobility, supplementation of calcium and vitamin D where necessary, with the addition of a bisphosphonate when there is evidence of fractures, may be helpful.

Puberty is the acquisition of secondary sexual characteristics, associated with a growth spurt, resulting in the attainment of reproductive function and final adult height. Delayed puberty is defined as the absence of any pubertal development at an age 2 standard deviations (SD) more than the mean, which corresponds to an age of approximately 14 years for boys and 13 years for girls. The degree to which growth and pubertal development are affected in chronic illness depends on the disease itself, as well as factors such as age of onset, duration and severity; the earlier the onset and the more severe the disease, the greater the effect on growth and pubertal development. Most children with severe types of epidermolysis bullosa have abnormal growth and pubertal delay. The possible pathophysiology is discussed.

Among the severe genetic disorders of the skin that are suitable for gene and cell therapy, most efforts have been made in the treatment of blistering diseases including dystrophic epidermolysis bullosa. This condition can be recessively or dominantly inherited, depending on the nature and position of the mutation or mutations in the gene encoding type VII collagen. At present, there is no specific treatment for recessive dystrophic epidermolysis bullosa, and gene and cell therapy approaches hold great promise. This article discusses the different gene therapy approaches that have been used for the treatment of this disease and the new perspectives that they open.

Dystrophic epidermolysis bullosa (DEB) is a severe skin fragility disorder associated with trauma-induced blistering, progressive soft tissue scarring, and increased risk of skin cancer. DEB is caused by mutations in the COL7A1 gene which result in reduced, truncated, or absent type VII collagen, and anchoring fibrils at the dermal-epidermal junction (DEJ). Because no topical wound-healing agents have shown unequivocal benefit in the treatment of DEB, alternative approaches are needed. The purpose of cell therapy for recessive DEB is to increase the amount of collagen VII in the basement membrane zone in order to heal wounds and prevent further wound formation. Fibroblast-based cell therapy is safe and easy to work with, has few side effects, can dramatically restore stable collagen VII at the DEJ, and can normalize the substructure changes of DEB for at least a few months. Even though the mechanism and the duration of newly produced collagen VII at the DEJ are still unknown, this form of cell therapy provides a new effective approach to the treatment of recessive DEB.

Recessive dystrophic epidermolysis bullosa (RDEB) is a severe inherited blistering disease caused by mutations in the type VII collagen gene, resulting in defective anchoring fibrils at the epidermal-dermal junction. At present, no curative treatment for RDEB exists. Mounting evidence on reprogramming of bone marrow stem cells into skin has prompted the authors and others to develop novel strategies for treatment of RDEB. The rationale for bone marrow stem cell therapies for RDEB is based on the evidence that bone marrow–derived cells are guided into becoming skin cells, given the right microenvironment. Preclinical studies in mouse models have shown that wild-type bone marrow–derived cells can ameliorate the phenotype of RDEB and improve survival by restoring the expression of type VII collagen and the anchoring fibrils. At present, several clinical studies are ongoing around the world to study the therapeutic effects of bone marrow stem cell transplantation for RDEB. These studies provide a framework for future development of standardized, effective methods for stem cell transplantation to cure severe inherited skin diseases, including RDEB.

An interdisciplinary team approach, in which the treatment can be individualized to each patient and his or her family and tailored to the severity of the disease, is most beneficial to the patient with epidermolysis bullosa (EB). In the Netherlands, the Center for Blistering Diseases in Groningen provides a large interdisciplinary EB team that performs at a high level to provide the best EB-patient care for both children and adults. The possibility of rapid diagnosis, the efficient carrousel-like clinics, and the continuity in care are typical elements of the Dutch method of delivering interdisciplinary EB care.

EPIDERMOLYSIS BULLOSA AROUND THE WORLD

There is a wide range of health care delivery systems within the United States for patients with epidermolysis bullosa (EB). They range from nonexistent, primarily because of remote geographic locations, to 4 comprehensive interdisciplinary EB centers. This article lists the subspecialties available at each of the 4 centers.

Based on the described prevalence and size of the population, approximately 300 to 500 patients with epidermolysis bullosa (EB) reside in Canada. There are specific challenges faced by patients and families as well as the practitioners looking after patients with EB.

Epidermolysis bullosa (EB) in Mexico continues to be a rare genodermatosis that is still unknown for most of the health care professionals in the country. The spirit of DebRA MEXICO was born in 1994 when the Mexican health care team started to see patients with the main purpose to provide medical care, genetic counseling, and advice to patients with EB and their families; to promote collaboration and exchange information among people with EB; to research and find new therapeutic approaches; and finally, to diffuse knowledge and raise awareness of the issues of EB in general public and health care professionals.

article discusses the clinical services and coordinated multidisciplinary management of EB in Italy.

Epidermolysis Bullosa in Japan

431

Satoru Shinkuma, Ken Natsuga, Wataru Nishie, and Hiroshi Shimizu

> Epidermolysis bullosa (EB) is a group of hereditary disorders characterized by mechanical stress-induced blistering of the skin and mucous membranes. This article discusses the prevalence among and genetic studies of Japanese patients with EB.

Epidermolysis Bullosa in Australia and New Zealand

433

Dédée F. Murrell

> This article describes the clinical services for EB in Australia and New Zealand. The history and epidemiology of EB in Australia is described. Current treatment and research achievements are described.

Erratum to "Plectin Gene Defects Lead to Various Forms of Epidermolysis Bullosa Simplex" [Dermatol Clin 28 (2010) 33–41]

439

Erratum to "Nail Involvement in Epidermolysis Bullosa" [Dermatol Clin 28 (2010) 153–157]

443

Index

445

Dermatologic Clinics

THE CLINICS ARE NOW AVAILABLE ONLINE!

Access your subscription at:
www.theclinics.com

Preface

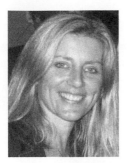

Dédée F. Murrell, MA, BMBCh, FAAD, MD
Guest Editor

When invited to edit a special issue of *Dermatologic Clinics of North America* on epidermolysis bullosa (EB) by Bruce Thiers, I was delighted and honored to accept.

Apart from two previous textbooks devoted to EB, there was no other single source for a dermatologist to access for an overview of the latest on this complex subject.

Unlike a textbook, where the articles may be a year or two out of date by the time the book is published, these articles have been written in the last 9 months by respected leaders in the particular aspects of EB. The first issue dealt with pathogenesis and clinical features of EB. This second issue has been organized into a section on the basics of how to diagnose different subtypes of EB, and then aspects of management.

Diagnosis goes from the basics of how to take a skin biopsy to how to organize prenatal diagnosis. Management covers basic bathing techniques and dressings, to the complications of the severe forms of EB, to the latest in gene, cell, and protein therapies. Lastly, there is a section on how EB is managed in different centers around the world, with information about the contributions from these centers and how they have managed to provide a service despite different levels of health care.

The experts who have contributed to this second issue are from all corners of the globe and collectively have hundreds of patient-years of experience. They include dermatologists Alan Arbuckle, Leena Bruckner-Tuderman, Christine Bodemer, Robin Eady, Helmut Hintner, Alain Hovnanian, Marcel Jonkman, Sarolta Kárpáti, Anne Lucky, John McGrath, Jemima Mellerio, Jean-Paul Ortonne, Elena Pope, Julio Salas-Alanis, Hiroshi Shimizu, Eli Sprecher, Anders Vahlquist,

Rosemarie Watson, and Giovanna Zambruno; geneticist Ginna Sybert; pediatrician Anna Martinez; pain specialist Richard Goldschneider; anesthetist Richard Howard; hand surgeon Catina Bernardis; pediatric surgeon Richard Azizkhan; endocrinologist Jeremy Allgrove; dentist Suzanne Krämer; scientists Daniele Castiglia, Angela Christiano, Trish Dopping-Hepenstal, Jim Meneguzzi, and Gabi Pohla-Gubo; podiatrist Tariq Khan; EB nurses Jacqui Denyer and José Duipmans; and pediatric dietician Lesley Haynes.

Unlike a textbook, these articles can be found on MEDLINE and PubMed and are accessible online, and the individual issues of the journal may be purchased for much less cost than either a textbook or buying the articles individually.

I thank all the contributors for their time and effort in writing these articles at relatively short notice and in a succinct manner with excellent color photographs and figures.

It is hoped that these two issues will be educational not only for dermatologists but for all clinicians who interact with patients with EB, as well as scientists, family members, and the patients themselves. Understanding what is so far known about a disease leads to improved clinical practice, better research, and improved compliance with therapy.

Dédée F. Murrell, MA, BMBCh, FAAD, MD
Department of Dermatology
St George Hospital
University of New South Wales
Gray Street
Sydney, NSW 2217, Australia

E-mail address:
d.murrell@unsw.edu.au

Dermatol Clin 28 (2010) xix
doi:10.1016/j.det.2010.02.023

derm.theclinics.com

How to Take Skin Biopsies for Epidermolysis Bullosa

Lizbeth Ruth A. Intong, MD[a],
Dédée F. Murrell, MA, BMBCh, FAAD, MD[b],*

KEYWORDS

• Epidermolysis bullosa • Biopsy • Diagnosis

The definitive diagnosis of inherited epidermolysis bullosa (EB) is best made with positive immunofluorescence (IF) antigenic mapping (IFM), transmission electron microscopy (EM), and EB-related monoclonal antibody studies,[1–4] the IF microscopy being faster to complete and more sensitive and specific than EM for subtyping of EB.[5] These are key diagnostic tools that not only confirm the clinical diagnosis but also help to identify the particular subtype of EB. This information ultimately sheds light on the likely prognosis and level of care required and provides a basis for genetic testing.

People who are afflicted with EB have varying degrees of severity depending on the structural protein involved. However, major subtypes of EB may be indistinguishable clinically, especially in the neonatal period. It is therefore essential that a proper diagnosis be made as soon as possible, and skin biopsies, when properly performed, can aid us in this.

This article provides information on the correct way of obtaining skin biopsies in EB, collecting and storing skin samples, and transporting specimens for analysis.

MATERIALS NEEDED
Basic Materials

Rubber eraser or pencil with rubber eraser (to induce a new blister)
Suture set containing tissue forceps, needle holder, and scissors

Biopsy punches (2 mm, 3 mm)
Suture material (4-0 or 5-0 nonabsorbable or absorbable sutures)
Antiseptic, nonstick dressings.

Transport Media
IF mapping

Normal saline (0.9% sodium chloride) solution or liquid nitrogen (for storage <24 hours) is ideal[6]
Michel medium (for storage from 24 hours to 6 weeks).[6,7]

Electron microscopy

2.5% glutaraldehyde or appropriate fixative.

PREPARING THE PATIENT

As in all surgical procedures, before any biopsy, informed consent must be taken from the patients or from parents in case the patient is a minor.

Choose an area of skin that seems clinically unaffected but preferably adjacent to the site where the patient usually gets blisters (ie, on the arms or legs). In neonates with more extensive forms of EB, a nonblistered site that has been freshly rubbed, such as the lower abdomen or the upper inner arm just above the elbow, is usually suitable. Skin should not be obtained from the palms or soles, as the overall thickness of the tissue will make it difficult to demonstrate skin cleavage.[8] If possible, choose an area where the resulting scar will not be so obvious.

[a] Department of Dermatology, St George Hospital, Gray Street, Kogarah, Sydney, NSW 2217, Australia
[b] Department of Dermatology, St George Hospital, University of New South Wales, Gray Street, Sydney, NSW 2217, Australia
* Corresponding author.
E-mail address: d.murrell@unsw.edu.au

Dermatol Clin 28 (2010) 197–200
doi:10.1016/j.det.2009.12.002

The best areas to take skin biopsies in EB patients are fresh blisters, as these will yield better results. Blisters that are more than 12 hours old, especially those with bloodstained contents, are not ideal because these may have false immunostaining caused by proteolytic antigen degradation and reepithelialization under the roof of the blister, resulting in multiple cleavage planes.[8,9] An area of nonblistered skin, which has been gently rubbed to produce mild erythema, is ideal because this will contain a cleavage plane without secondary changes.

In general, attempts at inducing microscopic cleavage should be done before the biopsy. Exceptions would be in the case of severe junctional and recessive dystrophic EB, where there is such inherent mechanical fragility that skin cleavage planes are readily demonstrable just with a routine punch biopsy technique.[8] The biopsy site should be identified, prepared in a sterile manner (ie, cleaned with an alcohol swab), and encircled. Rubbing is performed by applying firm downward pressure with a pencil eraser and then rotating it laterally (at least 180° each way).[8]

In newborns or infants, the selected area on the skin is rubbed with an eraser or pencil eraser at least 20 times at first (**Fig. 1**). The area may turn red but you should ideally wait for at least 5 minutes for a blister to develop microscopically before taking the biopsy.[10]

In cases of adults or children with less-severe forms of EB, such as EB simplex or dominant dystrophic EB, after identifying and marking the target area with a pen, have the patient or parent take the eraser or pencil eraser and rub on the area many times until it turns red (**Fig. 2**). They should stop rubbing if the skin starts to tear or peel off. They may need to arrive early at the clinic to be instructed to do this and leave the clinic for a few hours with the eraser, to return later for the biopsy. Alternatively, they can do whatever exercise induces their blisters the day before to ensure that the blisters are fresh.[10]

THE SKIN BIOPSY PROCEDURE

Clean the selected area of skin with an antiseptic or alcohol and drape it. Anesthetize with 1% lignocaine (and adrenaline to minimize bleeding) to raise a bleb (**Fig. 3**). When this procedure is preplanned in a child, a cream of a eutectic mixture of local anesthetics may be applied under occlusion to the site for 2 hours beforehand to minimize the discomfort.[10]

Perform a 3-mm punch biopsy using a twisting movement from the rubbed area (**Fig. 4**) and place it in Michel's solution (the same transport media used for IF specimens). If you can get the specimen to the diagnostic laboratory within 24 hours, then liquid nitrogen or normal saline is preferable. Take a 2-mm punch biopsy from the (same) rubbed area and place it in 2.5% glutaraldehyde solution for EM.

It is also useful to take a 3-mm punch biopsy from an unaffected nonrubbed area, usually the inner upper arm, because the reduction of protein staining, if present, is more easily assessed on skin that has not actually blistered. This sample would be transported in a similar manner to the other IFM specimen, in a separate Michel's media container, labeled as normal nonrubbed skin and the site of the biopsy.

Suture with 4-0 or 5-0 nonabsorbable sutures (ie, Ethilon or Prolene [Ethicon Inc, Somerville, NJ, USA]) depending on the site (**Fig. 5**), and apply

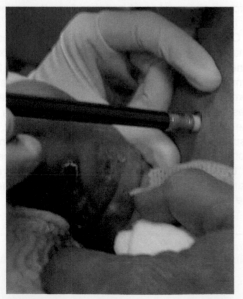

Fig. 1. Rub the selected area with an eraser at least 20 times.

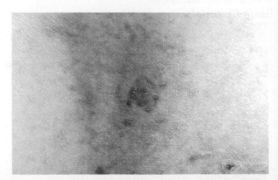

Fig. 2. Blister and erythema appear after rubbing with an eraser.

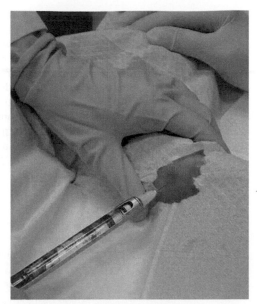

Fig. 3. Local anesthetic being infiltrated.

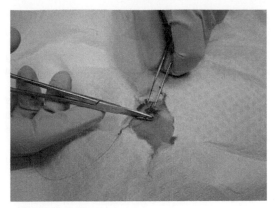

Fig. 5. Suture the biopsy.

a topical antibiotic ointment to the site and dress with nonstick dressings (ie, Mepitel or Mepilex [Mölnlycke Health Care, Norcross, GA, USA]). Sutures are taken out in a week. Alternatively, absorbable sutures (ie, catgut) that fall out on their own can be used.[10]

In some institutions, where it is considered more convenient for nurses to travel to outlying hospitals to take biopsies from newborn infants, as the ones in the United Kingdom, the nurses are instructed to insert a needle horizontally through the rubbed area and then use a scalpel blade to take a superficial biopsy, not suture it, and just apply a nonstick dressing. These very thin biopsies are more difficult for the IF laboratory to mount and cut than the ones taken by the punch technique. In the past, in the United States for instance, it was felt that incisional biopsies were the best way to

collect the skin specimens by inverting the skin and cutting it across with a scalpel blade. However, the European groups have shown that the punch technique works just as well and leaves less of a scar.

Arrange for specimen collection and processing.

INSTRUCTIONS FOR PATIENTS POSTPROCEDURE

As with any skin biopsy procedure, advise the patient to keep the area dry for the first 24 hours. The biopsy site may be dressed daily with an antibiotic ointment and nonstick dressing. The sutures are to be removed in a week's time if nonabsorbable sutures were used. Arrange to see the patients again when the results are available, usually in 1 or 2 weeks postprocedure.

REFERENCES

1. Fine JD. Laboratory tests for epidermolysis bullosa. Dermatol Clin 1994;12(1):123–32.
2. Hintner H, Stingl G, Schuler G, et al. Immunofluorescence mapping of antigenic determinants within the dermal-epidermal junction in the mechanobullous diseases. J Invest Dermatol 1981;76(2):113–8.
3. Black MM, Bhogal BS, Willsteed E. Immunopathological techniques in the diagnosis of bullous disorders. Acta Derm Venereol Suppl (Stockh) 1989;151: 96–105.
4. Jaunzems AE, Woods AE, Staples A. Electron microscopy and morphometry enhances differentiation of epidermolysis bullosa subtypes. With normal values for 24 parameters in skin. Arch Dermatol Res 1997;289:631–9.
5. Yiasemides E, Walton J, Marr P, et al. A comparative study between the transmission electron microscopy and immunofluorescence mapping in the

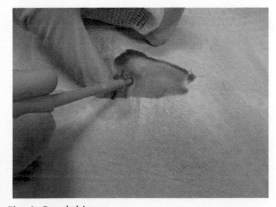

Fig. 4. Punch biopsy.

diagnosis of epidermolysis bullosa. Am J Dermato-pathol 2006;28:387–94.

6. Vodegel RM, de Jong MC, Meijer HJ, et al. Enhanced diagnostic immunofluorescence using biopsies transported in saline. BMC Dermatol 2004;4:10.

7. Vaughan Jones SA, Palmer I, Bhogal BS, et al. The use of Michel's transport medium for immunofluorescence and immunoelectron microscopy in autoimmune bullous diseases. J Cutan Pathol 1995;32:365–70.

8. Fine JD. Hereditary epidermolysis bullosa (EB) biopsy sites. Available at: http://www.beutnerlabs. com/request/biopsy-sites.php. Accessed January 20, 2010.

9. Eady RAJ, Fine JD, Burge SM. Genetic blistering diseases. In: Burns DA, Breathnach S, Cox N, et al, editors. Rook's textbook of dermatology. 7th edition. Oxford (UK): Blackwell Science Ltd; 2004. p. 1–24.

10. Murrell DF. Collection and transport of specimens for epidermolysis bullosa diagnosis. St. George hospital department of dermatology. Available at: http://www.blisters.org.au/AEBDL.html 2006; Ver 1. Accessed January 20, 2010.

Immunofluorescence Mapping for the Diagnosis of Epidermolysis Bullosa

Gabriela Pohla-Gubo, PhD[a],*, Rodrigo Cepeda-Valdes, MD[b],
Helmut Hintner, MD[a]

KEYWORDS

- Immunofluorescence mapping
- Epidermolysis bullosa • Classification of subtypes

What is the diagnosis for a baby born with severe blisters and erosions (**Fig. 1**)? With an uninformative medical and family history, an experienced dermatologist considers an infectious, immunobullous, traumatic, or less frequently, an inherited disorder. The spectrum of differential diagnoses is extensive, and distinction can be difficult.[1] Diagnostic routine tests such as microbial testing should be performed first, frequently followed by skin biopsy for routine histologic, immunohistochemical and, sometimes, ultrastructural assessment. In epidermolysis bullosa (EB), microscopic results first show an unremarkable routine histology, except for a split formation in distinct layers of the skin and a negative routine immunohistochemistry. As the newborn develops more blisters every day, especially on sites of mechanical trauma, the diagnosis of inherited EB has to be considered.

The challenges in the diagnosis of EB are identical worldwide. To achieve a correct diagnosis and classification of the disease, the first laboratory tool to be used successfully was transmission electron microscopy (TEM), and this has been the gold standard laboratory test for many years (see the article by Eady and Dopping-Hepenstal elsewhere in this issue for further exploration of this topic). However, TEM is time-consuming and expensive, and the results are, to a high degree,

operator-dependent and sometimes inaccurate. In addition, there are only a few laboratories with appropriate experience and skills to analyze and interpret EB samples in TEM. In 1981, the authors described the method of Immunofluorescence (antigen) mapping (IFM), which is based on the detection of structural proteins of keratinocytes or of the dermo-epidermal junction using specific poly- or monoclonal antibodies.[2] Using this method, the level of split formation can be determined by investigating the location of a given antigen (eg, type 4 collagen) in a natural or induced blister. This method also allows testing for the normal expression, reduction or absence of various structural proteins depending on the antibodies used.

Based on the localization of the level of blistering in the skin as determined by immunohistochemistry and/or TEM, the hereditary mechanobullous diseases are classified into 3 major groups: EB simplex (EBS), junctional EB (JEB), and dystrophic EB (DEB). A fourth group, the Kindler syndrome, was added according to the new classification published in 2008.[3]

There are various poly- or monoclonal antibodies that recognize structural proteins of keratinocytes or of the dermo-epidermal basement membrane zone (BMZ), which is known to be involved in the pathogenesis of EB. Fortunately,

[a] Department of Dermatology, Laboratory for Immunology, Allergology and Molecular Diagnostics, Paracelsus Medical University, Muellner Hauptstrasse 48, A-5020 Salzburg, Austria
[b] Department of Dermatology, Escuela de Medicina del Instituto Tecnológico y de Estudios Superiores de Monterrey, Monterrey NL, México
* Corresponding author.
E-mail address: g.pohla-gubo@salk.at

Dermatol Clin 28 (2010) 201–210
doi:10.1016/j.det.2009.12.005
0733-8635/10/$ – see front matter © 2010 Elsevier Inc. All rights reserved.

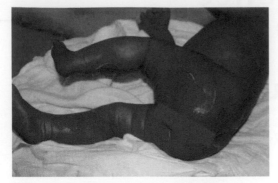

Fig. 1. Baby born with extensive blistering.

these antibodies are available worldwide for the frequently used IFM. IFM has widely replaced TEM and is now used as the first laboratory test to prove the clinical diagnosis of EB and to distinguish subtypes of EB. It is also the base for distinguishing the target proteins for mutation analysis.

In this article, IFM as a crucial diagnostic tool is described and the possibility of a worldwide cooperation in the diagnosis of EB is discussed.

MATERIALS AND METHODS
Biopsy

The method for taking a biopsy for EB is reviewed elsewhere in this issue (see the article by Intong and Murrell elsewhere in this issue for further exploration of this topic). A biopsy of patient skin, including parts of a fresh blister and of normal-appearing skin (Fig. 2), facilitates the determination of the split formation and allows conclusions about the major types of EB.[2,4]

Transport to the Specialized Laboratory

The biopsy sample should be immediately placed into Michel medium as originally described by Michel and colleagues[5] in 1973 and modified by

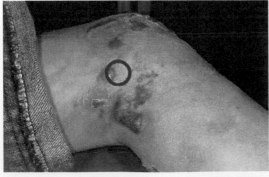

Fig. 2. Biopsy for IFM including part of a fresh blister.

Vaughan and colleagues[6] in 1995: 1 M citrate buffer pH 7.4, 2.5 mL; 0.1 M magnesium sulfate, 5 mL; 0.1 M N-ethylmaleimide, 5 mL; ammonium sulfate 55 g; distilled water, 87.5 mL; total volume 100 mL adjusted to pH 7.4 with 1 M sodium hydroxide. In this medium, the samples can be stored up to 28 days at room temperature and sent worldwide to any specialized laboratory that performs IFM. On receipt, the sample has to be rinsed immediately in phosphate buffered saline (PBS) for a few hours to reduce background staining and improve diagnostic sensitivity. Then the sample can be processed by cutting cryostat sections or snap frozen in liquid nitrogen or stored in a plastic tube without any liquid in a freezer at −20°C (or better, at −80°C) until further processing.

In a recent cooperation between an EB group in Mexico and the EB House at the Department of Dermatology in Salzburg, Austria, 48 biopsy samples were sent from Mexico to Austria. It was confirmed that the above-mentioned conservation and transport methods allow an excellent IFM quality leading to an appropriate classification (manuscript in preparation).

Antibodies

The primary antibodies for IFM are generated from different animal sources and bind to specific structural proteins of the skin that are relevant in the pathogenesis of various types of EB (Table 1). According to the proteins targeted for mutation analysis, we use IgG antibodies against cytokeratin 5, cytokeratin 14, plectin, α6 integrin, β4 integrin, type 17 collagen (180 kDa BPAG2), laminin 332, and type 7 collagen. We also use anti-type 4 collagen (present in the lamina densa of the dermoepidermal BMZ) antibodies for better visualization of the level of split formation, especially in patients with DEB. All primary antibodies are IgG class, and most of them are monoclonal, raised in mice. Therefore, the second antibody has to be a mouse-specific anti-IgG antibody, usually conjugated to the fluorescent dye, fluorescein isothiocyanate (FITC). An exception is the antibody against α6 integrin where rat is the source, and thus the second antibody has to be anti-rat IgG. The FITC bound to the second antibody produces a specific fluorescent signal at 450 to 490 nm and allows the visualization of specific antibody binding under the IF microscope. Depending on the frequency of requested IFMs and the final dilution necessary for IFM, different amounts of the original primary and secondary antibodies should be divided into aliquots and kept in the refrigerator until expiry date given on the bottle of the stock solution.

Table 1
List of antibodies and dilutions currently used for IFM in the laboratory of the Department of Dermatology, Paracelsus Medical University, Salzburg, Austria, and associated EB subtypes

1st Antibodies	Dilution	Host	Company	Catalog Number	EB Subtype
Cytokeratin 5	1:50	Mouse	Millipore	MAB 3224	EBS
Cytokeratin 14	1:100	Mouse	Millipore	MAB 3232	EBS
Plectin (5B3)	1:2	Mouse	Wiche (personal communication)		EBS, JEB
α6 integrin	1:50	Rat	Millipore	MAB 1378	EBS, JEB
β4 integrin	1:50	Mouse	Millipore	MAB 1964	EBS, JEB
Collagen 17	1:20	Mouse	In-house (EB laboratory)		JEB
Laminin 332[a]	1:50	Mouse	Millipore	MAB 1949	JEB
Collagen 4	1:50	Mouse	Millipore	MAB 3326	
Collagen 7	1:50	Mouse	Millipore	MAB 1345	DEB
2nd Antibodies					
IgG	1:100	Goat anti-mouse	Millipore	AP 124F	
IgG	1:100–400	Rabbit anti-rat	Dako	F 0234	

[a] Formerly laminin 5.

Working dilutions are always prepared fresh from these aliquots and are not reused.

Staining Procedure

To prepare the glass slides for IFM, we put 3 to 4 cryosections (4–6 μm thick) of the patient sample and 1 or 2 sections of healthy normal human skin (NHS) onto the slides (**Fig. 3**). The source for the NHS samples are normal parts of cutaneous biopsies and excision material from the Dermatosurgery Unit of the Department of Dermatology, where patients have given their informed consent for use. These samples are then used as NHS positive controls to prove the appropriate staining of the respective structural protein (as described earlier). For a complete IFM analysis, we prepare 11 slides: 9 for staining with the different primary antibodies according to the antigens (structural proteins) we are looking for and 2 for negative controls. The 2 negative controls are incubated with PBS instead of the primary antibody and are

then exposed to the secondary antibodies (FITC-conjugated anti-mouse or -rat IgG) to exclude nonspecific staining caused by the second antibody. Each slide is incubated with the appropriate dilution of the primary antibody (or PBS as negative control) for 30 minutes in a moist chamber at room temperature. After washing the sections in PBS (2 × 15 minutes), the appropriately diluted secondary antibody is overlaid followed by incubation for 30 minutes under the same conditions. The sections then have to be washed again twice in PBS for 15 minutes. They are covered with glycerol and a cover slip, viewed under the IF microscope and photographed for a permanent record. The stained slides are stable for some weeks when kept in a refrigerator at 4°C.

PATTERNS OF STAINING

Using IFM it is possible to visualize the localization and expression of structural proteins involved in the pathology of EB skin (**Fig. 4A, B**). However, the intensity of staining of the proteins is influenced by several factors, including the body site of the biopsy (normal or affected skin, sun-exposed skin) and age of the patient. To allow a comparison with normal conditions, it is advisable to take the NHS control from patients of similar age and similar body locations. In addition, the time of storage in the Michel medium (a maximum of 28 days is recommended) or the transport conditions (hot or

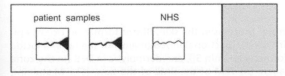

Fig. 3. Slide preparation for IFM. Frozen sections of patient's skin and normal human skin (NHS) on one slide.

freezing temperatures) can influence the results, as can repeated freezing and thawing of the diluted antibody. To compare the staining results of the patient sample with NHS, it is helpful to make a scale from 1 to 4 according to the brightness of the antibody reaction. It is important to have a blister (or split formation) in the sample, because this allows classification according to the main types of EB. For example, using an antibody to type 4 collagen (present in the lamina densa of the dermo-epidermal BMZ) in the case of intraepidermal blistering (EBS), the fluorescence is found on the blister floor. In JEB, the reaction can also be found on the

blister floor, whereas in DEB the antibody binds to the blister roof (see **Fig. 4C, a, b**).

Each EB subtype can also be distinguished by alterations in different skin proteins. With IFM, the expression of structural proteins can be normal, reduced in intensity, or completely lacking.

EBS

In patients with EBS (**Fig. 5A**), one of the proteins, cytokeratin 5 and 14, plectin, α6 integrin and β-4 integrin, is involved in the pathology, and the split formation occurs within the epidermis by cytolysis

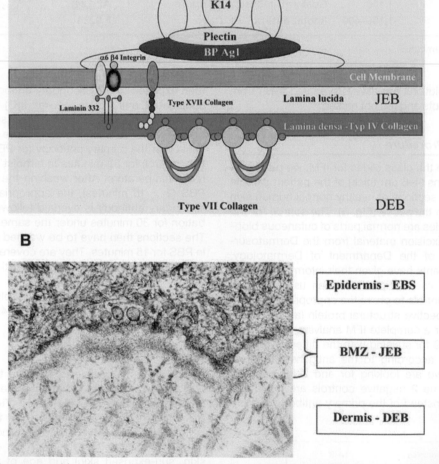

Fig. 4. (*A*) Ultrastructural localization of EB-relevant structural proteins in the skin. Blister formation occurs epidermolytic in EBS (in areas of K5, K14, plectin, and integrins α6β4), junctional in JEB (mainly in the lamina lucida at the sites of type 17 collagen [BPAG2] and laminin 332 [formerly laminin 5]), and dermolytic in DEB (in the zone of the lamina densa and below) at the site of type 7 collagen. (*B*) TEM of the BMZ of the skin. (*C*) IFM staining with anti-type 4 collagen to distinguish the level of blistering: (*a*) junctional blistering in a patient with JEB, type 4 collagen on blister floor (*arrow*); (*b*) dermolytic blistering in a patient with DEB, type 4 collagen on blister roof (*arrow*).

C

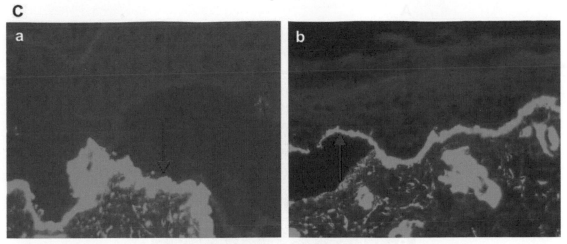

Fig. 4. *(continued)*

of basal keratinocytes (intraepidermal) (see Fig. 5B). In general, the proteins are expressed normal, except in autosomal recessive EBS,[7] when patients may have no cytokeratin 14 (see Fig. 5C, D). In patients with EBS-muscular dystrophy (EBS-MD), plectin is mostly absent, and in the rare case of EBS Ogna,[8] it is markedly reduced. In EB subtypes with pyloric atresia (either

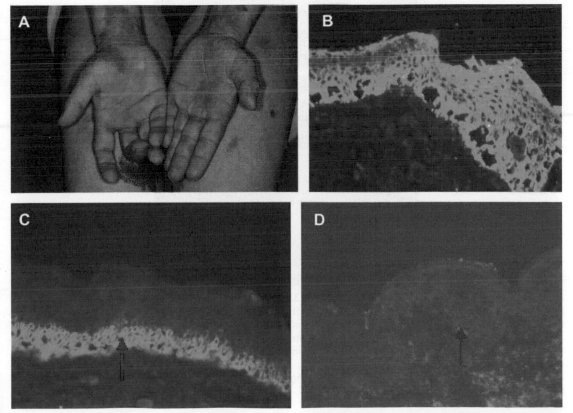

Fig. 5. IFM results in EBS. (*A*) Clinical picture of a patient with autosomal recessive EBS. (*B*) EBS patient's skin stained with anti-cytokeratin 5 antibody revealing normal expression but intraepidermal (epidermolytic) blistering (*arrow*). (*C*) NHS section stained with anti-cytokeratin 14 antibody (*arrow*). (*D*) Patient with autosomal recessive EBS. IFM negative with anti-cytokeratin 14 antibody.

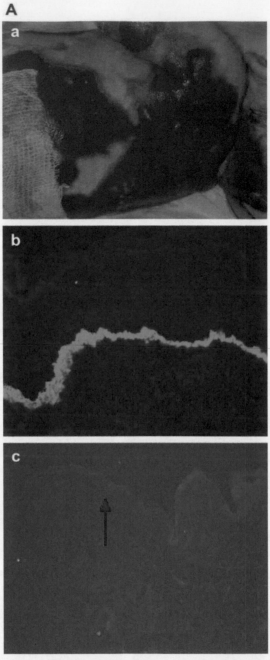

Fig. 6. IFM results in JEB. (*A*) Severe JEB-H (laminin 332 absent): (*a*) large denuded skin areas on the back of a newborn with JEB-H; (*b*) laminin 332 staining positive on NHS control; (*c*) laminin 332 absent on patient's skin (*arrow*). (*B*) Generalized JEB-nH (laminin 332 reduced): (*a*) nonhealing wound of a patient with generalized JEB-nH; (*b*) laminin 332 staining positive on NHS control; (*c*) laminin 332 reduced on patient's skin (*arrow*); (*d*) laminin 332 reduced on patient's skin showing junctional blistering with laminin 332 on the blister floor (*arrow*). (*C*) Generalized JEB-nH (formerly known as GABEB; type 17 collagen absent): (*a*) generalized blistering of a newborn with JEB-nH; (*b*) type 17 collagen staining positive in NHS control; (*c*) type 17 collagen absent in patient's skin.

B

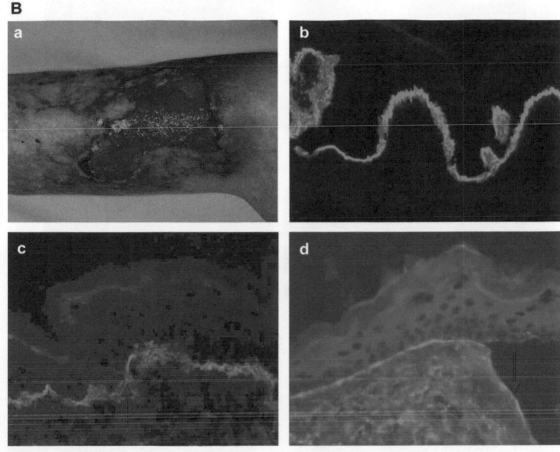

Fig. 6. *(continued)*

EBS or JEB), plectin, $\alpha6$ integrin and $\beta4$ integrin are reduced or absent.[9]

JEB

The main target proteins in JEB are type 17 collagen (BPAG2) and laminin 332. These proteins can be expressed normally or are reduced or absent.[10] In a junctional blister, they appear on the blister roof or floor depending on the subtype of the JEB (Fig. 6B, d).

In the severe JEB-Herlitz (JEB-H) subtype (see Fig. 6A, a–c), laminin 332 is mostly absent or markedly reduced. In cases with generalized JEB–non-Herlitz (JEB-nH gen), either laminin 332 or type 17 collagen is altered. In most cases of JEB-nH, laminin 332 is reduced (see Fig. 6B, a–d), and type 17 collagen is absent (see Fig. 6C, a–c) or reduced in a few cases. Laminin 332 remains normal in the latter set of patients, who

were previously classified as having generalized atrophic benign JEB (formerly GABEB).

DEB

The DEB subtypes are caused by type 7 collagen mutations. In patients with severe generalized recessive DEB (RDEB), the IFM shows mostly an absence of type 7 collagen (Fig. 7A, c). In these cases, the type 4 collagen antibody is used to visualize the level of blister formation. A reaction on the blister roof indicates dermolytic blistering (see Fig. 7A, d) and confirms DEB. On the other hand, a JEB or EBS has to be considered when type 4 collagen staining appears on the blister floor (see Fig. 6B, d). Other generalized or localized subtypes of DEB can show a reduced (see Fig. 7B, a–c) or normal expression of type 7 collagen.[11]

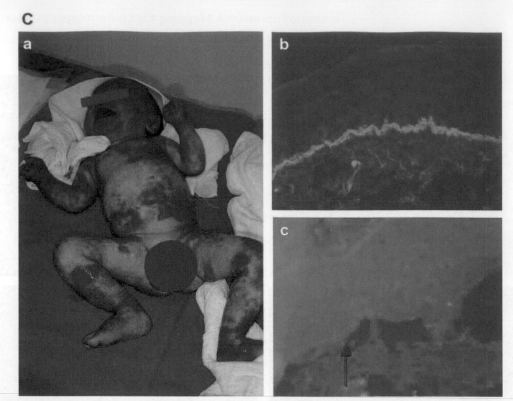

Fig. 6. (*continued*)

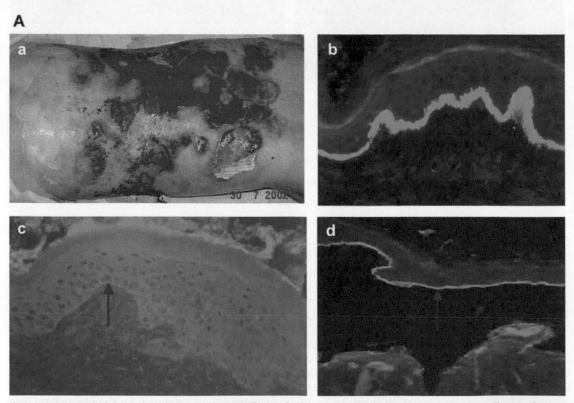

Fig. 7. IFM in DEB. (*A*) Severe generalized RDEB (formerly known as Hallopeau-Siemens, type 7 collagen absent): (*a*) large nonhealing wounds in a patient with severe generalized RDEB; (*b*) type 7 collagen staining positive on NHS control; (*c*) type 7 collagen absent on patient skin (*arrow*); (*d*) dermolytic split formation in the BMZ with anti-collagen 4 staining on the blister roof (*arrow*). (*B*) Generalized DEB (type 7 collagen reduced): (*a*) extensive milia formation in a child with generalized DEB; (*b*) type 7 collagen staining positive on NHS control; (*c*) reduced type 7 collagen on patient's skin mainly on the blister roof (dermolytic, *arrow*).

B

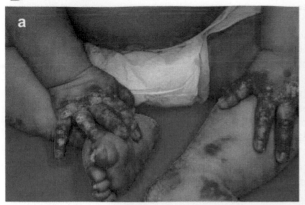

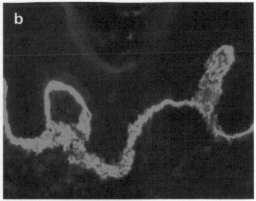

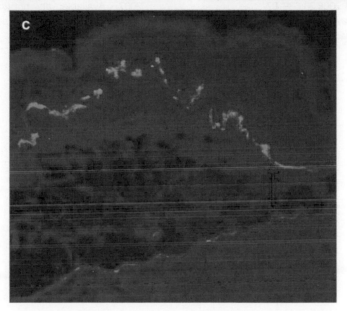

Fig. 7. (*continued*)

SUMMARY

IFM is the procedure of choice for a preliminary final diagnosis and classification of subtypes of EB. The immunofluorescence patterns (for the determination of the level of blister formation and visualization of the expression of the respective protein) identify proteins involved in the pathology and help to focus on the genes to be investigated by mutation analysis to establish the final diagnosis. IFM is a useful first instrument for counseling the patients and parents about the prognosis of the disease, and it takes only half a day to obtain the results. Using the Michel medium for storage and transport of skin samples to a specialized laboratory, IFM can comfortably be used in collaborations between different countries worldwide.

REFERENCES

1. Nischler E, Klausegger A, Hüttner C, et al. Diagnostic pitfalls in newborns and babies with blisters and erosions. Dermatology Research and Practice 2009;2009. DOI: 10.1155/2009/320403. Available at: http://www.hindawi.com/journals/drp/contents.html. Accessed December 22, 2009.
2. Hintner H, Stingl G, Schuler G, et al. Immunofluorescence mapping of antigenic determinants within the dermal-epidermal junction in mechanobullous diseases. J Invest Dermatol 1981;76:113–8.
3. Fine JD, Eady RA, Bauer EA, et al. The classification of inherited epidermolysis bullosa (EB): report of the third international consensus meeting on diagnosis and classification of EB. J Am Acad Dermatol 2008;58(6):931–50.
4. Fine JD, Hintner H, editors. Life with epidermolysis bullosa (EB). Etiology, diagnosis,

multidisciplinary care and therapy. Wien: Springer-Verlag; 2009. p. 338.

5. Michel B, Milner Y, David K. Preservation of tissue-fixed immunoglobulins in skin biopsies of patients with lupus erythematosus and bullous diseases. J Invest Dermatol 1973;59:449.

6. Vaughan Jones SA, Bhogal BS, Black MM. The use of Michel's transport media for immunofluorescence and immunoelectron microscopy in autoimmune bullous diseases. J Cutan Pathol 1995;22:365–70.

7. Yiasemides E, Trisnowati N, Su J, et al. Clinical heterogeneity in recessive epidermolysis bullosa due to mutations in the keratin 14 gene, KRT14. Clin Exp Dermatol 2008;33:689–97.

8. Koss-Harnes D, Høyheim B, Anton-Lamprecht I, et al. A site-specific plectin mutation causes dominant

epidermolysis bullosa simplex ogna: two identical de novo mutations. J Invest Dermatol 2002;118:87–93.

9. Pfendner Ellen G, Lucky Anne W. Epidermolysis bullosa with pyloric atresia. In: GeneReviews. Last revision, 2009. Available at: http://www.ncbi.nlm.nih.gov/bookshelf/br.fcgi?book=gene&part=eb-pa#eb-pa. Accessed November 13, 2009.

10. Pfendner Ellen G, Lucky Anne W. Junctional epidermolysis bullosa. In: GeneReviews, Initial posting, 2008. Available at: http://www.ncbi.nlm.nih.gov/bookshelf/br.fcgi?book=gene&part=ebj. Accessed November 13, 2009.

11. Pfendner Ellen G, Lucky Anne W. Dystrophic epidermolysis bullosa. In: GeneReviews, Last revision, 2007. Available at: http://www.ncbi.nlm.nih.gov/bookshelf/br.fcgi?book=gene&part=ebd. Accessed November 13, 2009.

Transmission Electron Microscopy for the Diagnosis of Epidermolysis Bullosa

Robin A.J. Eady, DSc, FRCP[a],*,
Patricia J.C. Dopping-Hepenstal, BSc[b]

KEYWORDS

- Electron microscopy • Epidermolysis bullosa
- Dermal-epidermal junction • Hemidesmosome
- Anchoring fibril • Keratin intermediate filament
- Desmosome

Since the early application of transmission electron microscopy (TEM) to the study of epidermolysis bullosa (EB),[1–3] TEM has for many years retained the premier position among diagnostic techniques for establishing or confirming the diagnosis of the major types of EB. Even today, TEM remains the most powerful method for determining the levels of skin separation which underlie the current classification of EB and certain related disorders.[4] Other laboratory techniques, including immunofluorescence (IF) microscopy and DNA analysis, have become increasingly important in EB diagnosis. However, no single method has yet fully superseded TEM, although it is now used mainly in a reference laboratory and is less applicable as a primary diagnostic procedure.

This article aims to provide a summary of the main TEM findings in the major types of EB and to describe briefly the ultrastructural features of some of the disorders that have been recently added to the EB classification.[4] Finally, it includes a short discussion on the current advantages and disadvantages of using TEM for EB diagnosis.

KEY STEPS FOR OPTIMIZING TISSUE PREPARATION FOR TEM

Compared with other laboratory applications such as routine diagnostic histopathology, TEM is very costly and time-consuming. The specialized equipment is expensive to purchase and maintain, and the laboratory staff is required to spend several hours of highly skilled technical work in the preparation of each specimen for analysis. Adherence to a few key guidelines helps avoid wasting time, effort, and expense in obtaining and processing skin biopsies for TEM diagnosis. All skin samples are precious and often it is possible to have only one attempt at procuring a suitable diagnostic biopsy from an EB patient, especially in the case of a neonate or young infant. It is usually preferable not to contemplate taking the biopsy unless all the appropriate steps are known to be available and achievable beforehand.

Laboratory Preparation

As soon as the biopsy is planned, it is essential to ensure that the laboratory is notified and the

We would like to thank DebRA (UK) for longstanding interest in our work and for generous financial support.
[a] St John's Institute of Dermatology, St Thomas' Hospital, London SE1 7EH, UK
[b] National Diagnostic Epidermolysis Bullosa Laboratory, GSTS Pathology, St John's Institute of Dermatology, St Thomas' Hospital, London SE1 7EH, UK
* Corresponding author.
E-mail address: robin.eady@kcl.ac.uk

Dermatol Clin 28 (2010) 211–222
doi:10.1016/j.det.2009.12.001

necessary reagents, mainly the TEM fixative, are available. An effective primary fixative for TEM contains 2.5% glutaraldehyde and 2% formaldehyde in 0.1M phosphate buffer at pH 7.4.[5] This fixative can be stored conveniently in a −20°C freezer as premeasured aliquots of double-strength buffer and double-strength aldehyde solutions, ready for thawing and mixing before use. The reactivity of the aldehydes is preserved better if kept separate from the buffer. Upon notification of an imminent biopsy, the laboratory can supply the clinician with this prepared fixative, with a disposable plastic minipipette for mixing the solutions. The fixative is adequately preserved during overnight transport at ambient temperature.

If a sample for IF antigen mapping is to be taken at the same time, the biopsy can usually be subdivided with minimal trauma by placing it, epidermis down, on the inverted lid of a 5cm plastic Petri dish and cutting it using a large (no. 22) scalpel blade with a rocking motion, thus minimizing shearing forces. For preservation of antigenicity, it is essential to avoid contamination of the IF sample with TEM fixative. Alternatively, a separate sliver of skin can be taken from the patient for IF studies. Once the TEM sample has been immersed in fixative, it can be dispatched to the laboratory at ambient temperature, suitably packaged to comply with local regulations for the transport of biologic material. If not dispatched on the day of the biopsy, the sample should be refrigerated (2–8°C).

Biopsy Site

Biopsies from established blisters or lesions more than an hour old will usually produce conflicting results arising from tissue necrosis and repair. Therefore, the authors recommend that the clinician induce skin separation (a clinically obvious blister is not necessarily best) by gently rubbing the skin in the proposed biopsy site. Ideally, the biopsy should contain the edge of a new lesion so that split and unseparated skin can be examined in the microscope. In extremely fragile skin, as encountered, for example, in Herlitz junctional EB, the very act of cutting the skin during the biopsy procedure is often sufficient to cause shearing of the epidermis from the dermis. In contrast, in certain subtypes of EB, notably localized EB simplex (EBS) (formerly called EBS-Weber-Cockayne), it can be very difficult to induce a blister, even after subjecting the skin to localized warming and extensive rubbing, so diagnostically useful biopsies are usually impractical and often unobtainable. Fortunately, in most cases of mild localized EBS a strong family and personal medical history, and relevant clinical features, are sufficient to support the diagnosis.

Biopsy Method

TEM fixatives, containing the powerful cross-linking agent glutaraldehyde, penetrate dense tissue such as skin relatively poorly. The addition of formaldehyde, a smaller molecule that diffuses into the tissue more rapidly, improves the penetration rate, but the biopsy sample still has to be subdivided to allow for adequate fixation. Shave biopsy samples are usually preferred since only shallow skin samples are required and the shearing motion that often accompanies the punch biopsy technique may result in total separation of the dermis from the epidermis if the skin is very fragile.

Specimen Processing

The sample should be immersed immediately in the TEM fixative since any delay will cause it to dry out and result in irreversible cellular and tissue damage, rendering it partly or totally useless for

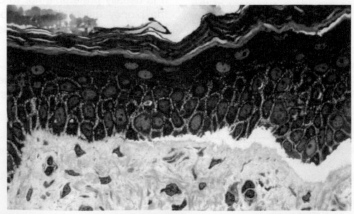

Fig. 1. Semithin plastic embedded section showing a clean split between the dermis and epidermis in junctional EB. Methylene blue and azure II stain. Original magnification 100×.

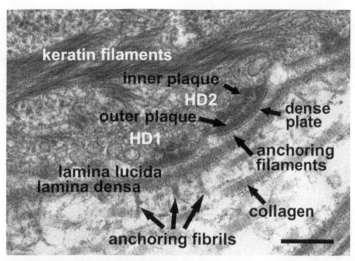

Fig. 2. Electron micrograph illustrating key components of an anchoring complex. HD1 and HD2 represent hemidesmosomes. Bar = 0.25 μm.

subsequent TEM analysis. The divided sample or subsamples must be small enough for adequate fixation and should also be large enough to allow for the provision of informative semithin (~0.5–1.0 μm thick) sections for light microscopy (see below), an essential step before trimming the resin blocks further for ultramicrotomy and TEM examination. Semithin sections will enable the level of blistering or tissue splitting to be ascertained (Fig. 1), thus complementing IF-antigen mapping, which will often be undertaken concurrently.

TEM ANALYSIS
Normal Versus Abnormal

A major prerequisite to performing TEM diagnosis is for the microscopist to be able to distinguish normal from abnormal. Where the level of tissue separation or blister formation can be seen clearly in well-prepared sections, the possibility of error is considerably reduced. However, this important feature may be less than clear, and thus equivocal. The figures provide examples of the ultrastructural features of different EB types. Fig. 2 shows the details of certain key structures of the dermal-epidermal junction that are relevant to EB diagnosis. These structures, conveniently incorporated in an "anchoring complex," can be linked to a number of molecules[6] that are important in normal skin function, including adhesion between the epidermis and dermis, and possible molecular interactions in the upper dermis.[7] All major types of EB will result from mutations in one or more of

Table 1 TEM features in EBS		
EBS Subtype	**Level of Split**	**Other Features**
EBS Weber-Cockayne	Lower epidermis	Basal cell lysis
EBS Koebner	Lower epidermis	Basal cell lysis
EBS Dowling-Meara	Lower epidermis	Tonofilament clumps
EBS-muscular dystrophy (plectin deficiency)	Lower epidermis	Small hemidesmosome plaques
EBS mottled pigmentation	Lower epidermis	Abnormal clustering of melanosomes
EBS pyloric atresia	Lower epidermis, just above hemidesmosomes	Diminutive hemidesmosomes lacking normal sub-basal dense plates
EBS autosomal recessive, generalized	Lower epidermis	Absence or severe reduction of normal tonofilaments
EBS superficialis	Upper epidermis	Cleavage present usually at interface between stratum granulosum and stratum corneum

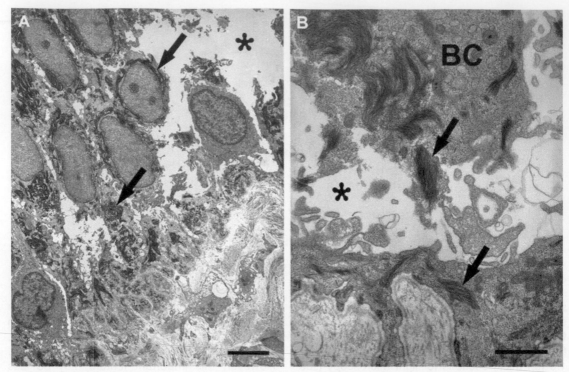

Fig. 3. EBS Dowling-Meara. Note extensive split through basal epidermis (*A*); shown in greater detail (*B*). Split (*asterisks*), tonofilament clumps (*arrows*). Bars (*A*) = 5 μm; (*B*) = 1 μm. BC: basal cells.

the 10 known genes encoding these proteins (see **Figs. 1** and **2**).

TEM Features of Major Types of EB

EBS

In all the major subtypes of EBS, including localized EBS, the split occurs through the lower part

of the epidermis, usually at a level starting beneath the basal cell nuclei[8,9]; whereas, in EBS superficialis the blister level is at the interface between the stratum corneum and stratum granulosum (**Table 1**).[10] In EBS Dowling-Meara, in addition to the intraepidermal cleavage (**Fig. 3A**), abnormal clumps of tonofilaments (keratin intermediate filaments) can be seen, mainly within basal

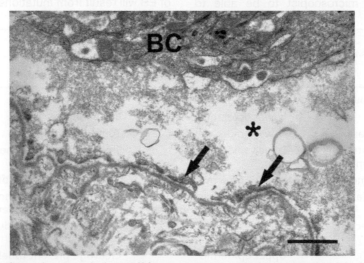

Fig. 4. EBS-Muscular dystrophy. The split (*asterisk*) has occurred through the lower pole of the basal epidermal cells, leaving the cell membrane and diminutive hemidesmosome plaques with the basement membrane at the base (*arrows*). Bar = 1 μm. BC: basal cells.

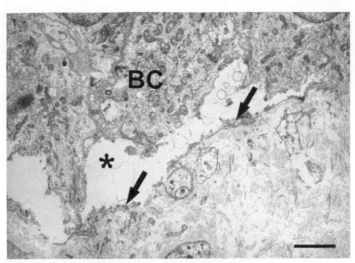

Fig. 5. EB-Pyloric atresia. The ultrastructural features are almost identical to those shown in **Fig. 4**. Note the low intraepidermal split (*asterisk*) with cell fragments at the base (*arrows*). Bar=2.5 μm. BC: basal cells.

keratinocytes[11–13] (see **Fig. 3**). This finding, which is thought to be pathognomonic, provided an early clue to the underlying molecular abnormality.[14] In the form of EBS with plectin deficiency, also known as EBS with muscular dystrophy, the split is just above the level of the hemidesmosomes, which are frequently diminutive[15–18] (**Fig. 4**). A similar type of split may also occur in EB-pyloric atresia (**Fig. 5**), which may not have been foreseen, since EB-pyloric atresia is normally thought to be a subtype of junctional EB.[19] Rarely, non-Herlitz junctional EB caused by mutations in collagen XVII may also be associated with an intraepidermal split.[20,21]

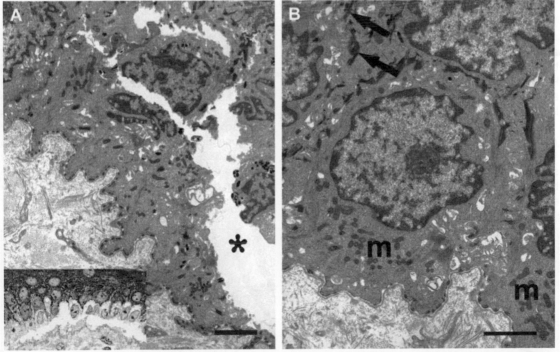

Fig. 6. EBS-generalized (autosomal recessive). The main feature is the striking lack of recognizable tonofilaments in the basal cells, shown at low magnification (A) and in greater detail (B). Split (*asterisk*). Grouped mitochondria (m), normal-appearing tonofilaments in keratinocyte in first suprabasal layer (*arrows*). Bars (A) = 2.5 μm; (B) = 2 μm. Inset: Light micrograph of semithin section showing paucity of staining of the basal epidermal cells. Original magnification 100x.

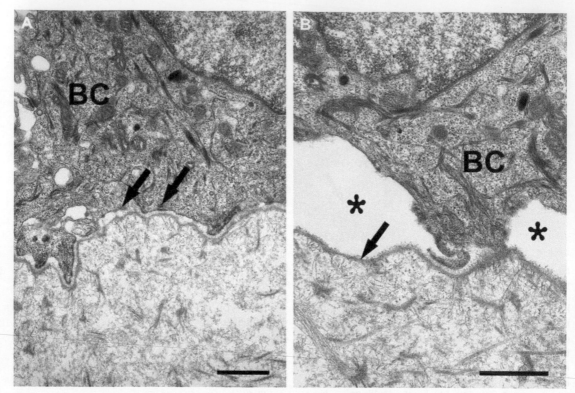

Fig. 7. Herlitz junctional EB. (*A*) Unsplit skin showing small hemidesmosomes (*arrows*) at bottom surface of a basal cell (BC). (*B*) A clean split (*asterisks*) is present through the lamina lucida, between the lower plasma membrane of a basal cell (BC) and a continuous lamina densa (*arrow*). Bars (*A*) = 1 μm; (*B*) = 1 μm.

Finally, in the rare form of generalized, autosomal recessive EB simplex caused by null mutations in the keratin 14 gene, the basal epidermal keratin filament network is severely compromised and normal tonofilaments are sparse in the basal layer or totally absent[22,23] (**Fig. 6**).

Junctional EB
The features of Herlitz junctional EB are usually straightforward, with a clean split at the level of the lamina lucida, usually accompanied by small and reduced numbers of hemidesmosomes[2,24–26]

(**Fig. 7**; **Table 2**). However, it is not uncommon to find the split extending into the lower portion of the basal cells, presumably because the normal structural integrity formed by the molecular binding of the keratin filaments and the hemidesmosome plaques may be compromised.[27] These features are also seen in EB pyloric atresia.[19] In non-Herlitz junctional EB resulting from mutations in laminin 5 (laminin 332) or collagen XVII, hemidesmosomes may be small and reduced in size or normal in number and appearance.[23,28] The authors know of no systematic study showing qualitative or

Table 2
TEM features in Junctional EB

Junctional EB (JEB) Subtype	Level of Split	Other Features
JEB Herlitz	Lamina lucida	Diminutive hemidesmosomes; absent or attenuated sub-basal dense plates; reduced anchoring filaments
JEB non-Herlitz	Lamina lucida	Hemidesmosomes diminutive or normal size. Sub-basal dense plates normal or attenuated.
JEB pyloric atresia	Lamina lucida	Diminutive hemidesmosomes; absent or attenuated sub-basal dense plates

quantitative ultrastructural differences between these two major genetic subtypes of non-Herlitz junctional EB (see **Fig. 7**).

Dystrophic EB

The cleavage plane is consistently immediately below the lamina densa. The next most useful diagnostic indicator is that in the generalized autosomal recessive (or Hallopeau-Siemens) form, normal anchoring fibrils are absent[29] (**Fig. 8; Table 3**). In the dominant and more localized recessive forms, anchoring fibrils are present but fewer than normal. A detailed quantitative analysis failed to find differences in anchoring fibrils between these different genetic subtypes.[29] The disorder known as (transient) bullous dermolysis of the newborn is characterized by an apparent delay in collagen VII

secretion, and the presence of membrane-bound inclusions containing a stippled or otherwise amorphous material in basal keratinocytes[30,31] (**Fig. 9**), which has been shown immunohistochemically to label for collagen VII[29].

TEM OF OTHER DISORDERS RECENTLY CLASSIFIED AS TYPES OF EB
Kindler Syndrome

Unlike any other form of EB, the tissue level of early blister formation in Kindler syndrome may vary, and appear within the epidermis (**Fig. 10A**) or the lamina lucida, or beneath the lamina densa[32,33] (**Table 4**). All three cleavage levels may be seen, even within the same section. Other characteristic findings include multilayering of the lamina densa (see

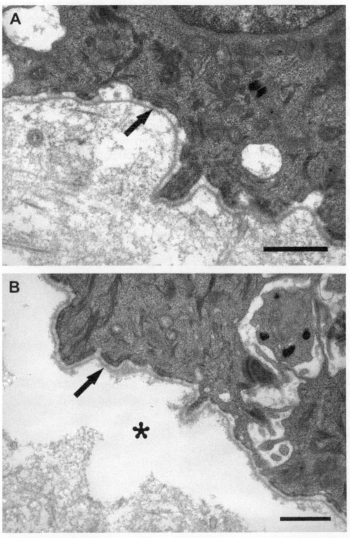

Fig. 8. Recessive dystrophic EB (Hallopeau-Siemens). (*A*) Normal anchoring fibrils are absent beneath the lamina densa (*arrow*) in unsplit skin. (*B*) A split (*asterisk*) is seen between the lamina densa (*arrow*) and upper dermal matrix. Bars (*A*) = 1 μm; (*B*) = 1 μm.

Table 3
TEM features of Dystrophic B

Dystrophic EB (DEB) Subtype	Level of Split	Other Features
DEB autosomal recessive, generalized	Sublamina densa	Absence of normal anchoring fibrils
DEB autosomal recessive, localized	Sublamina densa	Anchoring fibrils reduced in number
DEB autosomal dominant	Sublamina densa	Anchoring fibrils reduced in number
Bullous dermolysis of newborn	Sublamina densa	Intracytoplasmic inclusions in basal cells; reduced anchoring fibrils

Fig. 10B), the presence of dermal colloid bodies, apparent gaps in the dermal matrix (see **Fig 10B**), especially surrounding fibroblasts, and numerous melanophages in the superficial dermis.

Desmosome Disorders

The major clue to the first genetic desmosome disorder, ectodermal dysplasia with skin fragility, caused by mutations in plakophilin 1, was the striking epidermal cell separation and widening of the intercellular space, associated with diminutive desmosomes in the suprabasal layers[34,35] (**Fig. 11A**). Additionally, there is marked perinuclear condensation of the keratin filament network with only sparse peripheral connections with the desmosomes. The cell-cell detachment appears to be caused by the fracture of finger-like cellular projections, proximal to the desmosome plaques (**Fig. 11B**). Similar features have been reported in the more recently described "lethal acantholytic EB simplex" resulting from a deletion in the tail domain of desmoplakin.[36]

Laryngo-onycho-cutaneous Syndrome

Patients with this rare disorder caused by an N-terminal deletion in laminin alpha 3a isoform[37] rarely have true blisters, but do suffer with highly characteristic erosions on the face and elsewhere.

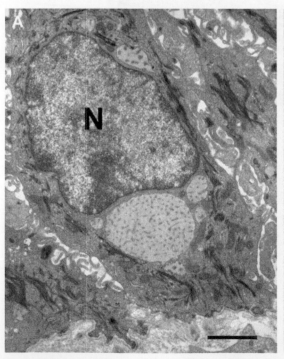
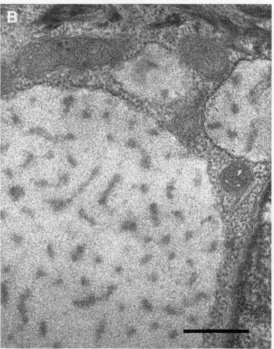

Fig. 9. Bullous dermolysis of the newborn. (*A*)The highly characteristic intracytoplasmic inclusions (*arrows*) are present beneath the nucleus of a basal cell (N). (*B*) Higher magnification of an inclusion showing the electron-dense, irregularly shaped rod-like structures over an amorphous background. Bars (*A*) = 2.5 μm; (*B*) = 0.5 μm.

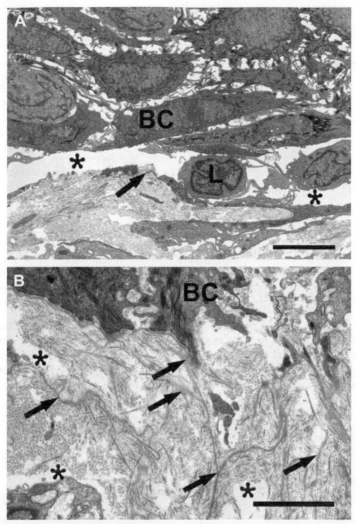

Fig. 10. Kindler syndrome. (*A*) The precise level of split (*asterisks*) is often difficult to determine, and appears to be within the basal epidermis just above the basement membrane (*arrow*). A lymphocyte (L) is present in the basal cell (BC) layer. (*B*) Note the pronounced reduplication of the lamina densa (*arrows*) extending into the upper reticular dermis and associated electron-lucent areas (*asterisks*) often in a pericellular distribution. Bars (*A*) = 5 μm; (*B*) = 2.5 μm.

TEM has shown a focal widening of the lamina lucida associated with small hemidesmosomes.[37]

STRENGTHS AND WEAKNESSES OF TEM VERSUS OTHER METHODS

In mild forms of EB, the IF results may be normal, whereas TEM enables the identification of microsplits and other ultrastructural abnormalities at the dermal-epidermal junction. However, the changes may be subtle, so extensive experience in interpretation is necessary. TEM is essential for the diagnosis of EBS Dowling-Meara, especially in the neonate before the typical herpetiform blisters are evident. IF may show no abnormality, apart from an intraepidermal split, but TEM is able to demonstrate the characteristic tonofilament abnormality in basal cells. Similarly, TEM is useful for the diagnosis of bullous congenital ichthyosiform erythroderma (or epidermolytic hyperkeratosis) where the tonofilament clumps are located in the upper epidermis, in the distribution of keratins K1 and K10. For some disorders, TEM is required because the antibody needed for IF diagnosis is not widely available or not reliable.

TEM has led to the recognition of pathology and provided essential clues to the causative genes underlying certain novel genodermatoses. For example, the first clue to the first human hereditary desmosomal disorder, caused by a deficiency of

Table 4
TEM features of various disorders recently classifies as variants of EB

Disorder	Level of Split	Other Features
Kindler syndrome	Variable; intraepidermal, intralamina lucida, or sublamina densa	Reduplication of lamina densa; presence of upper dermal colloid bodies and melanophages
Ectodermal dysplasia with skin fragility	Mid-epidermis	Widening of intercellular spaces in spinous layer; cleavage through cytoplasm proximal to small desmosomes; condensation of tonofilaments to perinuclear region
Lethal acantholytic EB simplex	Mid-epidermis	Widening of intercellular spaces in spinous layer; cleavage through cytoplasm proximal to desmosomes; contraction of tonofilaments to perinuclear region
Laryngo-onycho-cutaneous syndrome	Splitting not usually present	Focal widening of lamina lucida, some hemidesmosomes small with attenuated sub-basal dense plates

plakophilin 1, came from TEM analysis of a patient's skin. There are several further examples where TEM has been essential in contributing to our knowledge of the structure and function of cells and subcellular components in the skin and other organs. As its role in the diagnosis of EB and other genodermatoses diminishes with time, it is worth remembering that even today it continues to provide a gold standard on which to base the EB classification.

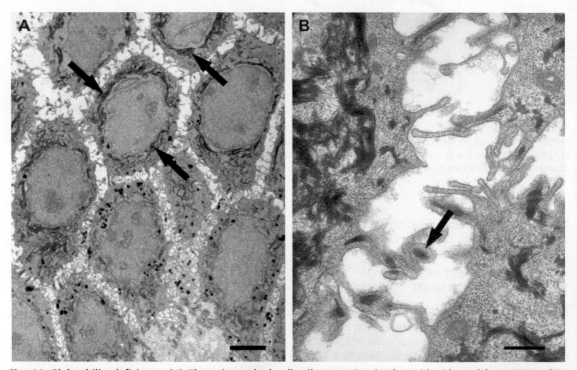

Fig. 11. Plakophilin deficiency. (*A*) There is marked cell-cell separation in the midepidermal layer. Note thin, finger-like processes projecting from the cell surfaces, some of which bear abnormally small desmosomes. The keratin filament network appears to have lost normal connections at the cell periphery and are condensed around the nuclei (*arrows*). (*B*) At higher magnification, the peripheral cell processes appear to have ruptured proximal to the diminutive desmosomes (*arrows*). Bars (*A*) = 2.5 μm; (*B*) = 0.5 μm.

SUMMARY

TEM has been immensely important for EB diagnosis and in laying down markers for the classification of EB, even in its wider, current context. It has also provided invaluable clues to the genetic causes of different types of EB[38] and related desmosomal disorders. In addition, it contributes to translational research that may lead to new treatments, for example, aiming to improve healing of lesions in recessive dystrophic EB.[39]

REFERENCES

1. Pearson RW. Studies on the pathogenesis of epidermolysis bullosa. J Invest Dermatol 1962;39:551–75.
2. Arwill T, Bergenholtz A, Thilander H. Epidermolysis bullosa hereditaria. 5. The ultrastructure of oral mucosa and skin in four cases of the letalis form. Acta Pathol Microbiol Scand 1968;74(3):311–24.
3. Pearson RW, Potter B, Strauss F. Epidermolysis bullosa hereditaria letalis. Arch Dermatol 1974;109:349–55.
4. Fine JD, Eady RA, Bauer EA, et al. The classification of inherited epidermolysis bullosa (EB): report of the Third International Consensus Meeting on Diagnosis and Classification of EB. J Am Acad Dermatol 2008; 58(6):931–50.
5. Wan H, Dopping-Hepenstal PJ, Gratian MJ, et al. Desmosomes exhibit site-specific features in human palm skin. Exp Dermatol 2003;12(4):378–88.
6. McMillan JR, Akiyama M, Shimizu H. Epidermal basement membrane zone components: ultrastructural distribution and molecular interactions. J Dermatol Sci 2003;3:169–77.
7. Villone D, Fritsch A, Koch M, et al. Supramolecular interactions in the dermo-epidermal junction zone: anchoring fibril-collagen VII tightly binds to banded collagen fibrils. J Biol Chem 2008; 283(36):24506–13.
8. Anton-Lamprecht I. Ultrastructural identification of basic abnormalities as clues to genetic disorders of the epidermis. J Invest Dermatol 1994;103:6S–12S.
9. Haneke E, Anton-Lamprecht I. Ultrastructure of blister formation in epidermolysis bullosa hereditaria: V. Epidermolysis bullosa simplex localisata type Weber-Cockayne. J Invest Dermatol 1982; 78(3):219–23.
10. Fine J-D, Johnson L, Wright T. Epidermolysis bullosa simplex superficialis. A new variant of epidermolysis bullosa characterized by subcorneal skin cleavage mimicking peeling skin syndrome. Arch Dermatol 1989;125:633–8.
11. Anton-Lamprecht I, Schnyder UW. Epidermolysis bullosa herpetiformis Dowling-Meara. Report of a case and pathomorphogenesis. Dermatologica 1982;164:221–98.
12. Niemi KM, Kero M, Kanerva L, et al. Epidermolysis bullosa simplex: a new histological subgroup. Arch Dermatol 1983;119:138–41.
13. McGrath JA, Ishida Yamamoto A, Tidman MJ, et al. Epidermolysis bullosa simplex (Dowling-Meara). A clinicopathological review. Br J Dermatol 1992;126: 421–30.
14. Ishida-Yamamoto A, McGrath JA, Chapman SJ, et al. Epidermolysis bullosa simplex (Dowling-Meara type) is a genetic disease characterized by an abnormal keratin filament network involving keratins K5 and K14. J Invest Dermatol 1991;97:959–68.
15. Niemi KM, Sommer H, Kero M, et al. Epidermolysis bullosa simplex associated with muscular dystrophy with recessive inheritance. Arch Dermatol 1988;124: 551–4.
16. Fine J-D, Stenn J, Johnson L, et al. Autosomal recessive epidermolysis bullosa simplex. Generalized phenotypic features suggestive of junctional or dystrophic epidermolysis bullosa, and association with neuromuscular diseases. Arch Dermatol 1989; 125:931–8.
17. Gache Y, Chavanas S, Lacour JP, et al. Defective expression of plectin/HD1 in epidermolysis bullosa simplex with muscular dystrophy. J Clin Invest 1996;97:2289–98.
18. Smith FJD, Eady RAJ, Leigh IM, et al. Plectin deficiency results in muscular dystrophy with epidermolysis bullosa. Nat Genet 1996;13:450.
19. Valari MD, Phillips RJ, Lake BD, et al. Junctional epidermolysis bullosa and pyloric atresia: a distinct entity. Clinical and pathological studies in five patients. Br J Dermatol 1995;133:732–6.
20. Huber M, Floeth M, Borradori L, et al. Deletion of the cytoplasmatic domain of BP180/collagen XVII causes a phenotype with predominant features of epidermolysis bullosa simplex. J Invest Dermatol 2002;118:185–92.
21. Pasmooij AM, van der Steege G, Pas HH, et al. Features of epidermolysis bullosa simplex due to mutations in the ectodomain of type XVII collagen. Br J Dermatol 2004;151:669–74.
22. Rugg EL, McLean WHI, Lane EB, et al. A functional "knockout" for human keratin 14. Genes Dev 1994;8: 2563–73.
23. Chan Y, Anton-Lamprecht I, Yu Q-C, et al. A human keratin 14 "knockout": the absence of K14 leads to severe epidermolysis bullosa simplex and a function for an intermediate filament protein. Genes Dev 1994;8:2574–87.
24. Hashimoto I, Gedde-Dahl T Jr, Schnyder UW, et al. Ultrastructural studies in epidermolysis bullosa hereditaria. IV. Recessive dystrophic types with junctional blistering. (Infantile or Herlitz-Pearson type and adult type). Arch Dermatol Res 1976;26(257): 17–32.

25. Tidman MJ, Eady RAJ. Hemidesmosome heterogeneity in junctional epidermolysis bullosa revealed by morphometric analysis. J Invest Dermatol 1986; 86:51–6.

26. Smith LT. Ultrastructural findings in epidermolysis bullosa. Arch Dermatol 1993;129(12):1578–84.

27. McMillan JR, McGrath JA, Tidman MJ, et al. Hemidesmosomes show abnormal association with the keratin filament network in junctional forms of epidermolysis bullosa. J Invest Dermatol 1998;110:132–7.

28. Hintner H, Wolff K. Generalized atrophic benign epidermolysis bullosa. Arch Dermatol 1982;118:375–84.

29. Tidman MJ, Eady RAJ. Evaluation of anchoring fibrils and other components of the dermal–epidermal junction in dystrophic epidermolysis bullosa by a quantitative ultrastructural technique. J Invest Dermatol 1985;84:374–7.

30. Hashimoto K, Matsumoto M, Iacobelli D. Transient bullous dermolysis of the newborn. Arch Dermatol 1985;121:1429–38.

31. Fine J-D, Horiguchi Y, Stein DI, et al. Intraepidermal type VII collagen. Evidence for abnormal intracytoplasmic processing of a major basement membrane protein in rare patients with dominant and possibly localized recessive forms of dystrophic epidermolysis bullosa. J Am Acad Dermatol 1990;22:188–95.

32. Hovnanian A, Blanchet-Bardon C, de Prost Y. Poikiloderma of Theresa Kindler: report of a case with ultrastructural study, and review of the literature [review]. Pediatr Dermatol 1989;6(2):82–90.

33. Shimizu H, Sato M, Ban M, et al. Immunohistochemical, ultrastructural, and molecular features of Kindler syndrome distinguish it from dystrophic epidermolysis bullosa [review]. Arch Dermatol 1997; 133:1111–7.

34. McGrath JA, McMillan JR, Shemano CS, et al. Mutations in the plakophilin 1 gene result in ectodermal dysplasia/skin fragility syndrome. Nat Genet 1997; 17:240–4.

35. McMillan JR, Haftek M, Akiyama M, et al. Alterations in desmosome size and number coincide with the loss of keratinocyte cohesion in skin with homozygous and heterozygous defects in the desmosomal protein plakophilin 1. J Invest Dermatol 2003;121: 96–103.

36. Jonkman MF, Pasmooij AM, Pasmans SG, et al. Loss of desmoplakin tail causes lethal acantholytic epidermolysis bullosa. Am J Hum Genet 2005;77: 653–60.

37. McLean WH, Irvine AD, Hamill KJ, et al. An unusual N-terminal deletion of the laminin alpha 3a isoform leads to the chronic granulation tissue disorder laryngo-onycho-cutaneous syndrome. Hum Mol Genet 2003;12(18):2395–409.

38. Eady RAJ. Discovery of basement membrane zone ultrastructural entities by electron microscopy. J Invest Dermatol 2008;128:E1–2 [online].

39. Wong T, Gammon L, Liu L, et al. Potential of fibroblast cell therapy for recessive dystrophic epidermolysis bullosa. J Invest Dermatol 2008;128(9): 2179–89.

Molecular Testing in Epidermolysis Bullosa

Daniele Castiglia, PhD, Giovanna Zambruno, MD*

KEYWORDS

- Mutation detection • Mismatch screening
- DNA sequencing • Epidermolysis bullosa

The development of DNA technology and improved knowledge of the structure and function of the human genome have led to the identification of the causative genes responsible for the different forms of epidermolysis bullosa (EB) and provided the opportunity to determine the precise location and type of mutations present in EB patients, allowing the diagnosis of this disease at the level of the defective gene itself. The large genetic heterogeneity of EB, however, precludes the direct use of molecular testing for EB diagnosis. In addition, only a few diagnostic or research laboratories in the world are equipped to perform mutational screening, which is still labor intensive and associated with considerable costs, because most mutations are private (ie, unique to one or a few families). The laboratory diagnostic approach to EB involves at first the use of immunofluorescence epitope mapping (IFM) and transmission electron microscopy (TEM) examination of a skin biopsy to determine the level of skin cleavage and the presence of morphologic alterations of epithelial adhesion structures and the defective expression of specific protein components. IFM and TEM enable definition of the major EB type and, in most cases, the subtype and identification of the protein component targeted by the mutations. These analyses define the candidate genes for mutation screening and they must precede molecular testing, which should be primarily considered when (1) prenatal or preimplantation diagnosis is being planned, (2) the mode of genetic transmission cannot be delineated from the family pedigree in combination with IFM and TEM findings, and (3) a gene-replacement therapy protocol is foreseen (see the article by Sybert elsewhere in this issue for further exploration of this topic).[1]

Mutation identification in a given family is required for prenatal diagnosis, although linkage analysis using markers (either intragenic polymorphisms or tightly linked microsatellites) for the mutant gene may be an alternative method when the mutation is unknown (see the article by Sybert elsewhere in this issue for further exploration of this topic).[2,3] This approach cannot be applied, however, to EB types presenting locus heterogeneity (ie, junctional EB [JEB] and EB simplex [EBS]).[1,4] Prenatal testing by linkage analysis is restricted to dystrophic EB (DEB) families, because all DEB cases result from mutations in a single gene, COL7A1. Prenatal diagnosis by indirect DNA analysis requires the availability of DNA samples from several family members (at least of both parents and a previously affected child) to identify the marker allele that segregates with the mutant gene in the kindred.

Besides its crucial relevance for prenatal diagnosis, mutation identification is recommended to provide accurate genetic counseling regarding the mode of inheritance and the risk of disease recurrence in sporadic cases presenting with mild to moderate DEB, which can result from either dominant de novo or recessive inherited mutations.[1]

Molecular testing can also be an excellent way to confirm the diagnosis for very rare EB variants caused by mutations that invariably occur at the same nucleotide position. A typical example is the recurrent dominant missense mutation at nucleotide 74 (c.74C>T/p.P25L) of keratin 5 gene causing EBS with mottled pigmentation.[5]

This work is supported by grants from the Istituto Superiore di Sanità (No. 526D/4 and E-Rare 1, acronym Kindlernet).

Laboratory of Molecular and Cell Biology, IDI-IRCCS, Via dei Monti di Creta 104, 00167 Rome, Italy

* Corresponding author.

E-mail address: g.zambruno@idi.it

Dermatol Clin 28 (2010) 223–229

doi:10.1016/j.det.2009.12.003

Finally, patient genotyping can be required when Kindler syndrome is suspected. Kindler syndrome diagnosis is difficult to achieve in the newborn and infant because of the clinical overlap with other forms of EB. Moreover, TEM and IFM findings on a skin biopsy can be insufficiently specific to establish a diagnosis of Kindler syndrome. Mutational screening of the causal gene FERMT1/KIND1 represents the best technical option for Kindler syndrome diagnosis confirmation.[6]

When considering molecular testing in the diagnostic approach of an EB patient, it should be kept in mind that the sensitivity of any gene screening procedure is not 100%. The mutation detection rate in the most complex and frequently analyzed gene, COL7A1, can vary from 60% to 95% depending on the screening technique used.[7–9] The detection rate in other genes, such as those encoding for laminin-332 (LAMA3, LAMB3, and LAMC2), integrin α6β4 (ITGA6 and ITGB4), collagen XVII (COL17A1), and plectin (PLEC1), ranges from 83% to 95%, as deduced from mutational studies of large patient cohorts performed in molecular diagnostic laboratories worldwide.[10,11] The mutation detection rate seems to be lower (67%) in keratin genes.[12] Personnel involved in genetic counseling should inform affected families asking for molecular testing about the sensitivity of the mutation screening strategy performed. The inability to detect a mutation can be intrinsic to the resolving power of the chosen method or related to the mutation site, which could lie outside the coding exons and flanking intronic junctions (ie, within noncoding regulatory elements or deep intronic regions that are usually not screened). In addition, all the polymerase chain reaction (PCR)–based methods applied in routine diagnostics are unable to detect large deletions or duplications encompassing the entire gene or one or more exons.

This article reviews the most popular methods used in EB molecular analysis.

SOURCES OF GENETIC MATERIAL

Mutational and linkage analyses are performed using DNA from the proband and his or her relatives. Among the latter, the most important samples are those of the patient's parents. DNA can be extracted from any tissue. In EB diagnostics constitutional DNA is usually obtained from the white cells present in a blood draw, which is stored in tubes containing EDTA. Standard sampling is 5 mL of EDTA blood from adults and children and 2 to 3 mL from infants, although adequate DNA amount can be obtained from 0.2 mL of blood or less.

Whenever a blood draw cannot be performed, buccal swabs may represent an alternative source to obtain constitutional DNA. The DNA amount retrieved might be insufficient for the screening of large genes, however, such as COL7A1. DNA can also be extracted from the skin biopsy used for immunomapping investigations or from keratinocyte-fibroblast cell cultures derived from the skin biopsy. Cultured cells also represent a source of messenger RNA (mRNA), which in many circumstances is useful to verify mutation consequences on splicing of the pre-mRNA.[13] In addition, total RNA can be used as the target molecule for mutational screening procedures (see later). DNA extraction from lesional and nonlesional skin can be of interest if revertant or somatic mosaicism is suspected.[13] Sperm is the proper source of constitutional DNA to verify the presence of a known mutation in the proband's father when the occurrence of a paternal gonadal mosaicism has to be proved.

SCREENING OF UNKNOWN MUTATIONS

Mutational detection strategies have been developed for all genes involved in EB. Preliminary to mutation search is the choice of the gene to be analyzed. In particular, EB types showing locus heterogeneity, such as JEB and EBS, can require screening of more than one gene. IFM findings can allow identification of the defective protein (eg, laminin-332 or collagen XVII or α6β4 integrin in JEB) and guide mutation search. Nevertheless, IFM is not adequate to distinguish the mutant polypeptide subunit in altered multimeric proteins. In these cases, multistep testing can be devised. When a gene coding for a chain subunit of a multimeric protein is more frequently targeted by mutations compared with the genes coding for the other subunits, then that gene should be screened at first. In JEB with laminin-332 deficiency, molecular analysis should start with LAMB3 testing, thereafter continue with LAMC2, and terminate with LAMA3. In JEB with pyloric atresia, ITGB4 should be screened at first, followed by ITGA6, which is very rarely mutated.[11]

Mutation scanning techniques are based on PCR amplification of target DNA or RNA sequences. Because missense, nonsense, and splice site mutations represent the most common types of nucleotide changes underlying EB, the screening strategies have been designed to detect point mutations.[13–27] Selective and rapid amplification of each exon and intron-exon boundary is obtained using genomic DNA (gDNA) as a template and specific primer pairs that anneal on flanking intronic sequences. Alternatively, overlapping primer pairs that anneal on exons and cover the entire coding region can be used when reverse transcribed mRNA (complementary DNA [cDNA]) is chosen as a template. The latter strategy depends on the availability of an RNA source, which in turn implies laboratory facilities and tools for setting up primary keratinocyte-fibroblast cell cultures. Because mRNA comprises all the coding regions but does not contain intervening sequences, the advantage of a cDNA-based screening strategy resides in the amplification of a reduced number of PCR fragments.

Conversely, gDNA-based screening strategies imply, in case of genes with many large introns, the amplification of a greater number of PCR products, each encompassing one or a few exons and flanking sequences. Blood from which the gDNA is extracted is easy to obtain, however, whereas procedures for deriving primary cultured cells are time consuming and more expensive. Mutation search on gDNA is favored by most of the diagnostic laboratories.

Genomic DNA-based strategies are available for all genes involved in EB, whereas cDNA-based strategies have been developed for a limited number of genes, in particular the largest ones, such as COL7A1, ITGB4, ITGA6, LAMB3, and LAMC2.[15,16,19,28,29] Seventy-two primer pairs (72 PCRs) are commonly used to amplify all 118 COL7A1 exons using gDNA, whereas the entire COL7A1 coding region is comprised in only 22 cDNA amplicons.[18,19] To amplify ITGB4, ITGA6, LAMB3, and LAMC2 exons, 38, 26, 23, and 23 primer pairs are usually used with gDNA as a template, whereas 12, 9, 8, and 8 PCR fragments can be generated from cDNA, respectively.[15,16,21,22,28,29]

Molecular testing of keratin 14 gene (KRT14), which is involved in EBS, is complicated by the presence of two inactive pseudogenes, whose sequences could be coamplified with functional KRT14 sequences. Current gDNA-based strategies for KRT14 mutational screening have been conceived to avoid pseudogene amplification. These protocols imply single-step allele-specific PCR with primers that specifically anneal on functional KRT14 sequences, or exploit restriction sites on gDNA to exclude the pseudogene sequences from the subsequent PCR.[24–26]

Once chosen, the target molecule's gene segments are amplified using PCR; then, the most accurate way to characterize them is to obtain the exact DNA sequence. In this manner, aberrant variations can be identified and their presence confirmed in family members. Direct sequencing can be labor intensive because of the size of the gene but, especially when a cDNA-based strategy is used, it represents

a relatively simple and reliable technology endowed with high sensitivity (<95%).[10,11] Moreover, if a gene has been extensively screened and a large mutation database is already available, "priority" strategies based on gDNA amplification and direct sequencing of priority regions, which are defined according to the number and frequency of the reported mutations, can be devised.[30] Priority screening is a general principle that also works well in genotyping new patients belonging to specific populations with a well-characterized constellation of recurrent and unique mutations.[31,32] This strategy may speed diagnosis and improve the mutation detection rate in highly complex genes necessitating the generation and sequencing of many amplicons, such as LAMA3, LAMB3, LAMC2, and COL7A1 genes.[30,31]

Nevertheless, systematic DNA sequencing has the disadvantage of being expensive and time-consuming for analysis of genes with a large exon number, such as COL7A1. Alternative strategies have been developed over time with the purpose to identify a single amplicon for sequencing. These include single-strand conformation polymorphism (SSCP), denaturing gradient gel electrophoresis (DGGE), conformation sensitive gel electrophoresis (CSGE), denaturing high-performance liquid chromatography (DHPLC), and protein truncation test (PTT).[33–37] By using adapted apparatus, the first four methods are able to detect local mismatches within heteroduplex DNA molecules that form following hybridization between wild-type and mutant DNA (Fig. 1A). Their sensitivities vary greatly depending on the size of the amplicon screened. SSCP and CSGE have low detection levels (<70%–75%), but are easy to use. DGGE and DHPLC are more complex to set up, but once optimized they are very efficient with a mutation detection rate of up to 95%, approaching that of DNA sequencing. PTT is conceived for screening very big genes using either RNA or DNA and can detect only mutations that lead to protein truncation. It is important to consider that these methods allow the identification of point variations, which can be either true mutations or polymorphisms without any relation to the disease. The pathogenic role of a sequence variant can be obvious by looking at its nature, position within the gene, and frequency. If doubts remain, functional tests at the mRNA and protein levels should be considered.[13]

SSCP

This method works well with small PCR fragments (<150 bp), which need to be denatured, and then run in nondenaturing polyacrylamide gels.[38]

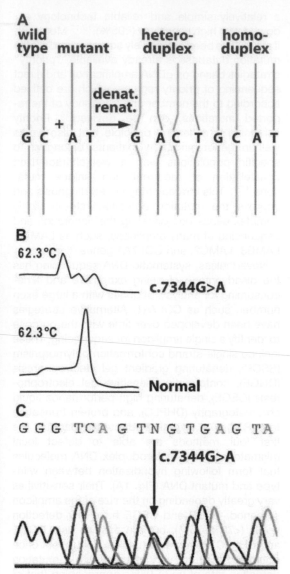

Fig. 1. (*A*) Schematic representation of heteroduplex formation, which results by mixing, denaturing, and reannealing of PCR fragments amplified from wild-type and mutant alleles that differ in sequence because of a point mutation. Current mutation screening strategies use a range of techniques to detect heteroduplexes. (*B*) Aberrant DHPLC profile of a COL7A1 PCR amplicon harboring the c.7344G>A mutation, which is recurrent in Italian recessive DEB patients. At an optimal running temperature (62.3°C), the PCR product amplified from a standard (*normal*) DNA shows only one chromatographic peak corresponding to homoduplex molecules, whereas a mixture of mutant and standard DNA reveals homoduplex (*right peak*) and early released heteroduplex traces (*left peaks*). (*C*) Subsequent identification of the c.7344G>A mutation by direct DNA sequencing of the aberrant amplicon. Overlapped G/A peaks at nucleotide position 7344 (highlighted by N) indicate the heterozygous status for the mutation.

During electrophoresis, the mobility and migration of single-stranded and reannealed double-stranded DNA molecules depend on both their size and the conformation assumed on the basis of nucleotide sequence composition. If two alleles differ for a point mutation, the PCR fragment spanning this variation is expected to result in four types of single-stranded and two types of double-stranded molecules that appear on a gel as four bands with a different migration speed. If the two alleles are identical, only two bands are observed. SSCP has been applied to mutational screening of COL7A1 in DEB families.[39]

DGGE

The method has the best performance with fragments of up to 500 bp.[35,40] It allows the detection of point variations within double-stranded DNA fragments (heteroduplex analysis) run on a gel containing an increasing denaturant concentration (gradient gel). In this condition, homoduplex PCR fragments resulting from the reassociation of complementary strands of one allele have different mobility and migration in respect to heteroduplex PCR fragments formed between two alleles, which are different for the presence of the mutation. Optimization of this method requires that the gradient of denaturing agent concentration be adapted to the sequence of the analyzed gene fragments. Also, this method is used for COL7A1 mutation detection.[40]

CSGE

This method is expected to have high sensitivity for fragments of up to 600 bp. Experimentally, it was shown to yield mutation detection rates of up to 75% when applied to COL7A1 screening.[7,8] CSGE was developed for heteroduplex analysis in a modified polyacrylamide gel electrophoresis that enhances the tendency of single mismatch to produce conformational changes in mildly denaturing environment. It allows one to discriminate homoduplexes from heteroduplexes of PCR fragments in virtue of their differential electrophoretic mobility. Protocols for mutation detection by CSGE have been reported for most EB genes.[8–11,15–17,20–22]

DHPLC

This is an efficient, semiautomatic, high-throughput system for fragments of up to 600 bp. For these reasons, DHPLC technology is being increasingly used in EB diagnostics. In particular, it has been optimized for molecular diagnosis of DEB and JEB.[9,11,31,41] The principle through which the DHPLC functions is the identification of heteroduplex DNA molecules formed by mixing, denaturing, and reannealing the PCR products amplified from alleles differing in sequence because of point mutations (see **Fig. 1**). The PCR fragments are automatically loaded on a polystirene column and eluted with an acetonitrile gradient buffer. Under partial denaturing conditions, fragments containing mismatches (heteroduplexes) are released from the column easier than perfectly matched fragments (homoduplexes). The DHPLC apparatus records the elution profiles of amplicons by an ultraviolet lamp and shows them as chromatographic peaks. By comparing the elution profile of an amplicon generated from the testing sample with the one from a standard homozygote, aberrant heteroduplex profiles can be easily recognized, and the corresponding PCR product sequenced to precisely identify the mutation.

PTT

This method consists of synthesizing a double-stranded cDNA by reverse transcription of the total RNA using primers that encompass specific regions of the studied gene. Using a forward primer that contains the phage T7 promoter as an extra sequence, the freshly synthesized cDNA fragment can be transcribed and then translated in vitro using a coupled rabbit reticulocyte lysate system in the presence of tRNA labeled with radioactive amino acids. The in vitro synthesized peptides are resolved according to their size by electrophoresis on a denaturing gel, and then transferred onto a membrane by Western blot. Finally, the membrane is autoradiographed and the size of the peptides corresponding to the screened sample is determined by comparison with control peptides synthesized by a wild-type gene. A DNA-based PTT protocol has been developed and widely used for the detection of truncating mutations within the large exon 32 (3.3 kb) and 33 (7.2 kb) of the PLEC1 gene in EBS with muscular dystrophy.[42,43] In addition, PTT has had a limited application for screening COL7A1 mutations in patients with recessive DEB.[7]

From what has been reviewed, it is evident that all currently available technologies have individual merits and limitations. Assessment of sensitivity degree of each method is in absolute not so obvious and the success in detecting a sequence variation often relies on the possibility for a given diagnostic laboratory to combine different scanning techniques. Future approaches that could ease EB mutation detection include the automated resequencing of entire genes using customized microarrays spotted with partially overlapping oligonucleotides spanning the sequence of the target genes. Customized genechips are suited for hybridization with gene segments PCR-amplified from the DNA sample to be tested. Appropriate software has been conceived to analyze the hybridization signals on chips and to convert them in DNA sequence. The advantage of the genechip approach consists of the possibility that a single array can assemble up to 300 kb of sequence, allowing the analysis of multiple genes (in theory all the EB genes).[44]

Current mutation scanning methods cannot detect large deletions or duplications encompassing the entire gene or involving gene segments. Such rare complex DNA rearrangements have been reported in a few EB patients.[10,31,45] For the characterization of these cases different screening strategies have been conceived. These make use of several research tools, which comprise Southern or Northern blots, long-range PCR amplifications, real-time quantitative PCRs, and fluorescent in situ hybridization analysis. A combination of these techniques is always needed to precisely define the mutation. They cannot be routinely used in diagnostics and their application remains confined to the research field of EB molecular genetics.

SCREENING OF KNOWN MUTATIONS

Knowledge of the mutations affecting EB patients is particularly valuable to determine the inheritance pattern. For these purposes, accurate carrier screening of the identified mutations has to be performed in the patient's parents and other relatives. The occurrence of a known mutation in a family member's gDNA samples may be verified sometimes by means of less expensive and more rapid tests and without the need for DNA sequencing. For instance, a mutation could alter the sequence recognized by a restriction enzyme, either abolishing the recognition site or creating a new one. In this case, digestion of the mutant PCR fragment with the appropriate enzyme results in a different band pattern on an agarose gel compared with that of a wild-type amplicon, helping mark the mutated allele and follow its inheritance among relatives.[8,10,15]

When the mutation does not alter a restriction site, an alternative method being used is an allele-specific amplification analysis, which exploits differences in the DNA sequence over the site of the mutation. Specifically, gDNAs from the proband and family members and other unrelated healthy subjects are amplified using a common sense (or antisense) primer in combination with an allele-specific antisense (or sense) wild-type primer (whose sequence perfectly matches that of the wild-type allele) or mutant primer (whose sequence perfectly matches that of the mutant allele). At appropriate annealing temperatures of the primer pairs, gDNA samples from heterozygous carriers of the mutation yield an amplified product, visible as a band on an agarose gel, with both primer combinations, whereas gDNAs of homozygous subjects for either wild-type or mutant allele yield only one fragment using the corresponding primer combination, the other one being not amplifiable.[5,46]

When applicable, these analyses are simple to perform and represent the gold standard for mutation carrier screening. Also, DNA-based prenatal diagnosis may involve screening by restriction enzyme digestion, which accelerates evaluation of the risk.[2,3] Moreover, restriction enzyme digestion and allele-specific amplification applied to the detection of recurrent mutations (as part of a priority strategy) speed up gene screening in new patients.

REFERENCES

1. Fine JD, Eady RA, Bauer EA, et al. The classification of inherited epidermolysis bullosa (EB): report of the third international consensus meeting on diagnosis and classification of EB. J Am Acad Dermatol 2008;58(6):931–50.
2. Pfendner EG, Nakano A, Pulkkinen L, et al. Prenatal diagnosis for epidermolysis bullosa: a study of 144 consecutive pregnancies at risk. Prenat Diagn 2003;23(6):447–56.
3. Fassihi H, Eady RA, Mellerio JE, et al. Prenatal diagnosis for severe inherited skin disorders: 25 years' experience. Br J Dermatol 2006;154(1):106–13.
4. Uitto J. Epidermolysis bullosa: the expanding mutation database. J Invest Dermatol 2004;123(4):xii–xiii.
5. Irvine AD, McKenna KE, Jenkinson H, et al. A mutation in the V1 domain of keratin 5 causes epidermolysis bullosa simplex with mottled pigmentation. J Invest Dermatol 1997;108(5):809–10.
6. Lai-Cheong JE, Tanaka A, Hawche G, et al. Kindler syndrome: a focal adhesion genodermatosis. Br J Dermatol 2009;160(2):233–42.
7. Whittock NV, Ashton GH, Mohammedi R, et al. Comparative mutation detection screening of the type VII collagen gene (COL7A1) using the protein truncation test, fluorescent chemical cleavage of mismatch, and conformation sensitive gel electrophoresis. J Invest Dermatol 1999;113(4):673–86.
8. Gardella R, Castiglia D, Posteraro P, et al. Genotype-phenotype correlation in Italian patients with dystrophic epidermolysis bullosa. J Invest Dermatol 2002; 119(6):1456–62.
9. Varki R, Sadowski S, Uitto J, et al. Epidermolysis bullosa. II. Type VII collagen mutations and phenotype-genotype correlations in the dystrophica subtypes. J Med Genet 2007;44(3):181–92.
10. Posteraro P, De Luca N, Meneguzzi G, et al. Laminin-5 mutational analysis in an Italian cohort of patients with junctional epidermolysis bullosa. J Invest Dermatol 2004;123(4):639–48.
11. Varki R, Sadowski S, Pfendner E, et al. Epidermolysis bullosa. I. Molecular genetics of the junctional and hemidesmosomal variants. J Med Genet 2006; 43(8):641–52.
12. Pfendner EG, Sadowski SG, Uitto J. Epidermolysis bullosa simplex: recurrent and de novo mutations in the KRT5 and KRT14 genes, phenotype/genotype correlations, and implications for genetic counseling and prenatal diagnosis. J Invest Dermatol 2005; 125(2):239–43.
13. Castiglia D, Zambruno G. Mutation mechanisms in epidermolysis bullosa. Dermatol Clin 2010;28(1):17–22.
14. Pulkkinen L, Uitto J. Mutation analysis and molecular genetics of epidermolysis bullosa. Matrix Biol 1999; 18(1):29–42.
15. Pulkkinen L, McGrath JA, Christiano AM, et al. Detection of sequence variants in the gene encoding the beta 3 chain of laminin 5 (LAMB3). Hum Mutat 1995;6(1):77–84.
16. Pulkkinen L, McGrath J, Airenne T, et al. Detection of novel LAMC2 mutations in Herlitz junctional epidermolysis bullosa. Mol Med 1997;3(2):124–35.
17. Pulkkinen L, Cserhalmi-Friedman PB, Tang M, et al. Molecular analysis of the human laminin alpha3a chain gene (LAMA3a): a strategy for mutation identification and DNA-based prenatal diagnosis in Herlitz junctional epidermolysis bullosa. Lab Invest 1998;78(9):1067–76.
18. Christiano AM, Hoffman GG, Zhang X, et al. Strategy for identification of sequence variants in COL7A1 and a novel 2-bp deletion mutation in recessive dystrophic epidermolysis bullosa. Hum Mutat 1997; 10(5):408–14.
19. Gardella R, Zoppi N, Ferraboli S, et al. Three homozygous PTC mutations in the collagen type VII gene of patients affected by recessive dystrophic epidermolysis bullosa: analysis of transcript levels in dermal fibroblasts. Hum Mutat 1999;13(6):439–52.
20. Gatalica B, Pulkkinen L, Li K, et al. Cloning of the human type XVII collagen gene (COL17A1), and detection of novel mutations in generalized atrophic benign epidermolysis bullosa. Am J Hum Genet 1997;60(2):352–65.
21. Pulkkinen L, Kim DU, Uitto J. Epidermolysis bullosa with pyloric atresia: novel mutations in the beta4 integrin gene (ITGB4). Am J Pathol 1998; 152(1):157–66.
22. Pulkkinen L, Kimonis VE, Xu Y, et al. Homozygous alpha6 integrin mutation in junctional epidermolysis

bullosa with congenital duodenal atresia. Hum Mol Genet 1997;6(5):669–74.

23. Pfendner E, Rouan F, Uitto J. Progress in epidermolysis bullosa: the phenotypic spectrum of plectin mutations. Exp Dermatol 2005;14(4):241–9.

24. Schuilenga-Hut PH, Vlies P, Jonkman MF, et al. Mutation analysis of the entire keratin 5 and 14 genes in patients with epidermolysis bullosa simplex and identification of novel mutations. Hum Mutat 2003;21(4):447.

25. Wood P, Baty DU, Lane EB, et al. Long-range polymerase chain reaction for specific full-length amplification of the human keratin 14 gene and novel keratin 14 mutations in epidermolysis bullosa simplex patients. J Invest Dermatol 2003;120(3):495–7.

26. Glász-Bóna A, Medvecz M, Sajó R, et al. Easy method for keratin 14 gene amplification to exclude pseudogene sequences: new keratin 5 and 14 mutations in epidermolysis bullosa simplex. J Invest Dermatol 2009;129(1):229–31.

27. Siegel DH, Ashton GH, Penagos HG, et al. Loss of kindlin-1, a human homolog of the *Caenorhabditis elegans* actin-extracellular-matrix linker protein UNC-112, causes Kindler syndrome. Am J Hum Genet 2003;73(1):174–87.

28. Vidal F, Aberdam D, Miquel C, et al. Integrin beta 4 mutations associated with junctional epidermolysis bullosa with pyloric atresia. Nat Genet 1995;10(2):229–34.

29. Ruzzi L, Gagnoux-Palacios L, Pinola M, et al. A homozygous mutation in the integrin alpha6 gene in junctional epidermolysis bullosa with pyloric atresia. J Clin Invest 1997;99(12):2826–31.

30. Kern JS, Kohlhase J, Bruckner-Tuderman L, et al. Expanding the COL7A1 mutation database: novel and recurrent mutations and unusual genotype-phenotype constellations in 41 patients with dystrophic epidermolysis bullosa. J Invest Dermatol 2006;126(5):1006–12.

31. Castori M, Floriddia G, De Luca N, et al. Herlitz junctional epidermolysis bullosa: laminin-5 mutational profile and carrier frequency in the Italian population. Br J Dermatol 2008;158(1):38–44.

32. Has C, Wessagowit V, Pascucci M, et al. Molecular basis of Kindler syndrome in Italy: novel and recurrent Alu/Alu recombination, splice site, nonsense, and frameshift mutations in the KIND1 gene. J Invest Dermatol 2006;126(8):1776–83.

33. Orita M, Suzuki Y, Sekiya T, et al. Rapid and sensitive detection of point mutations and DNA polymorphisms using the polymerase chain reaction. Genomics 1989;5(4):874–9.

34. Ganguly A. An update on conformation sensitive gel electrophoresis. Hum Mutat 2002;19(4):334–42.

35. Myers RM, Maniatis T, Lerman LS. Detection and localization of single base changes by denaturing gradient gel electrophoresis. Meth Enzymol 1987;155:501–27.

36. Xiao W, Oefner PJ. Denaturing high-performance liquid chromatography: a review. Hum Mutat 2001;17(6):439–74.

37. Roest PA, Roberts RG, Sugino S, et al. Protein truncation test (PTT) for rapid detection of translation-terminating mutations. Hum Mol Genet 1993;2(10):1719–21.

38. Sheffield VC, Beck JS, Kwitek AE, et al. The sensitivity of single-strand conformation polymorphism analysis for the detection of single base substitutions. Genomics 1993;16(2):325–32.

39. Dunnill MG, McGrath JA, Richards AJ, et al. Clinicopathological correlations of compound heterozygous COL7A1 mutations in recessive dystrophic epidermolysis bullosa. J Invest Dermatol 1996;107(2):171–7.

40. Hovnanian A, Hilal L, Blanchet-Bardon C, et al. Recurrent nonsense mutations within the type VII collagen gene in patients with severe recessive dystrophic epidermolysis bullosa. Am J Hum Genet 1994;55(2):289–96.

41. Posteraro P, Pascucci M, Colombi M, et al. Denaturing HPLC-based approach for detection of COL7A1 gene mutations causing dystrophic epidermolysis bullosa. Biochem Biophys Res Commun 2005;338(3):1391–401.

42. Dang M, Pulkkinen L, Smith FJ, et al. Novel compound heterozygous mutations in the plectin gene in epidermolysis bullosa with muscular dystrophy and the use of protein truncation test for detection of premature termination codon mutations. Lab Invest 1998;78(2):195–204.

43. Rouan F, Pulkkinen L, Meneguzzi G, et al. Epidermolysis bullosa: novel and de novo premature termination codon and deletion mutations in the plectin gene predict late-onset muscular dystrophy. J Invest Dermatol 2000;114(2):381–7.

44. Lebet T, Chiles R, Hsu AP, et al. Mutations causing severe combined immunodeficiency: detection with a custom resequencing microarray. Genet Med 2008;10(8):575–85.

45. Titeux M, Mejía JE, Mejlumian L, et al. Recessive dystrophic epidermolysis bullosa caused by COL7A1 hemizygosity and a missense mutation with complex effects on splicing. Hum Mutat 2006;27(3):291–2.

46. Shurman D, Losi-Sasaki J, Grimwood R, et al. Epidermolysis bullosa simplex with mottled pigmentation: mutation analysis in the first reported Hispanic pedigree with the largest single generation of affected individuals to date. Eur J Dermatol 2006;16(2):132–5.

Prenatal Diagnosis of Epidermolysis Bullosa

Hiva Fassihi, MD, MRCP(UK), John A. McGrath, MD, FRCP*

KEYWORDS

- Genodermatosis • Fetal skin biopsy
- Chorionic villus sampling
- Preimplantation genetic diagnosis
- Noninvasive prenatal testing

Recent progress in clinical and molecular genetics have helped refine the diagnosis and management of epidermolysis bullosa (EB), although the new discoveries have yet to lead to substantial advances in treatment through gene, protein, cell or drug therapies.[1,2] Disease prevention therefore remains the main option for couples at reproductive risk of EB and one of the major translational benefits of research has been the development of prenatal diagnostic testing.

The techniques have changed over the years, from being heavily reliant on analysis of fetal skin biopsy (FSB) samples acquired during the second trimester to the examination of DNA from first-trimester chorionic villus samples. Furthermore, efforts to design simpler, less-invasive methods of prenatal diagnosis that can be performed earlier in pregnancy, without compromising the sensitivity of the assay and the accuracy of the results, are ongoing. In the absence of a cure for EB, prenatal testing along with appropriate counseling is an integral part of the management of families at risk of some forms of EB.

HISTORY OF PRENATAL DIAGNOSIS

Before the availability of accurate prenatal diagnosis, couples at reproductive risk were faced with limited options. These options included normal conception and acceptance of the risk of having an affected offspring, avoidance of future pregnancies, adoption, artificial insemination with screened donor sperm, or egg donation and in vitro fertilization with the spouse's sperm.

The first prenatal diagnostic examination for a subtype of EB was reported in 1980.[3] These innovative prenatal tests involved the ultrastructural examination of FSBs but were only relevant to a limited number of disorders, including severe forms of junctional and recessive dystrophic EB. The early biopsies were performed during the second trimester with the aid of a fetoscope to visualize the fetus.[4] This involved the insertion of a fiberoptic endoscope into the uterus, under sedation and local anesthesia. However, with improvements in sonographic imaging, FSBs subsequently could be taken under ultrasound guidance.

FSB samples obtained during the early 1980s could only be examined by light microscopy and transmission electron microscopy.[4,5] For EB, the diagnosis was made by finding a split at the dermal-epidermal junction by light microscopy (**Fig. 1A, B**), and then the precise level of cleavage was determined by electron microscopy. The introduction of a number of monoclonal and polyclonal antibodies to various basement membrane components during the mid-1980s, however, led

The authors acknowledge the financial support from the Department of Health via the National Institute for Health Research (NIHR) comprehensive Biomedical Research Centre award to Guy's & St Thomas' NHS Foundation Trust in partnership with King's College London and King's College Hospital NHS Foundation Trust. Support for the authors' own studies on prenatal diagnosis has been provided by the Dystrophic Epidermolysis Bullosa Research Association (DebRA, UK).

Division of Genetics and Molecular Medicine, King's College London (Guy's Campus), St John's Institute of Dermatology Research Laboratories, Floor 9, Tower Wing, Guy's Hospital, Great Maze Pond, London, SE1 9RT, UK

* Corresponding author.
E-mail address: john.mcgrath@kcl.ac.uk

Dermatol Clin 28 (2010) 231–237
doi:10.1016/j.det.2010.02.001

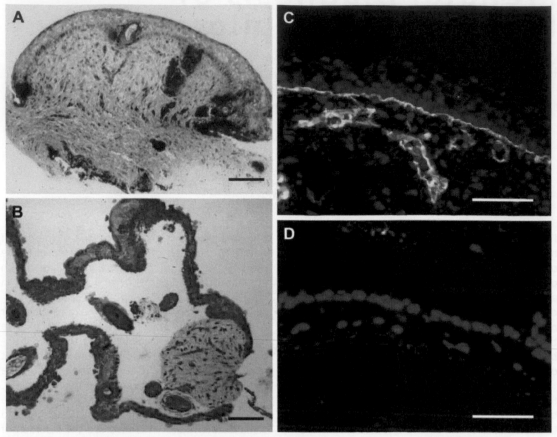

Fig. 1. FSB prenatal diagnosis. (*A*) Photomicrograph of a semi-thin section of normal fetal skin sampled at 18 weeks' gestation (Richardson's stain, bar = 50 μm). (*B*) Photomicrograph of a semi-thin section of fetal skin from an individual with severe generalized recessive dystrophic EB sampled at 18 weeks' gestation showing extensive epidermal detachment (Richardson's stain, bar = 50 μm). (*C*) Normal fetal skin (18 weeks' gestation) labeled with a fluorescently-labeled antibody to type VII collagen and orange propidium iodide nuclear counterstain, showing linear type VII collagen staining at the dermal-epidermal junction and around part of a cross-sectioned hair peg (bar = 50 μm). (*D*) Severe generalized recessive dystrophic EB fetal skin (18 weeks' gestation) labeled with a fluorescently-labeled antibody to type VII collagen, showing a complete absence of immunoreactivity and only the orange propidium iodide nuclear counterstain is evident (bar = 50 μm).

to the development of immunohistochemical tests to help complement ultrastructural analysis in establishing an accurate diagnosis (**Fig. 1C, D**).[6]

Although FSB has been largely superseded by DNA-based prenatal tests in the majority of cases, FSB may still be indicated if insufficient DNA data are available. Couples can be counseled that FSB sampling is an invasive procedure with an approximately 1% rate of fetal loss more than the background incidence of spontaneous abortion. Sampling error, inadequacy of samples for analysis, and difficulty in interpreting the morphologic and immunohistochemical features can pose problems and may necessitate repeat sampling.[7,8] From a practical perspective, FSBs cannot be performed before the 16th week of gestation, and the

prospect of a second-trimester termination of an affected pregnancy is often associated with considerable emotional and physical distress.[9] It is also important to note that there are few centers with the necessary experience and expertise to undertake FSB procedures and to adequately analyze the very small pieces of fetal skin.

Recently, it has also been demonstrated that immunohistochemical labeling of other fetal material, notably chorionic villi, can also be used for prenatal diagnosis. It has been shown that villous trophoblasts, sampled during the first trimester, display immunoreactivity to α6β4 integrin and plectin, thereby permitting diagnosis/exclusion of EB associated with pyloric atresia through tissue diagnosis.[10]

DEVELOPMENT OF MOLECULAR DIAGNOSTICS AND PROGRESS IN PRENATAL TESTING

As the molecular basis of EB has been elucidated, FSB has gradually been superseded by DNA-based diagnostic screening using fetal DNA from amniotic fluid cells or chorionic villi (Fig. 2).

After implantation of the embryo, the chorion, the outermost layer of the embryonic sac derived from the trophoblast layer of the blastocyst, attaches to the uterine wall. The chorion is lined by microscopic projections referred to as chorionic villi. These projections are the fetal components of the placenta and contain the same genetic material as the fetus; therefore, they are a useful source of fetal DNA.

Similarly, the cells within the amniotic fluid, surrounding the fetus, are derived from fetal epidermis as well as the gastrointestinal and genitourinary mucosae. Chorionic villus sampling (CVS) is usually performed between 10 and 12 weeks' gestation, whereas amniocentesis, the method for obtaining amniotic fluid and its cells, is conducted later, at approximately 16 weeks' gestation. Therefore, CVS is the favored method for DNA-based prenatal testing in many units.[11]

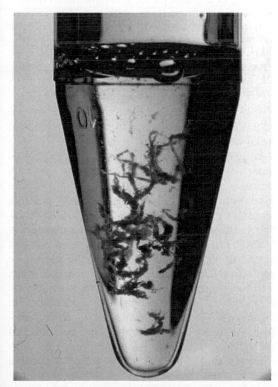

Fig. 2. Chorionic villi sampled at 11 weeks' gestation. Fetal DNA can be extracted from this material for DNA-based prenatal testing.

The most severe forms of EB are usually inherited in an autosomal recessive manner. Couples who have already had 1 affected child can be offered DNA-based prenatal testing in subsequent pregnancies if the causative gene is known and the pathogenic mutations have been identified. Indeed, initial reports of molecular prenatal testing for EB were published in 1995.[12–16]

Before any prenatal test, however, samples from both parents and any previous affected siblings are analyzed for pathogenic mutations. This initial screening is crucial for accurate genetic counseling and to establish the reliability of the prenatal test, as it determines the pattern of inheritance, tracing the transmission of the mutated gene(s) from generation to generation. In autosomal recessive EB, ideally both parents must be shown to be heterozygous carriers of the pathogenic mutation(s). The possibility of de novo mutations, nonpaternity, and uniparental disomy (the inheritance of both copies of a chromosome pair from just 1 parent) should be excluded before considering the suitability of the prenatal test. For DNA-based prenatal tests, fetal DNA is extracted from the chorionic villi or amniotic cells and analyzed for genetic mutations. After CVS, tissue obtained needs to be cleaned under a dissecting microscope to exclude maternal cells, such as decidua or blood, which could contaminate the sample and affect the accuracy of the results. The actual analysis of fetal DNA can usually be accomplished between 48 and 72 hours after its receipt in the laboratory. Couples can be counseled that the risk of fetal loss following these procedures is approximately 0.5% to 1%, depending on the expertise of the unit conducting the procedures.[11]

Since the initial DNA-based tests were introduced for EB, many more severe inherited skin disorders have been diagnosed or excluded prenatally in couples at reproductive risk,[15,16] including harlequin ichthyosis, tuberous sclerosis, congenital erythropoietic porphyria, Netherton syndrome, ectodermal dysplasia/skin fragility syndrome, and Ehlers-Danlos syndrome. With advances in molecular diagnostics, DNA-based prenatal testing is now feasible for any severe inherited skin disorder for which the causative gene is known and the pathogenic mutations and/or informative markers are defined.

Despite the advances in prenatal diagnostic techniques, reproductive choice and preventative options for couples at risk of EB are still limited. With all the prenatal tests mentioned so far, the diagnosis can only be made once pregnancy is established, with the subsequent option of terminating an affected pregnancy. This raises fundamental moral issues for many couples at risk. Moreover, some couples will not consider termination of pregnancy because of religious reasons or personal beliefs.

PREIMPLANTATION GENETIC DIAGNOSIS

Preimplantation genetic diagnosis (PGD) is an alternative to conventional DNA-based prenatal tests. It is a highly specialized procedure available in relatively few centers worldwide, involving the testing of cellular material from oocytes or early human embryos for specific genetic abnormalities before pregnancy has begun.[17,18] After stimulation of the ovaries with exogenous gonadotrophins, oocytes are collected by transvaginal ultrasound-guided aspiration. The individual oocytes are then fertilized by intracytoplasmic sperm injection, a procedure whereby a single spermatozoon is injected directly into a mature oocyte (**Fig. 3A**).[19] The embryos can then be sampled at various stages of development. A cleavage-stage biopsy is the preferred option for many PGD centers and is performed at the 8- to 12-cell stage (about 72 hours after fertilization), when the individual cells of the embryo are still totipotent.[20] The biopsy procedure involves breaching the zona pellucida, either by a laser beam or by a jet of acidified Tyrode solution. Following this, a sampling pipette is introduced into the embryo and a single nucleated blastomere is removed by suction for analysis (**Fig. 3B**). After genetic diagnosis using DNA from the single cell, suitable embryos can be transferred to the uterus on day 4 or day 5 of development. Couples should be counseled that the overall clinical pregnancy rate after PGD for monogenic disorders is about 25% per embryo transfer. In addition, PGD can be associated with generic complications of in vitro fertilization, such as ovarian hyperstimulation syndrome and multiple pregnancies, when more than 1 embryo is transferred per cycle. After a clinical pregnancy is achieved, confirmation of diagnosis by CVS at approximately 11 weeks' gestation is offered to all couples undergoing PGD. Because PGD is performed before pregnancy is established, it obviates termination of an affected pregnancy.

The first successful clinical application of PGD was in 1990,[21] and since then, several thousand cycles have been performed worldwide, resulting in the birth of hundreds of healthy children.[22] However, until recently, there had been no successful cases of PGD for severe inherited skin disorders. Two cases of PGD for Herlitz junctional EB (MIM226700) had been described,

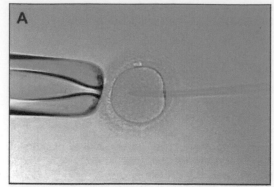

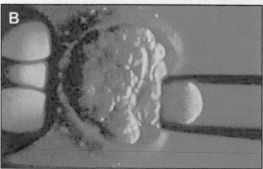

Fig. 3. In vitro fertilization and preimplantation genetic diagnosis. (*A*) A mature oocyte fertilized by intracytoplasmic sperm injection. (*B*) Single-cell sampling of a blastocyst for preimplantation genetic diagnosis. A cleavage-stage embryo at 72 hours post-fertilization is held stationary on a glass micropipette (left side of picture) by gentle suction. The zona pellucida is breached and a sampling pipette is introduced, removing a single nucleated blastomere by suction. The extracted single cell is then available for DNA analysis.

although pregnancy (beyond initial biochemical tests) was not established in either case.[23]

In 2006, the first case of successful PGD was reported for an intra-epidermal form of EB simplex, ectodermal dysplasia-skin fragility syndrome (MIM604536).[24] This is an autosomal recessive disorder that results from loss-of-function mutations in the gene encoding for plakophilin 1 (*PKP1*), a component of desmosome cell-cell junctions. For PGD in this case, the molecular screening involved a nested polymerase chain reaction protocol using DNA from a single cell with primers specific for the *PKP1* mutations in this family.[25] Pregnancy was established and progressed to term with delivery of an unaffected baby girl.

Efforts to make PGD more widely applicable have focused on the design of simpler and more generic protocols. In most cases of EB, pathogenic mutations are family-specific and, therefore, a mutation-detection approach to PGD is often too time-consuming. Consequently, most PGD tests now involve assessment of linkage markers, either microsatellites (variable polymorphic repeats of DNA) or single-nucleotide polymorphisms, that are close to or within the disease gene locus.[26] Nevertheless, designing robust PGD tests can be challenging because of the small amount of DNA available from a single cell (approximately 6 pg). In addition, because there are only 2 copies of each chromosome in a single cell, there may be a failure to amplify one (allele drop out) or both alleles of interest.

To counter these practical difficulties, recent technical innovations now permit amplification of the template DNA by whole genome amplification before any disease markers are assessed. One technique involves multiple displacement amplification, an isothermal whole genome amplification method using the bacteriophage φ29 DNA polymerase and results in approximately 1 million-fold amplification, thus increasing the template DNA from a single cell to approximately 6 μg.[27] Subsequently, the risk of *polymerase chain reaction* failure or allele dropout can be overcome by the use of multiple polymorphic linkage markers within and flanking the disease gene. This new approach is referred to as preimplantation genetic haplotyping (PGH)[28] and represents a major advance in reproductive technology applied to the prevention of EB. It has reduced the time taken to develop assays for other genetic disorders and will widen the scope and availability of preimplantation genetic testing, making it a practical reality for many more couples at risk for various forms of EB. Indeed, PGH protocols for Herlitz junctional EB have already been licensed and successfully used in clinical practice.[29]

NONINVASIVE METHODS OF PRENATAL DIAGNOSIS FOR EB

The methods of prenatal testing for EB that are currently available (FSB, CVS, and PGD/PGH) all involve invasive procedures. Strategies are being developed to assess whether it is possible to undertake prenatal testing by less-invasive approaches.

Ultrasound imaging of the fetus and other uterine contents can provide a considerable amount of information for some conditions.[30] Abnormalities in inherited skin disorders, however, are usually too subtle and beyond the resolution of this technique. Nevertheless, the snowflake sign in the amniotic cavity may be a marker of fetal skin sloughing in certain disorders, including junctional EB with pyloric atresia (MIM226730) and harlequin ichthyosis (MIM242500).[31] Nevertheless,

ultrasound imaging for the prenatal diagnosis of EB is not part of routine clinical practice.

Another noninvasive method that is still at a pre-clinical stage in the prenatal diagnosis of EB is the assessment of fetal DNA in the maternal circulation by means of a simple blood test.[32] In the 1960s, it was established that nucleated fetal cells could be detected in the maternal circulation. Indeed, numerous fetal cell populations have been reported in maternal peripheral blood, including erythrocytes, lymphocytes, and trophoblasts. However, these cells are infrequently found (only approximately 1 cell per milliliter of maternal blood), making their isolation and detection very difficult. In addition, nucleated fetal cells may persist in the maternal circulation for months or years, rendering their detection of dubious value for prenatal testing.[33]

In 1997, it was established that cell-free circulating fetal DNA was also present in the maternal circulation.[34] This fetal DNA constitutes about 5% of cell-free DNA in the maternal plasma[35] and consists mostly of short fragments (<200 base pairs). This fetal DNA is detectable as early as day 18 after embryo transfer by assisted reproduction,[36] and its concentration increases as gestation progresses. Unlike nucleated fetal cells, there is no long-term persistence of free fetal DNA in the maternal circulation. In fact, fetal DNA is cleared rapidly, with a mean half-life of 16 minutes.[37] The main source of fetal DNA in the maternal plasma is the placenta. The qualitative assessment of free fetal DNA can be used to obtain valuable information about the fetus. Once isolated, chromosomes, genes, or genetic polymorphisms and mutations inherited from the father can be targeted.

As free fetal DNA makes up a very small proportion of the total free DNA in the maternal circulation, it is technically very challenging to detect a DNA sequence that the fetus has inherited from its mother. To address this, there has been considerable interest in establishing epigenetic signatures of fetal DNA (eg, differential DNA methylation status) that will allow for the detection of both maternal and paternal markers.[38,39] Further technical advances in this field may lead to the introduction of maternal blood tests taken between 6 and 7 weeks' gestation as alternative approaches for the prenatal diagnosis of EB, but such tests are not yet part of current clinical practice.

SUMMARY

Over the last 30 years, there have been significant advances in prenatal testing options for couples at reproductive risk of severe forms of EB with the first FSB in 1980, the start of DNA-based tests in 1995 and the introduction of successful PGD in 2006. Laboratory protocols are becoming quicker and technically easier, and, therefore, counseling of couples at risk of recurrence of a specific disease should include mention of the significant and clinically relevant developments that are occurring in this field, such as PGH. Moreover, the quest for faster, more-reliable, and less-invasive tests continues. An attractive option in the future may be testing free fetal DNA in the maternal circulation, although this is currently not feasible for EB. Nevertheless, the development of prenatal tests for couples at reproductive risk of EB represents a significant benefit of translational research that is already providing options and choice for many couples.

REFERENCES

1. Irvine AD, McLean WH. The molecular genetics of the genodermatoses: progress to date and future directions. Br J Dermatol 2003;148:1–13.
2. Mavilio F, Pellegrini G, Ferrari S, et al. Correction of junctional epidermolysis bullosa by transplantation of genetically modified epidermal stem cells. Nat Med 2006;12:1397–402.
3. Rodeck CH, Eady RA, Gosden CM. Prenatal diagnosis of epidermolysis bullosa letalis. Lancet 1980; 1:949–52.
4. Rodeck CH, Nicolaides KH. Fetoscopy and fetal tissue sampling. Br Med Bull 1983;39:332–7.
5. Eady RA, Gunner DB, Tidman MJ, et al. Rapid processing of fetal skin for prenatal diagnosis by light and electron microscopy. J Clin Pathol 1984;37: 633–8.
6. Heagerty AH, Kennedy AR, Gunner DB, et al. Rapid prenatal diagnosis and exclusion of epidermolysis bullosa using novel antibody probes. J Invest Dermatol 1986;86:603–5.
7. Holbrook KA, Smith LT, Elias S. Prenatal diagnosis of genetic skin disease using fetal skin biopsy samples. Arch Dermatol 1993;129:1437–54.
8. Shimizu A, Akiyama M, Ishiko A, et al. Prenatal exclusion of harlequin ichthyosis; potential pitfalls in the timing of the fetal skin biopsy. Br J Dermatol 2005;153:811–4.
9. Broen AN, Moum T, Bodtker AS, et al. The course of mental health after miscarriage and induced abortion: a longitudinal, five-year follow-up study. BMC Med 2005;3:18.
10. D'Alessio M, Zambruno G, Charlesworth A, et al. Immunofluorescence of villous trophoblasts: a tool for prenatal diagnosis of inherited epidermolysis bullosa with pyloric atresia. J Invest Dermatol 2008;128: 2815–9.
11. Alfirevic Z, Sundberg K, Brigham S. Amniocentesis and chorionic villus sampling for prenatal diagnosis. Cochrane Database Syst Rev 2003;(3):CD003252.
12. Hovnanian A, Hilal L, Blanchet-Bardon C, et al. DNA-based prenatal diagnosis of generalized recessive dystrophic epidermolysis bullosa in six pregnancies at risk for recurrence. J Invest Dermatol 1995;104: 456–61.
13. Vailly J, Pulkkinen L, Miquel C, et al. Identification of a homozygous one-basepair deletion in exon 14 of the LAMB3 gene in a patient with Herlitz junctional epidermolysis bullosa and prenatal diagnosis in a family at risk for recurrence. J Invest Dermatol 1995;104:462–6.
14. Dunnill MG, Rodeck CH, Richards AJ, et al. Use of type VII collagen gene (COL7A1) markers in prenatal diagnosis of recessive dystrophic epidermolysis bullosa. J Med Genet 1995;32:749–50.
15. McGrath JA, Dunnill MG, Christiano AM, et al. First trimester DNA-based exclusion of recessive dystrophic epidermolysis bullosa from chorionic villus sampling. Br J Dermatol 1996;134:734–9.
16. Fassihi H, Eady RA, Mellerio JE, et al. Twenty-five years' experience of prenatal diagnosis for severe inherited skin disorders. Br J Dermatol 2006;154: 106–13.
17. Braude P, Pickering S, Flinter F, et al. Preimplantation genetic diagnosis. Nat Rev Genet 2002;3:941–53.
18. Renwick P, Ogilvie CM. Preimplantation genetic diagnosis for monogenic diseases: overview and emerging issues. Expert Rev Mol Diagn 2007;7: 33–43.
19. Devroey P, Van Steirteghem A. A review of ten years experience of ICSI. Hum Reprod Update 2004;10: 19–28.
20. Hardy K, Martin KL, Leese HJ, et al. Human preimplantation development in vitro is not adversely affected by biopsy at the 8-cell stage. Hum Reprod 1990;5:708–14.
21. Handyside AH, Kontogianni EH, Hardy K, et al. Pregnancies from biopsied human preimplantation embryos sexed by Y-specific DNA amplification. Nature 1990;344:768–70.
22. Harper JC, de Die-Smulders C, Goossens V, et al. ESHRE PGD consortium data collection VII: cycles from January to December 2004 with pregnancy follow-up to October 2005. Hum Reprod 2008;23: 741–55.
23. Cserhalmi-Friedman PB, Tang Y, Adler A, et al. Preimplantation genetic diagnosis in two families at risk for recurrence of Herlitz junctional epidermolysis bullosa. Exp Dermatol 2000;9:290–7.
24. Fassihi H, Grace J, Lashwood A, et al. Preimplantation genetic diagnosis of skin fragility-ectodermal dysplasia syndrome. Br J Dermatol 2006; 154:546–50.

25. Thornhill AR, Pickering SJ, Whittock NV, et al. Preimplantation genetic diagnosis of compound heterozygous mutations leading to ablation of plakophilin-1 (*PKP1*) and resulting in skin fragility ectodermal dysplasia syndrome: a case report. Prenat Diagn 2000;20:1055–62.

26. Fassihi H, Renwick PJ, Black C, et al. Single cell PCR amplification of microsatellites flanking the *COL7A1* gene and suitability for preimplantation genetic diagnosis of Hallopeau-Siemens recessive dystrophic epidermolysis bullosa. J Dermatol Sci 2006;42:241–8.

27. Hellani A, Coskun S, Tbakhi A, et al. Clinical application of multiple displacement amplification in preimplantation genetic diagnosis. Reprod Biomed Online 2005;10:376–80.

28. Renwick PJ, Trussler J, Ostad-Saffari E, et al. Proof of principle and first cases using preimplantation genetic haplotyping – a paradigm shift for embryo diagnosis. Reprod Biomed Online 2006;13:110–9.

29. Fassihi H, Renwick PJ, Pickering S, et al. Preimplantation genetic diagnosis for inherited skin disorders in the UK: from bench to bedside to birth. Br J Dermatol 2006;155(Suppl 1):3–4.

30. Sonek J. First trimester ultrasonography in screening and detection of fetal anomalies. Am J Med Genet C Semin Med Genet 2007;145:45–61.

31. Dolan CR, Smith LT, Sybert VP. Prenatal detection of epidermolysis bullosa letalis and pyloric atresia in a fetus by abnormal ultrasound and elevated α-fetoprotein. Am J Med Genet 1993;47:395–400.

32. Fu XH, Chen HP. Advances on circulating fetal DNA in maternal plasma. Chin Med J (Engl) 2007;120:1256–9.

33. Bianchi DW, Simpson JL, Jackson LG, et al. Fetal gender and aneuploidy detection using fetal cells in maternal blood: analysis of NIFTY I data. National Institute of Child Health and Development Fetal Cell Isolation Study. Prenat Diagn 2002;22:609–15.

34. Lo YM, Corbetta N, Chamberlain PF, et al. Presence of fetal DNA in maternal plasma and serum. Lancet 1997;350:485–7.

35. Lo YM, Tein MS, Lau TK, et al. Quantitative analysis of fetal DNA in maternal plasma and serum: implications for noninvasive prenatal diagnosis. Am J Hum Genet 1998;62:768–75.

36. Guibert J, Benachi A, Grebille AG, et al. Kinetics of SRY gene appearance in maternal serum: detection by real time PCR in early pregnancy after assisted reproductive technique. Hum Reprod 2003;18:1733–6.

37. Lo YM, Zhang J, Leung TN, et al. Rapid clearance of fetal DNA from maternal plasma. Am J Hum Genet 1999;64:218–24.

38. Poon LL, Leung TN, Lau TK, et al. Differential DNA methylation between fetus and mother as a strategy for detecting fetal DNA in maternal plasma. Clin Chem 2002;48:35–41.

39. Lo YM, Chiu RW. Prenatal diagnosis: progress through plasma nucleic acids. Nat Rev Genet 2007;8:71–7.

Genetic Counseling in Epidermolysis Bullosa

Virginia P. Sybert, MD[a,b,*]

KEYWORDS

- Recurrence • Prenatal diagnosis
- Epidermolysis bullosa • Genetic counseling

This article contains my views on genetic counseling in cases of epidermolysis bullosa (EB) syndrome. It is a synthesis of what I have been taught by my colleagues, my mentors, and my patients and their parents. It reflects generally accepted principles of counseling (nondirective) and my idiosyncratic views. There are many other sources of information on genetic counseling, which have been listed later in the article.

Genetic counseling is usually provided by a health care professional trained in medical genetics. This can be a physician, a genetics associate (having an MS in medical genetics), a medical geneticist with a PhD, or other appropriate providers. Dermatologists may also be called on to provide genetic counseling in cases of EB disorders because we are often most familiar with these disorders, involved early in their diagnosis, and continuously engaged in their treatment. For those who prefer not to be burdened with this time-intensive task, referral to a medical genetics clinic should be made.

The provision of genetic counseling entails several absolutes:

1. Diagnosis
2. Natural history
3. Treatment
4. Mode of inheritance
5. Recurrence risks/prenatal diagnosis
6. Referral.

These absolutes are no different from what we do for any disease, with the single exception that there may be other individuals in the family who are also at risk. Thus the patient is actually the family and not just the affected individual. The provision of genetic information during counseling needs to be nonpejorative while being supportive and informative.

The diagnosis must be correct. All information we provide is based on the diagnosis. Neither the natural history nor the recurrence risks will be correct if the diagnosis is incorrect. Molecular testing will be misdirected if the diagnosis is wrong. The natural history and management of the condition must be known. However, it may be inappropriate to provide all this information at once (eg, the lifetime risk for squamous cell carcinoma for a person with recessive EB may not be an important piece of information to provide to parents on the second day of their infant's life). The mode of inheritance and recurrence risks to affected individuals, parents, and other relatives must be established. The availability and reliability of molecular testing and prenatal diagnosis must be ascertained. The transmittal of all this information must be done in a nonjudgmental and nondirective manner, in stages if necessary, and on multiple occasions according to patients' needs.

The EB syndromes, like most single-gene disorders, are characterized by allelic and locus heterogeneity, somatic and germline mosaicism, and variable expression. These are factors that can complicate the process of diagnostic testing and genetic counseling. Penetrance, defined as the

[a] Division of Medical Genetics, University of Washington School of Medicine, Box 357720, 1959 NE Pacific, Seattle, WA 98195, USA
[b] Group Health Permanente, 125 16th Avenue East, Seattle, WA 98112, USA
* Corresponding author. Division of Medical Genetics, University of Washington School of Medicine, Box 357720, 1959 NE Pacific, Seattle, WA 98195.
E-mail address: flk01@u.washington.edu

Dermatol Clin 28 (2010) 239–243
doi:10.1016/j.det.2009.12.004

proportion of individuals who carry the necessary genes to express disease and yet do not express it, is not a significant issue.

CORRECT DIAGNOSIS

The clinical descriptions of EB and the methods of establishing a correct diagnosis are dealt within other articles in this issue (see the articles by Intong and Murrell, Pohla-Gubo and colleagues, and Eady and Dopping-Hepenstal elsewhere in this issue for further exploration of this topic.). It may be several weeks until the correct diagnosis can be made, and genetic counseling may take a back seat to immediate medical needs. Parents are always certain that they are somehow responsible for their infant's disease. Irrespective of the diagnosis, parents can be told that this is not true. Predictions of lethality may be over or understated. I have found that assurances of providing maximum support while waiting for information, despite the condition's possible fatality, are better received than the immediate hanging of crepe. I also make it clear that despite many tools providing medical support, much of what happens is not in the physician's or the parents' hands, and the infants have a say too. They will determine how they will do and may not survive despite best efforts.

The correct diagnosis is required before recurrence risks can be estimated. The diagnosis of epidermolysis bullosa simplex (EBS) Koebner type (generalized) implies an autosomal dominant cause, heterozygosity for a mutation in keratin 5 (KRT5) or keratin 14 (KRT14), and a 50% recurrence risk to offspring of an affected person. EBS with muscular dystrophy due to homozygosity for plectin mutations can look clinically identical to EBS until the muscular dystrophy manifests. These are autosomal recessive disorders, and the risk of transmission to offspring, although higher than the background risk, is absolutely small, whereas the risk for affected siblings is 25%. If the correct diagnosis is not established, bad medicine will be practiced.

The correct diagnosis is required before molecular testing can be performed efficiently. Mostly, molecular testing does not establish the diagnosis of EB but confirms it. Molecular testing is directed by clinical acumen. If one mistakes junctional disease for dystrophic disease and tests for mutations in COL7A1 (type 7 collagen), testing will be uninformative. Junctional disease is not due to mutations in COL7A1. If the diagnosis of dystrophic disease is correct, a negative test for COL7A1 does not rule out dystrophic disease. Sensitivity of molecular testing is almost never 100%; technologic limitations and the creative packaging of DNA can make some mutations undetectable. Allelic heterogeneity (where different versions or alterations in the same gene can cause the disorder) can also complicate molecular testing. Molecular testing may be limited to common or hotspot mutations, thus missing mutations that are due to alterations elsewhere in the gene. Locus heterogeneity (where mutations in different genes can result in clinically indistinguishable disorders) also limits the utility and accuracy of molecular testing. For simplex disease, both KRT5 and KRT14 must be analyzed. In junctional disease, mutations in the pair of 1 of at least 6 different genes (LAMB3, LAMC2, LAMA3, COL17A1, ITGB4, ITGA6) may be causal, and testing needs to be performed in a stepwise fashion.

The correct diagnosis is required before a prognosis can be generated and is necessary to determine the likely natural history for the condition. It is not enough to tell affected individuals or parents what the diagnosis and recurrence risks are and whether prenatal diagnosis is available and appropriate. They need to know about the disorder, how to care for the skin, what to expect, and how to manage complications. All this is also part of genetic counseling. Parents of babies with severe junctional EB need to know about the possibility of respiratory arrest. They should know that no matter how vigilant they are, the infants may slough their respiratory mucosa and succumb. If they want to learn how to resuscitate, we need to teach them. But they need to understand that even the most vigorous of interventions may fail. We should address pain control, blister care, and feeding. The medical geneticist is also involved in this and must be able to discuss these issues knowledgeably. The dermatologist and the intensivist must understand the genetic aspects of these conditions. Genetic counseling needs to be provided by all the professionals involved in the care of the patient because the information is overwhelming, confusing, easily forgotten or misunderstood, and bears repeating. Listen to the patients and the parents. Hear their overt questions and respond to their tacit concerns. Be prepared to sideline some discussions and to deal with others based on what the patients or parents are telling you. Ask them what their questions are, what they understand, and what is important to them.

NATURAL HISTORY

It is important to be able to give some guidance about the future to the affected individuals. What can they expect? What do we know and don't know? People, including physicians, have an unreasonable expectation that a specific diagnosis allows for specific predictions. But we do not have crystal balls; each person is different, and the spectrum of expression of a disorder is broad. Will this baby succumb to infection? Will this one experience amelioration of signs and symptoms? Will that one be run over by a car at age 7? We need to be informative without overstepping our knowledge. Patients with recessive dystrophic EB (DEB) need to know about skin cancer surveillance and an increased risk for squamous cell carcinoma. At the same time, we cannot tell them that they will inexorably develop it. We can only paint with a broad brush.

TREATMENT

Discussions on treatment are a part of the genetic counseling experience. Although a full discussion may not be required, there will always be questions, so the counselor needs to be prepared with information about treatment. In the twenty-first century, families will also ask about gene therapy. The counselor needs to be able to explain where things stand and what the limitations and chances are. The patients may wish to be informed if there are experimental protocols. The counselor should try to find out if there are trials that the patients might consider. Providing genetic counseling is hard work, and there are no shortcuts.

MODE OF INHERITANCE, RECURRENCE RISKS, AND PRENATAL DIAGNOSIS

The EB syndromes are single-gene disorders inherited in a Mendelian fashion. To all intents and purposes, X-linked inheritance does not play a role in EB. All forms of EB are either autosomal dominant or autosomal recessive conditions.

EBS is almost always autosomal dominant, resulting from heterozygosity for a mutation in 1 of the 2 *KRT5* alleles or 1 of the 2 *KRT14* alleles. DEB can also be autosomal dominant, usually presenting with localized involvement without pseudoamputation. An individual with autosomal dominant EBS or autosomal dominant DEB could have inherited the gene from an affected parent, or the mutation may have newly occurred in the sperm or egg that made that person.

The offspring of a person having an autosomal dominant condition have a 50% risk of inheriting the mutation. The severity of expression depends on the specific mutation. Irrespective of the sex of the offspring, the likelihood is 50% with each conception. If the affected individuals are the first in the family to be affected, and it seems that the disorder is due to a new mutation, then the recurrence risk to the individuals' parents and siblings is

negligible because the mutation is believed to be a one-time event. For the affected persons, however, the risk to their offspring is 50%. A child may rarely have what seems to be a new dominant mutation when one parent carries the gene but does not show it. This lack of expression is either because they carry it only in their gonads or they have such low levels of somatic mosaicism that they do not express the condition, or the affected individuals themselves may be mosaic for the mutation. Mosaicism for single-gene mutations results from events occurring after fertilization. In this instance, the recurrence risk is higher than that of the general population. This situation is uncommon, and although it must be mentioned when providing risk figures, its likelihood can be minimized. There have been rare instances of EBS resulting from homozygosity (2 of the same mutations or deletions of the 2 *KRT5* or *KRT14* alleles) or compound heterozygosity (2 different mutations in the 2 *KRT5* or *KRT14* alleles). In this situation, there is a 25% recurrence risk for the subsequent offspring to be affected. For a family with more than one affected generation with EBS, molecular testing is not necessary to establish recurrence risks, but in a family with an isolated affected individual, molecular testing may help to determine the mode of inheritance and the reproductive risks.

Autosomal recessive inheritance is the primary mode of inheritance for EB disorders caused by mutations in plectin (EB with muscular dystrophy and EBS with pyloric atresia). It is also the primary mode of inheritance for the junctional forms of EB and for the generalized severe (formerly Hallopeau-Siemens) and inverse forms of EB dystrophica. In autosomal recessive conditions, both copies of the causal gene must be mutated. The mutations may be the same (homozygosity) or different (compound heterozygosity), but they are always in the same gene pair. Compound heterozygosity for mutations in 2 different genes would not result in disease because the other normal allele would always "rescue" the phenotype. Each parent of a child with autosomal recessive EB is a carrier of a mutated allele (gene) and a normal allele (gene). The normal gene provides enough gene product to maintain normal skin integrity. Each child born to them (ie, siblings to the affected child) has a 25% chance to inherit both abnormal alleles and be affected. The children have a 25% chance to inherit both normal alleles and 50% likelihood to inherit one or the other abnormal allele and a second normal allele, that is, to be carriers. Carriers and affected individuals with autosomal recessive EB have an increased relative risk but low absolute risk to have affected offspring. (In mathematical terms, offspring of the affected person will inherit an abnormal allele from the latter. The likelihood that the spouse of the affected person would carry a mutation in the same gene is no greater than 1 in 50 [based on the disease frequency and estimates of carrier frequency in the general population], unless the spouse is a relative. [This is not unheard of in many cultures. If the spouse is a relative, the risk to be a carrier of the same mutation is higher than in the general population, and the specific risk must be calculated from the coefficient of inbreeding, which is a job for professionals.] The chance that the offspring would also inherit the abnormal allele from the spouse is 50%, resulting in an overall recurrence risk of 1 in 100. This risk is much higher than that in the general population, estimated at 1 in 10,000 or less, but still does not add appreciably to the baseline risk for birth defects of 3% to 5% that every pregnancy carries. The unaffected siblings of a person with autosomal recessive EB each have a two-third risk to be carriers. If they are carriers, their offspring have a 50% chance to inherit the abnormal allele, and, as discussed, a 50% chance to inherit an abnormal allele from the sibling's spouse who has a 1 in 50 chance to be a carrier. Hence, there is a risk of 1 in 300 for nieces or nephews of an affected person to also be affected, which, similarly, is absolutely low but relatively high compared with the general population.)

Sometimes, these risks can seem unbelievably complicated and difficult to understand and explain, but anyone can understand Mendelian risks through simple mathematics. Each of us has 2 copies of every gene (except for those on the X chromosome, not considering the X chromosome in EB), and each of our children inherits 1 of those 2 copies from each parent. In recessive conditions, the gene from each parent must be abnormal, and in dominant conditions, only 1 abnormal gene is needed. In dominant conditions, the presence of a normal gene does not protect you; the abnormal allele is stronger or dominant. In recessive conditions, the normal gene does protect you, and if you only have 1 abnormal gene, you are a carrier. The abnormal gene is recessive. I personally do not find using diagrams and charts helpful; you can see patients' eyes glaze over. But if you have 4 fingers (it is useful to have someone else, such as parents, helping you in the counseling) you can do it all. Holding up a finger for each of the alleles (one of you plays eggs and the other plays sperm; the sperm get to move, so it is a better role to have) you can graphically show the different possible outcomes at fertilization. The concepts are simple, but it is our jargon that obscures. I

have also found that humor in counseling is not unwelcome. Using hands and keeping it simple humanizes you and goes a long way in relieving the anxiety of patients that they aren't smart or knowledgeable enough to understand the terms.

Molecular studies can obviate mathematical calisthenics. If the mutations are identified, spouses and at-risk carriers can be tested.

In the provision of recurrence risks, it is really important to emphasize that genetic disorders and mutations are common, that all of us carry potentially deleterious alleles, and that parents have not done or failed to do anything to have caused this condition in their child. Parents at risk may choose to reproduce, but they do not choose the genes that their children inherit. Couples at risk may choose to use prenatal diagnosis to prevent or prepare for the birth of an affected child, or they may forego the opportunity. Prenatal detection of the mutant alleles can be done as part of a preimplantation protocol whereby eggs and sperm from the couple are harvested, fertilization is done in the laboratory, and molecular testing is performed at the 8-cell stage. Unaffected zygotes are then reimplanted into the recipient mother. This service is available only at certain centers and must be arranged in advance. Prenatal diagnosis can also be done by testing of chorionic villous cells, usually at about 10 weeks, or by amniocentesis, usually at about 16 weeks. Each method has its pros and cons. There is ongoing research looking at the feasibility of prenatal diagnosis using fetal cells present in maternal circulation. Prenatal diagnosis requires knowledge of the mutations present in the affected individual. Cells/tissue for DNA banking should be obtained from any individual with EB to ensure that prenatal testing is feasible in the future, if parents or individuals desire it.

In my practice, I have been consistently surprised by the decisions that families make, and I learned long ago that my job is to provide information and to support families in their usage of this information. Couples at high risk have chosen to reproduce without prenatal testing, whereas couples at low risk have eschewed further reproduction. People often don't act in reality as they had expected to. Although I hold strong personal opinions about these choices, I do not let them leak into my professional actions. Above all, I want to be a good doctor, and that means being there for these families and not for myself. If you cannot, in good faith, provide nondirective genetic counseling to families, you should gracefully delegate the job to someone who can.

Usually, results obtained from molecular testing are straightforward. The causal mutations will have been identified, and this information can be easily transmitted to families. In autosomal recessive conditions, once the mutations have been found, siblings can be tested for carrier status, if desired. Carrier testing of minor children is arguable, and it may be recommended that families consider deferring testing until the child is of the age of consent. Testing can also be offered to other relatives at risk (eg, aunts and uncles of the proband). Prenatal testing can be offered. Occasionally, testing is not informative. None or only 1 of 2 mutations may be identified in the case of autosomal recessive disease. No mutation may be identified in autosomal dominant disease. Such cases may be because the mutation is not accessible to testing or because the entire gene is deleted and the method of testing used misses deletions. It may also be because the diagnosis is wrong and the wrong gene has been tested. Each of these situations requires communication with the testing laboratory and a knowledge of the current state of the art. Occasionally, a mutation or alteration in a gene is identified, but its significance is unknown. This may be a mutation that has not been reported before or that is in a region of the gene believed not to be important. Some molecular changes are polymorphisms, which are believed to be unimportant alterations common in the general population. Interpretation of molecular results is not always simple.

REFERRAL

The diagnosis of an EB syndrome is only the beginning. Families need to know where to go for help and be informed about support groups. Sometimes, parents are too overwhelmed to reach out actively but welcome an extended helping hand. I have several veteran parents in my area who have volunteered to be "go-to" people for the new parent. If other specialists are needed, which may be the case for more severe forms of EB, parents need to be helped in finding them. Ancillary services such as social work, wound care, respite care, respiratory services, occupational and physical therapy, and school services may all be required.

Genetic counseling is more than a recitation of recurrence risks. The genetic counselor needs to be informed and informative. The complete provider answers all the needs of the patients and their families, not always single-handedly or in one session, but inevitably and reliably over the course of the patient's life. The privilege of being able to be woven into these families' lives more than rewards the efforts involved. I realize how smarmy this may read, but there is nothing that is more gratifying than being there for these patients and their families. Although we have limited treatment for these disorders, our knowledge can be a great comfort to them. We can reduce fear of the unknown and face it with them. Providing such help is what genetic counseling is all about.

RESOURCES

http://www.ncbi.nlm.nih.gov/sites/GeneTests/clinic?db= genetests gives a list of medical genetics clinics in the United States.

http://www.ncbi.nlm.nih.gov/sites/GeneTests/review?db= GeneTests contains reviews of genetic/molecular information for single-gene disorders and for laboratories offering testing.

http://clinicaltrials.gov/ gives a list of clinical trials in the United States.

http://www.nsgc.org/client_files/GuidetoGeneticCounseling. pdf is a lay guide to genetic counseling from the National Society of Genetic Counselors.

Epidermolysis Bullosa Simplex with Muscular Dystrophy

C. Chiavérini, MD, PhD[a,b],*, A. Charlesworth, MSc[a,b,c],
G. Meneguzzi, PhD[c], J.P. Lacour, MD[a,b],
J.P. Ortonne, MD, PhD[b]

KEYWORDS
- Epidermolysis bullosa simplex • Muscular dystrophy
- Pyloric atresia • Ogna form

Epidermolysis bullosa simplex (EBS) is an inherited skin disorder characterized by separation of the epidermis from the underlying dermis, with the cleavage plane lying within the basal cell layer of the epithelium.[1] The major clinical subtypes of EBS have a dominant inheritance and have been associated with genetic defects in specific domains of keratins K5 and K14 that result in abnormal organization of the keratin network and cell disruption. Autosomal recessive forms of EBS associated with extracutaneous manifestations, such as muscular dystrophy (EBS-MD) (MIM 226670) or pyloric atresia (EBS-PA) (MIM 612138), have been linked to genetic mutations in the gene for plectin (PLEC).[2–5] PLEC mutations have also been found in 2 families with the rare dominant Ogna form of EBS.[6,7] PLEC encodes for plectin, a versatile cytoskeletal linker protein abundantly expressed in several cell types. Plectin is associated with intermediate filaments, and various subplasma membrane–cytoskeleton and membrane-cytoskeleton junctional complexes in epithelia, muscles, and fibroblasts. Consistent with its numerous binding partners, plectin mutation results in pleiotropic phenotypes.[8]

EBS WITH MD
Dermatologic Findings

Patients reported in literature with EBS-MD are usually born at term after an uneventful pregnancy (Table 1). Consistent with an autosomic recessive inheritance, parents are often found to be related and are asymptomatic. At birth or soon after (15 days) the affected newborn develops blisters and erosions on the extremities, the back, and the face, which recur at the sites of mechanical trauma. Blisters are tense and can be hemorrhagic. Healing occurs without scarring but occasionally with mild residual atrophy. No congenital cutis aplasia (CCA) is present. One patient developed a few milia on the fingers.[9] In all cases, no improvement of skin involvement has been described with time and skin fragility seems to be mild. Nail involvement is constant, with congenital onychodystrophy (pachyonychia) of the fingers and toes, although loss of nails is uncommon (Fig. 1). Four patients had a focal plantar hyperkeratosis with crusted lesions.[2,9,10] Dental anomalies such as premature tooth decay have been reported in 64% of cases.[4,5,11–14] Some patients have presented from a few months of age with

The authors have no conflicts of interest to declare.
[a] French Reference Center of Hereditary Epidermolysis Bullosa, Nice, France
[b] Department of Dermatology, Archet 2 Hospital, 151 Route Saint Antoine de Ginestière, 06202 Nice Cedex 3, France
[c] INSERM U634, Faculty of Medicine, 28 Avenue Valombrose, 06107 Nice Cedex 2, France
* Corresponding author. Department of Dermatology, Archet 2 Hospital, 151 Route Saint Antoine de Ginestière, 06202 Nice Cedex 3, France.
E-mail address: Chiaverini.c@chu-nice.fr

Dermatol Clin 28 (2010) 245–255
doi:10.1016/j.det.2010.01.001

Table 1
Summary of clinical and molecular features of patients with EBS-MD and published plectin mutations

Patient	Sex/Age (Years)	Consanguinity	Origin	Skin Involvement Age Onset	Mucosa	Nail	Teeth	Focal Plantar Keratoderma	Muscle Involvement Age of Onset (Years)	Evolution	Other	Mutation 1	Type	Exon	Mutation 2	Type	Exon	Refs.
P1	F/49	1	Japan	Birth	0	1	1	0	19	Artificial ventilation		Q1450X	ptc	32	Q1450X	ptc	32	14
P2	M/33	0	Malta	Birth	1	1	NA	0	2		Cerebral and cerebellar atrophy	R2465X	ptc	32	R2465X	ptc	32	15
P3	F/10	1	Italy	Neonatal	1	NA	NA	0	0 at 10			(5905del2) 5854del2	ptc	32	(5905del2) 5854del2	ptc	32	15
P4	NA	1	Malta	Birth	0	NA	NA	0	Teens			R2465X	ptc	32	R2465X	ptc	32	19
P5	M/24	1	Spain	Neonatal	0	1	1	0	10	Unable to walk age 13		(5148del8) 5085del8	ptc	32	(5148del8) 5085del8	ptc	32	4
P6	NA	NA	NA	Neonatal	0	NA	NA	0	13 months			5309insG*	ptc	32	5309insG*	ptc	32	19
P7	NA	NA	NA	Neonatal	0	NA	NA	0	Teens			E1614X	ptc	32	E1614X	ptc	32	19
P8	NA	NA	NA	Neonatal	0	NA	NA	0	Childhood			R2421X	ptc	32	NA	ptc	NA	19
P9	F/46	1	Japan	Neonatal	0	1	0	0	30	Able to walk and carry out routine activity		(2719del9) 2668del9	In-frame del3aa	22	(2719del9) 2668del9	In-frame del3aa	22	5
P10	M/38	0	Japan	Neonatal	1	1	1	0	30	Unable to walk in mid-30s		(5866delC) 5815delC	ptc	32	(5866delC) 5815delC	ptc	32	5
P11	F/5.5	1	England	Birth	1	1	0	0	0 at 5,5			(5069del19) 5018del19	ptc	32	(5069del19) 5018del19	ptc	32	9
P12	M/40	0	NA	Neonatal	1	1	1	0	20	Considerable muscle weakness		(4416delC) 4365delC	ptc	32	(4359ins13) 4308ins13?	ptc	32	13
P13	M/9	1	Japan	Birth	1	1	1	0	Infancy	Major difficulties in walking at 9	Partial scarring alopecia	Q1936X	ptc	32	(Q1053X) Q1054X?	ptc	24	11

Patient	Sex/Age		Ethnicity	Onset					Age	Clinical	Clinical	Mutation 1		Exon	Mutation 2		Exon	Ref
P14	M/33	0	Japan	Neonatal	0	1	1	0	5		Partial scarring alopecia	R2421X	ptc	32	(12633ins4) 12582ins4	ptc	33	11
P15	M/4	0	NA	Neonatal	1	1	0	0	0-4	Unable to walk at 22		Q1713X	ptc	32	R2351X	ptc	32	10
P16	F/52	0	Japan	Birth	0	1	1	0	25	Unable to walk age 46		R2319X	ptc	32	R2319X	ptc	32	12
P17	F/3	1	Lebanon	Birth	1	1	0	0	0-3			(5588insG) 5258insG	ptc	32	(5588insG) 5258insG	ptc	32	16
P18	M/NA	0	Germany	NA	0	NA	NA	0	NA			E1914X*	ptc	32	E1914X*	ptc	32	32
P19	F/5 months	1	France	Neonatal	1	NA	1	1	0-5 months			(2745-9 del21) 2769del21	In-frame del7aa	22	(5083del(G) 5032delG	ptc	32	10
P20	F/29	1	Italy	Birth	0	1	0	1	Childhood			Q1910X	ptc	32	Q1910X	ptc	32	2
P21	NA	NA	NA	Birth	0	NA	NA	0	1			(5907ins8) 5854ins?	ptc	32	(5907ins8) 5854ins8?	ptc	32	18
P22	M/6 months	0	Spain	Birth	0	1	0	0	0-6 months		Extensive cleft lift and palate	E2005X	ptc	32	K4460X	ptc	33	10
P23	M/4	0	White	Birth	0	1	0	0	0-6 years			1287ins3*/957ins3	In-frame ins1aa	9	Q1518X	pct	31	22
P24	F/25	0	White	Birth	0	1	0	0	11 years	Facial weakness, ptosis, exophthalmia, dysphonia, weakness, and atrophy of trunk and limbs	Mental retardation, bilateral cataract, cardiac hypertrophy, MAV left leg, cerebral atrophy	(13803ins16) 13474ins16?	pct	33	(13803ins16) 13474ins16?	pct	33	20
P25	NA	NA	NA	NA	NA	NA	NA	NA	42 years			1541ins36*	In-frame ins12aa	14	(677del9) 2637del9?	In-frame del3aa	22	17

Numbering of *PLEC* mutations on the nucleotide and protein level has been adjusted to begin at the start codon ATG, which is located in the second exon. The position of each mutation was confirmed based on the published sequence chromatograms, and when necessary corrected with the ATG as +1. When the numbering has been corrected the published mutation is in parentheses. An asterisk has been added at the end of a mutation when the precise localization of the mutation could not be confirmed.

Abbreviations: del, deletion; F, female; ins, insertion; M, male; MAV, arteriovenous malformation; NA, not available.

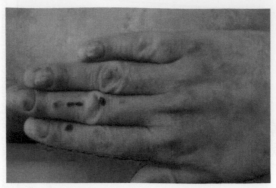

Fig. 1. Nail dystrophy (pachynychia) and blood-filled blisters of the hand in a patient with EBS-MD.

severe mucous membrane involvement with a hoarse cry, episodes of inspiratory stridor, recurrent and severe respiratory tract infections, and occasional bouts of severe respiratory insufficiency caused by swelling of the laryngeal mucosa.[5,9–11,13,15,16] Laryngoscopic examination typically reveals blisters, erosions, and strictures of epiglottis and laryngeal mucous membranes with fusion of the arytenoid cartilages; the appearance of the infraglottic airway is normal. Oral lesions were noted in only 1 case and involved the tongue in particular, but clinical descriptions of patients are not always clear. Treatment of the laryngeal complications required a tracheotomy for 3 patients varying in age from 20 months to 3 years; for another patient, repeated balloon dilatations led to stabilization of respiratory problems. One patient also had urethral strictures in infancy and another patient had only urethral stricture without oral involvement. The presence of severe mucous lesions does not indicate an early onset of MD, but all patients with an early onset of MD have mucous involvement. No ophthalmologic findings have been reported and hair has been described as normal, although 2 patients had partial congenital alopecia of the scalp.

Muscular Findings

In most cases, muscle weakness is first observed during the latter part of the first decade of life or during the teens, and muscle involvement often leads to progressive disabling muscular atrophy with ptosis and subsequent premature demise of the patient in their third decade of life because of weakened intercostal muscles. In some families, however, the onset of muscle weakness is considerably delayed (until 42 years) and the progression of MD is slow.[5,12,17] By contrast, very early onset of MD (infancy) has been reported.[15,18,19]

Other Findings

Although developmental milestones are usually normal, 2 patients showed cerebral atrophy on magnetic resonance imaging.[20] One of them had delayed motor milestones, bilateral cataract, mild left ventricular hypertrophy of the heart, and an arteriovenous malformation of the left leg.[20]

Immunochemistry and Electron Microscopy

Skin

To determine the level of cleavage in the skin and verify the involved gene/protein, a skin biopsy is taken at the edge of a blister. If no blister is available, a biopsy must be taken after strongly rubbing the skin. Histopathology with routine hematoxylin and eosin staining reveals tissue separation at the dermal-epidermal junction. Subsequently, immunofluorescence analysis using antibodies specific to the plectin protein is used to show the reduction or absence of plectin in the basal membrane zone (BMZ) (Fig. 2). Reports of a few antibodies against human plectin have been published[21]; the most common are HD1-121 (Dr Owaribe, University of Nagoya, Japan) (no longer available), 10F6 (commercial), and 5B3 (Dr Wiche, University of Vienna, Austria), which are all monoclonal antibodies (mAbs) and are directed against the rod domain. Immunofluorescence staining of other proteins in the skin, namely the collagens IV, VII, and XVII, 332 laminin and $\alpha_6\beta_4$ integrin subunits usually show normal staining and are on the floor of the patient's blisters. When it is tested, immunostaining against the 230-kDa bullous pemphigoid antigen has been reduced in more than 50% of cases,[4,5,9,15] although 1 publication reports the staining of BP230 split to the roof and floor of blister.[2] Cytokeratins 5 and 14 are detected on the floor and the roof of the blister, indicating that the cleavage plane is intracellular. To date no clear relation between immunofluorescence results and prognosis has been established.

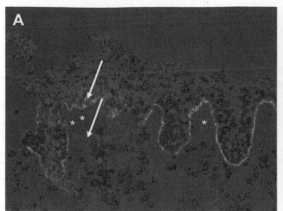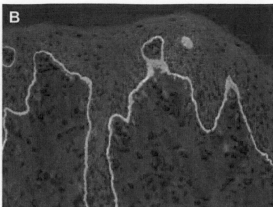

Fig. 2. Altered expression of plectin in patients with EBS. Immunofluorescence analysis of frozen sections of involved skin samples obtained from patient (*A*) and from a healthy control (*B*) using mAb HD121 specific to human plectin shows in the proband a reduced immunoreactivity of plectin that is present at the roof and the floor (*arrows*) of blisters (*asterisk*) compared with control. Magnification 20×.

Electron microscopy of skin biopsy reveals a cleavage within the basal keratinocytes, just above the cell basement membrane, indicated by cytoplasmic vacuoles. The overall frequency of hemidesmosomes is reduced. Hemidesmosomes are poorly formed along the roof of the blister, with the outer plaque generally normal in size and remaining attached to the base of the blister; the extracellular subbasal dense plates are present but attenuated. The inner plaque is absent or reduced. Keratin filaments show no contact with the reduced hemidesmosomes and are condensed in the perinuclear zone. Otherwise desmosomes are normal and the desmosome-keratin association appears intact in basal and suprabasal keratinocytes. Dermal anchoring filaments and anchoring fibrils are structurally normal.

Muscle

Light microscopy of muscle biopsy shows features of chronic myopathy with wide variation in striated muscle-fiber size, involving individual and grouped atrophic fibers with an increased amount of endomysial and perimysial connective and fatty tissue. Picnotic nuclear clumps and multiple internal nuclei can be present. There is evidence of continuing muscle-fiber necrosis with few regenerating fibers. Around muscular fibers, muscular nerves can be involved. Immunofluorescence analysis shows reduced or absent plectin staining.[2,15,20]

The most striking ultrastructural changes in EBS-MD muscle are the increased space between the plasma membrane and the muscle sarcomere, areas of focal myofibrillar disorganization, and focal loss of normal sarcomere organization with focal loss of or variation in normal Z-line size and alignment. The width of the sarcomere unit and length of Z-lines are often thinner and smaller. There is little uniformity between sarcomeres; thick and thin filaments are regularly seen running at a tangent to the plasma membrane. These filaments are observed at the edge of the sarcomere and often become extruded into the spaces between the sarcomeres. Where sarcomeres remain intact, they are incomplete or misaligned with their neighboring sarcomeres. Z-line smearing is apparent in focal areas of sarcomere disorganization but is not associated with any abnormal storage material within the myocyte. The loss of myofibrils is replaced by amorphous material, glycogen, and swollen sarcoplasmic reticulum cisternae. The number and position of mitochondria at the cell periphery adjacent to the sarcomeres is within normal limits, occasionally showing a mild disruption. There is extensive reduplication of the basement membrane caused by successive fiber necrosis and regeneration.[15,20] Immunostaining with antibodies against dystrophin, α-dystroglycan, sarcoglycan, and vinculin gives normal results. Plectin immunostaining is variable from normal[20] with the characteristic cross-striated pattern in longitudinal sections reduced,[9] abnormal,[2,15] or absent.[22,23] Immunostaining with desmin antibodies can reveal marked abnormalities, including cytoplasmic and sarcolemnal desmin-positive deposits in essentially all muscle fibers. The normal striated pattern of the intermediate filament protein desmin and α-actinin in longitudinal sections is attenuated or abolished.[2,15,20] Patients without clinical myopathy can have morphologic changes but the time between the onset of histologic and clinical manifestations is not known.

EBS WITH PA

Epidermolysis with pyloric atresia (EB-PA) is a genetically heterogeneous entity related to *PLEC1* or *ITGA6/B4* mutations. EB-PA related to *ITGA6/B4* mutation is not the subject of this article. This article focuses only on EBS-PA caused by plectin mutations.

Dermatologic Findings

Often cases of EBS-PA were initially detected in prenatal ultrasound examination showing suspicion of PA (polyhydramnios) (Table 2). Babies were usually born prematurely with a low birth weight and poor general condition. All newborn babies were reported to have generalized blisters, erosions, and skin fragility. Four patients had oral mucous membrane involvement.[14,24] Healing generally occurred without scarring or milia formation. Extensive CCA of the trunk, face, scalp, or limbs was reported in 60% of the cases.[3,25] Extremities of limbs were affected, with an abrupt transition to normal skin. Onychodystrophy was noted by investigators in only 2 cases, but no nails were seen when CCA involved limb extremities. No hair involvement has been reported. In 3 patients who survived more than 1 month, cutaneous involvement seems to improve with age.[3,14] One neonate had a dysmorphic syndrome with dysmature aspect with a relative macrocephaly, deep-set eyes, hypoplastic ears with helices fused with the skin of the skull, an upturned hypoplastic nose, and fingers and toes in hyperextension.[24] Two additional patients had hypoplastic ears.[25] Clinical features of EBS-PA are similar to those which results from integrin $\alpha_6\beta_4$ mutations.

Other Findings

PA was diagnosed antenatally or within the first days of life and was surgically corrected in the first week when possible. Laparostomy revealed a severely distended stomach, with a membrane at the pylorus. The treatment consisted of an excision of the membrane and pyloroplasty.

Consistent with the low birth weight and poor general conditions, 80% of patients died within the first month of life as a result of respiratory distress or systemic infection. Moreover, most families had a history of 1 or more previous children with the same clinical manifestations at birth and who also died in the first days of life.[3,24,25] These data highlight the lethal prognosis of this condition.

Only 3 patients in the world are known to have survived past infancy and are alive. They did not develop MD until 6, 16 months, and 7 years old,

respectively[3,14] (Chiavérini and colleagues, personal data, 2010). The 2 patients in apparently good general condition had no CCA.[14]

Immunochemistry and Electron Microscopy

Immunohistochemical studies using mAbs HD1-121, 10F6, and 5B3 against plectin showed a markedly attenuated or completely negative signal. Immunostaining for other BMZ proteins including the α_6 and β_4 integrins, laminin 332, type VII and IV collagens, BPAG1 and BPAG2 were normal. In 1 case staining was negative for BP180[25] and in another keratin 15 was reduced.[3]

Ultrastructural changes are similar to EBS-MD with a plane of separation within the basal keratinocytes, just above the HD inner plaque, and hypoplastic and reduced in frequency HD.

EBS-OGNA

This peculiar form of EBS was first described in 1970 in a Norwegian family, then in a second family of German descent. This autosomal dominant disorder is characterized by a generalized epidermal fragility from birth, tendency to bruising, small traumatic blood blebs (usually localized at extremities), and onychogriphosis.[1,6,7] No additional symptoms (muscular or digestive) have been described in these patients.

Electron microscopy shows features similar to EBS-MD and EBS-AP. Immunofluorescence analysis shows that patients' skin consistently lacks immunoreactivity at the basal cell layer with the 2 antibodies 10F6 and 5B3 that are directed against epitopes in the rod domain of plectin. Antibodies against the other BMZ proteins show an immunoreactivity similar to control. Staining of muscle biopsy is instead normal with all antiplectin antibodies.[7]

GENOTYPE-PHENOTYPE CORRELATIONS

As discussed earlier, plectin mutations are associated with 3 different phenotypes and severity can vary considerably for each phenotype.[26]

Plectin has a multidomain structure that makes it well suited for cross-linking functions with other proteins. It comprises N- and C-terminal domains that contain multiple protein-protein interaction sites, separated by an elongated central rod domain that is predicted to mediate self-association via coil-coil interactions. The N-terminal region contains an actin-binding domain (ABD) that binds to the first pair of fibronectin type III (FnIII) domains of the integrin β_4 cytoplasmic domain in hemisdesmosomes. Adjacent to the ABD, the plakin domain binds to regions of integrin β_4 downstream of the

Table 2
Summary of clinical and molecular features of patients with EBS-PA and published plectin mutations

Patient	Sex/Age (Months)	Consanguinity	Origin	Dermatologic Features					Mutations						Other Familial Cases	Refs.
				Evolution	CCA	Mucosa	Nails	Other	Mutation 1	Type	Exon	Mutation 2	Type	Exon		
1	F/0	1	Pakistan	Death	0	0	0		1563del4	ptc	15	1563del4	ptc	15	2 dead	JID04[17]
2	M/0	1	Lebanon	Death	1	0	1	War anomalies	Q305X	ptc	10	Q305X	ptc	10		JID04[17]
3	F/0	1	Saudi Arabia	Death	0	0	0		R3029X	ptc	33	R3029X	ptc	33	1 dead	JID04[17]
4	M/0	1	Europe	Death	1	0	1		2769del21	del7aa	23	2769del21	del7aa	23		JID04[17]
5	M/16	0	Japan	Intensive care	1	0	1		1344G>A	Splice loss exon 13?	13	Q305X	ptc	10	1 dead	JMD05[3]
6	M/0	0	Japan	Death	1	0	1		R1189X	ptc	28	R1189X/ Q2538X	ptc	28		JMD05[3]
7	F/0	1	Turkey	Death	1	1	1	Ears and nose anomalies, contracture of the limbs	(2727del14) 2676del14	ptc	22	(2727del14) 2676del14	ptc	22	2 dead	JID03[24]
8	M/6	0	NA	Amelioration of the skin	0	1	0		Q2466X	ptc	32	Q2545X	ptc	33		JID07[14]

Numbering of *PLEC* coding sequence initiates at the ATG codon of the second exon. Plectin mutations have been checked and if necessary corrected using this numbering. An asterisk has been added at the end of the mutation when precise localization of the mutation could not be confirmed. When numbering has been corrected the published mutation is in parentheses.
Abbreviations: del, deletion; F, female; ins, insertion; M, male; NA, not available.

second FnIII domain. The plakin domain also harbors a binding site for the type XVII collagen. The C-terminal region of plectin contains 6 plakin repeat domains and harbors binding sites for intermediate filaments (desmin, vinculin) and integrin β_4.[8,27,28]

Pleomorphic Phenotypes of Plectin Mutations

Analysis of plectin mutations (**Fig. 3**) reveals that

- **EBS-MD** is usually a result of nonsense, insertion, or deletion mutations in exon 32, which encodes for the second rod domain. No missense mutation has been published. These 3 types of mutations generally cause a premature termination codon (PTC) during protein translation, which results in truncated polypeptides and downregulation of the corresponding mRNA through nonsense-mediated mRNA decay. In Malta 3 unrelated families have the

same plectin mutation but with variable severity, suggesting the possibility of other regulator genes.[15,19]

- **EBS-PA** is usually a result of nonsense, insertion, or deletion mutations in the N-terminal region of plectin, which is responsible for the interaction with integrin β_4, another protein that is associated with PA when defective, and the first rod domain. These mutations result in a PTC during translation or loss or gain of amino acids.

The absence of PA in patients with EBS-MD and mutations in the rod domain can be explained by the normal synthesis in keratinocytes of a splice variant of plectin without the rod domain,[29,30] which can rescue the inefficiency of the mutated plectin to link correctly with $\alpha_6\beta_4$ and intermediate fibrils. Some patients with EBS-MD have mutations in the N-terminal domain of plectin. These mutations are compound heterozygous insertion/

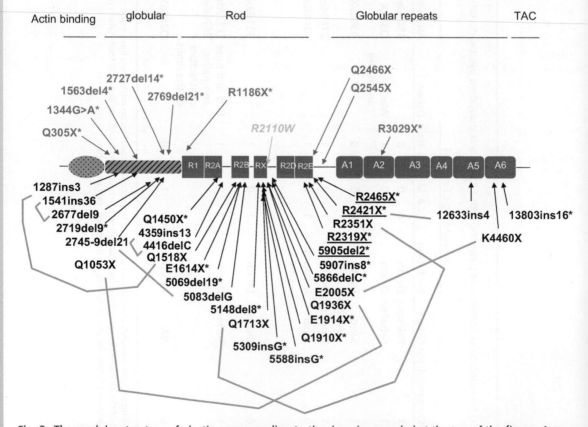

Fig. 3. The modular structure of plectin corresponding to the domains encoded at the top of the figure. Arrows indicate the positions of the published mutations. Those identified in families with EBS-MD, or with characteristic skin lesions and mutations and at the risk of muscle involvement, are shown below the schematic structure of plectin. The positions of mutations in the plectin gene (PLEC1) in patients with EBS-PA are shown above. The specific R2110W mutation associated with EBS-Ogna is shaded in gray. Recurrent mutations are underlined. Homozygous mutations are followed by an asterisk, and compound heterozygous mutation combinations are linked by a line.

deletion of 1 to 12 amino acids. Analysis of the sequence in this region shows that mutations associated with EBS-PA involve the second tandem pair of spectrin repeats, whereas mutations associated with EBS-MD do not involve this kind of sequence (**Figs. 3** and **4**).[31] These data suggest that mutations associated with EBS-MD allow an interaction of plectin with integrin β_4, but alter other properties of plectin necessary for its proper function, in particular in muscle. Plectin has been shown to interact with a wide range of proteins in muscle like intermediate filaments (desmin, vinculin), actin, and dystrophin-glycoprotein complexes.[32,33]

An observation regarding phenogenotype consequences can be made with 2 patients with EBS-PA with mutations in exon 32 and 33, which usually lead to an EBS-MD phenotype. The first patient (patient 8) is compound heterozygous for 2 nonsense mutations, 1 in exon 32 coding for the second rod domain of the protein and the other in exon 33, which codes for the transitory domain between the rod domain and C-terminal globular domain; this second mutation is near to a homozygous nonsense mutation, which is associated with EBS-MD.[14] The second patient (patient 3) has a homozygous nonsense mutation in exon 33 in a region coding for the second plakin repeat domain C-terminal globular domain.[25] Contrary to the reported cases of EBS-PA, the first patient has a mild phenotype and is still alive, whereas the

second one died a few days after birth. Neither of them had CCA. Immunofluorescence analysis showed a reduced but not absent plectin in patient 1 and was not available for patient 2. In these patients it can be hypothesized that the rodless isoform of plectin is also affected and therefore cannot rescue a normal interaction with $\alpha_6\beta_4$, hence leading to PA.

One patient with EBS-MD has a homozygous insertion mutation in exon 33 in a region coding for the 3′ end of the last plakin repeat domain (patient 24). This mutation causes a frame shift and premature termination 48 amino acids downstream of the insertion site, thus leading to a truncated protein lacking the last 35 amino acids. This patient has weak residual protein expression in the skin and an unusual and severe phenotype with skin, muscle, cardiac, ocular, and brain involvement, suggesting that the distal part of plectin is important for proper function.[20] The R6 domain is believed to be important in the packaging of the C-terminal domain. EBS of Ogna is caused by a missense mutation (R2110W) in the rod domain.

Variable Severity of Phenotype in Patients with EBS-MD

In patients with EBS-MD, the type of mutation (PTC-causing mutations vs in-frame insertions/deletions) influences the phenotypic severity and timing of the onset of MD. Thus, identification of

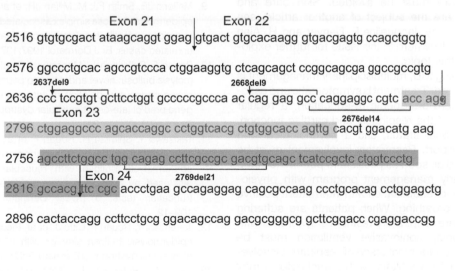

Exon 21 | Exon 22

2516 gtgtgcgact ataagcaggt ggag|gtgact gtgcacaagg gtgacgagtg ccagctggtg

2576 ggccctgcac agccgtccca ctggaaggtg ctcagcagct ccggcagcga ggccgccgtg

2637del9   2668del9

2636 ccc tccgtgt gcttcctggt gcccccgccca ac cag gag gcc caggaggc cgtc acc agg
Exon 23
2676del14
2796 ctggaggccc agcaccaggc cctggtcacg ctgtggcacc agttg cacgt ggacatg aag

2756 agccttctggcc tgg cagag ccttcgccgc gacgtgcagc tcatccgctc ctggtccctg

Exon 24   2769del21
2816 gccacg ttc cgc accctgaa gccagaggag cagcgccaag ccctgcacag cctggagctg

2896 cactaccagg ccttcctgcg ggacagccag gacgcgggcg gcttcggacc cgaggaccgg

helix C SR5   ↓   Start of exon

helix A SR6

Fig. 4. cDNA sequence of the spectrin repeats (SR) 5 and 6 of the N-terminal plakin domain of human plectin. Colored boxes localize the α-helices C of SR5 and A of SR6. Mutations of EBS-MD patients are above the sequence and those of EBS-AP below. Nucleotides involving deletions are underlined in black.

the type of mutations in a person with neonatal blistering of the hemidesmosomal type can serve as a prognostic indicator of the severity of the MD later in life. However, no correlation between the localization of the mutation and the phenotype severity has been shown.

Clinical Implications

The pleiomorphic consequences of PLEC mutations emphasize the importance of screening by means of immunofluorescence for plectin deficiency in patients with EBS-PA and EBS with or without signs of MD, in particular if there is ultrastructural evidence of tissue separation at the hemidesmosomal level, which is clearly distinct from the classic EBS cases caused by mutations in keratin 5 or 14.

Plectin mutations should be considered as the underlying cause of apparently sporadic cases of EBS, which, in the case of PLEC1 mutations, may represent a recessive disease rather than de novo dominant mutations such as with the keratin genes.

Treatment

Management of EBS requires a multidisciplinary approach with a pediatrician, dermatologist, anesthetist, surgeons, geneticist, and nurses. Patients must be handled with care because of the extreme fragility of their skin. Adhesives, friction or pressure must be avoided. Skin care and dressing are the subject of another article, see the articles by Jacqueline E. Denyer and H. Alan Arbuckle elsewhere in this issue for further exploration of this topic.

Regarding MD, multidisciplinary management is also required. Treatment is symptomatic and associates neuro-orthopedic re-education, a regular follow-up of the respiratory and cardiac function, the nutritional status, and a psychological and social support. Respiratory involvement must be diagnosed as soon as possible to permit the setup of an early management program with physiotherapy and rehabilitation with intermittent positive pressure breathing. When patients are suffering from severe respiratory restrictive syndrome with hypercapnia, noninvasive ventilation must be started. At a terminal stage of respiratory involvement invasive ventilation with a tracheotomy may be necessary.

REFERENCES

1. Fine JD, Eady RA, Bauer EA, et al. The classification of inherited epidermolysis bullosa (EB): report of the third international consensus meeting on diagnosis and classification of EB. J Am Acad Dermatol 2008;58:931–50.

2. Gache Y, Chavanas S, Lacour JP, et al. Defective expression of plectin/HD1 in epidermolysis bullosa simplex with muscular dystrophy. J Clin Invest 1996;97:2289–98.

3. Nakamura H, Sawamura D, Goto M, et al. Epidermolysis bullosa simplex associated with pyloric atresia is a novel clinical subtype caused by mutations in the plectin gene (PLEC1). J Mol Diagn 2005;7:28–35.

4. McLean WH, Pulkkinen L, Smith FJ, et al. Loss of plectin causes epidermolysis bullosa with muscular dystrophy: cDNA cloning and genomic organization. Genes Dev 1996;10:1724–35.

5. Pulkkinen L, Smith FJ, Shimizu H, et al. Homozygous deletion mutations in the plectin gene (PLEC1) in patients with epidermolysis bullosa simplex associated with late-onset muscular dystrophy. Hum Mol Genet 1996;5:1539–46.

6. Koss-Harnes D, Jahnsen FL, Wiche G, et al. Plectin abnormality in epidermolysis bullosa simplex Ogna: non-responsiveness of basal keratinocytes to some anti-rat plectin antibodies. Exp Dermatol 1997;6:41–8.

7. Koss-Harnes D, Hoyheim B, Anton-Lamprecht I, et al. A site-specific plectin mutation causes dominant epidermolysis bullosa simplex Ogna: two identical de novo mutations. J Invest Dermatol 2002;118:87–93.

8. Wiche G. Role of plectin in cytoskeleton organization and dynamics. J Cell Sci 1998;111(Pt 17):2477–86.

9. Mellerio JE, Smith FJ, McMillan JR, et al. Recessive epidermolysis bullosa simplex associated with plectin mutations: infantile respiratory complications in two unrelated cases. Br J Dermatol 1997;137:898–906.

10. Rouan F, Pulkkinen L, Meneguzzi G, et al. Epidermolysis bullosa: novel and de novo premature termination codon and deletion mutations in the plectin gene predict late-onset muscular dystrophy. J Invest Dermatol 2000;114:381–7.

11. Takizawa Y, Shimizu H, Rouan F, et al. Four novel plectin gene mutations in Japanese patients with epidermolysis bullosa with muscular dystrophy disclosed by heteroduplex scanning and protein truncation tests. J Invest Dermatol 1999;112:109–12.

12. Takahashi Y, Rouan F, Uitto J, et al. Plectin deficient epidermolysis bullosa simplex with 27-year-history of muscular dystrophy. J Dermatol Sci 2005;37:87–93.

13. Dang M, Pulkkinen L, Smith FJ, et al. Novel compound heterozygous mutations in the plectin gene in epidermolysis bullosa with muscular dystrophy and the use of protein truncation test for detection of premature termination codon mutations. Lab Invest 1998;78:195–204.

14. Sawamura D, Goto M, Sakai K, et al. Possible involvement of exon 31 alternative splicing in

phenotype and severity of epidermolysis bullosa caused by mutations in PLEC1. J Invest Dermatol 2007;127:1537–40.

15. McMillan JR, Akiyama M, Rouan F, et al. Plectin defects in epidermolysis bullosa simplex with muscular dystrophy. Muscle Nerve 2007;35:24–35.

16. Schara U, Tucke J, Mortier W, et al. Severe mucous membrane involvement in epidermolysis bullosa simplex with muscular dystrophy due to a novel plectin gene mutation. Eur J Pediatr 2004;163:218–22.

17. Uitto J. Compound heterozygosity of unique in-frame insertion and deletion mutations in the plectin gene in a mild case of epidermolysis bullosa with very late onset of muscular dystrophy. J Invest Dermatol 2004;122:A86.

18. Hovnanian A, Pollack E, Hilal L, et al. A missense mutation in the rod domain of keratin 14 associated with recessive epidermolysis bullosa simplex. Nat Genet 1993;3:327–32.

19. Pfendner E, Rouan F, Uitto J. Progress in epidermolysis bullosa: the phenotypic spectrum of plectin mutations. Exp Dermatol 2005;14:241–9.

20. Schroder R, Kunz WS, Rouan F, et al. Disorganization of the desmin cytoskeleton and mitochondrial dysfunction in plectin-related epidermolysis bullosa simplex with muscular dystrophy. J Neuropathol Exp Neurol 2002;61:520–30.

21. Foisner R, Feldman B, Sander L, et al. A panel of monoclonal antibodies to rat plectin: distinction by epitope mapping and immunoreactivity with different tissues and cell lines. Acta Histochem 1994;96:421–38.

22. Bauer JW, Rouan F, Kofler B, et al. A compound heterozygous one amino-acid insertion/nonsense mutation in the plectin gene causes epidermolysis bullosa simplex with plectin deficiency. Am J Pathol 2001;158:617–25.

23. Smith FJ, Eady RA, Leigh IM, et al. Plectin deficiency results in muscular dystrophy with epidermolysis bullosa. Nat Genet 1996;13:450–7.

24. Charlesworth A, Gagnoux-Palacios L, Bonduelle M, et al. Identification of a lethal form of epidermolysis bullosa simplex associated with a homozygous genetic mutation in plectin. J Invest Dermatol 2003;121:1344–8.

25. Pfendner E, Uitto J. Plectin gene mutations can cause epidermolysis bullosa with pyloric atresia. J Invest Dermatol 2005;124:111–5.

26. Shimizu H, Takizawa Y, Pulkkinen L, et al. Epidermolysis bullosa simplex associated with muscular dystrophy: phenotype-genotype correlations and review of the literature. J Am Acad Dermatol 1999; 41:950–6.

27. de Pereda JM, Lillo MP, Sonnenberg A. Structural basis of the interaction between integrin alpha6-beta4 and plectin at the hemidesmosomes. EMBO J 2009;28:1180–90.

28. Koster J, Geerts D, Favre B, et al. Analysis of the interactions between bp180, bp230, plectin and the integrin alpha6beta4 important for hemidesmosome assembly. J Cell Sci 2003;116:387–99.

29. Andra K, Kornacker I, Jorgl A, et al. Plectin-isoform-specific rescue of hemidesmosomal defects in plectin (-/-) keratinocytes. J Invest Dermatol 2003;120: 189–97.

30. Elliott CE, Becker B, Oehler S, et al. Plectin transcript diversity: identification and tissue distribution of variants with distinct first coding exons and rodless isoforms. Genomics 1997;42:115–25.

31. Sonnenberg A, Rojas AM, de Pereda JM. The structure of a tandem pair of spectrin repeats of plectin reveals a modular organization of the plakin domain. J Mol Biol 2007;368.1379–91.

32. Hijikata T, Nakamura A, Isokawa K, et al. Plectin 1 links intermediate filaments to costameric sarcolemma through beta-synemin, alpha-dystrobrevin and actin. J Cell Sci 2008;121:2062–74.

33. Hijikata T, Murakami T, Ishikawa H, et al. Plectin tethers desmin intermediate filaments onto subsarcolemmal dense plaques containing dystrophin and vinculin. Histochem Cell Biol 2003;119:109–23.

Wound Management for Children with Epidermolysis Bullosa

Jacqueline E. Denyer, RGN, RSCN, RHV[a,b,*]

KEYWORDS

• Epidermolysis bullosa • Wounds • Dressings • Atraumatic

Skin and wound care in EB is specific both to the type of EB and to individual wounds within each child. Availability of dressings and personal preference are also paramount in the selection of materials. The ideal dressing is yet to be developed, although there are now a variety of suitable dressings available. Wound healing is challenging and chronic wounds often feature. Factors adversely affecting healing include anemia, malnutrition,[1] infection, and pruritus.

CARE AND MANAGEMENT OF NEONATES

Appearance at birth may not necessarily indicate the type of EB or its severity. Factors such as mode of delivery and level of intrauterine movements are reflected in the amount of skin loss at birth, and those delivered by cesarean section may appear deceptively mildly affected but have a severe form of EB.[2]

To minimize further damage to this vulnerable group it is recommended that term infants are not nursed in an incubator, as the hot and humid environment can encourage blistering. Wounds should be covered with a nonadherent dressing such as Mepitel (Mölnlycke Healthcare, Sweden)[3] or Urgotul (Urgo, France)[4] (**Tables 1–3**) with secondary foam dressings used for absorption of exudate and protection from baby movements such as kicking. Where two raw surfaces are adjacent to each other, dressings should be placed between the digits to prevent fusion (**Fig. 1**). This procedure is of particular importance in those with dystrophic forms of EB, but fusion is possible in all types if digits are dressed without due care. It

may be necessary to apply dressings in such a way to minimize deformity, for example, exerting a slight pull in the opposite direction to a rotated foot.

Umbilical venous catheters are rarely necessary and attempted insertion of these can cause major skin damage (**Fig. 2**). Prophylactic antibiotic cover is not indicated, and oral feeding should be possible provided a specialized teat such as a Haberman/Special Needs Feeder is used in conjunction with topical analgesia. Breast feeding may also be possible.

If intravenous access is necessary, the cannula should be secured using silicone-based, rather than adhesive tapes (Mepitac, Mölnlycke Healthcare or Siltape, Advancis, Nottinghamshire, UK). Cannulae must be well padded to avoid damage to the skin from baby movements and in particular the risk of corneal abrasions if the cannula is sited in the hand. Periumbilical damage is common from trauma caused by plastic cord clamps, and it is recommended that these be removed and replaced by a ligature.

To minimize trauma from handling the baby should be nursed on a soft mattress recommended for infants, such as an incubator pad. The infant can be lifted onto this. When it is necessary to handle the baby off the mattress employ a "roll and lift" technique: roll the baby onto his or her side, place one hand flat behind the head and the other under the buttocks, press down onto the cot surface, and allow the baby to roll back onto your hands and lift.

Bathing should be delayed until the interuterine and birth damage have healed, because it is

a Department of Dermatology, Great Ormond Street Hospital, London WC1N 3JH, UK
b DebRA UK, 13 Wellington Business Park, Dukes Ride, Crowthorne, RG5 6LS, UK
* Department of Dermatology, Great Ormond Street Hospital, London WC1N 3JH, UK.
E-mail address: Jackie.denyer@debra.org.uk

Dermatol Clin 28 (2010) 257–264
doi:10.1016/j.det.2010.01.002

Table 1
Recommended dressings for EB simplex

Type	Brand	Manufacturer	Indication	Contraindication/ Comments
Primary	Mepitel	Mölnlycke Healthcare	Wound	Dowling-Meara
	Urgotul	Urgo	Wound	Very moist (problems with retention)
Foam	Mepilex/Mepilex Lite/Mepilex Transfer	Mölnlycke Healthcare	Protection	Heat-related blistering
Hydrogel	Intra site Conformable	Smith & Nephew	Cooling; pain reduction	
Biosynthetic cellulose	SuprasorbX	Activa	Cooling; pain reduction	
Bordered dressings	Mepilex Border/ Border Lite	Mölnlycke Healthcare	Protection	May require removal assisted by Silicone Medical Removers such as Appeel (Clinimed) or Niltac (Trio Healthcare) to avoid skin stripping
	Allevyn Gentle Border	Smith & Nephew		
	Urgotul Duo Border	Urgo		
Hydrofiber	Aquacel	Convatec	Dowling-Meara	
Powder	Cornflour		Apply following lancing of blister	Nappy area
	Catrix	Cranage Healthcare		

Table 2
Recommended dressings for junctional EB

Type	Brand	Manufacturer	Indication	Contraindication	Wear Time
Hydrogel	Intra Site Conformable	Smith & Nephew	Infant Herlitz junctional EB		Change daily or when dry
Hydrofiber	Aquacel	Convatec	Very moist wounds where difficult to keep dressing in place	Lightly exuding or dry wounds	Change every 3–4 d
Primary dressing	Urgotul	Urgo	Primary dressing		Change every 3–4 d
Soft silicone foam	Mepilex/Mepilex Lite/Mepilex Transfer	Mölnlycke Healthcare	Protection; absorption		As determined by exudate level
Polymeric membrane	PolyMem	Ferris	Chronic wounds; critical colonization/ infection		As determined by exudate level

Table 3
Recommended dressings for dystrophic EB; for antimicrobial management please see Table 4

Type	Brand	Manufacturer	Indication	Contraindication/Comments	Wear Time
Soft silicone primary dressing	Mepitel Silflex	Mölnlycke Healthcare Advancis Medical	Moist wound	Silicone sensitivity	3–4 d depending on presence of infection and patient choice
Lipidocolloid Primary dressing	Urgotul	Urgo	Moist wound, drier wounds and protection of vulnerable skin	Where retention is difficult	
Foam dressings Soft silicone	Mepilex Mepilex Lite Mepilex Transfer	Mölnlycke Healthcare	Absorption of exudate Protection Lightly exuding wounds To transfer exudate to absorbent dressing Where conformability required—digits, axillae	Overheating May need to apply over recommended atraumatic primary dressing such as Mepitel or Urgotul	Every 3–4 d
Foam dressings	Alleyvn Urgocell	Smith & Nephew Urgo	Absorption Protection	May need to apply over recommended atraumatic primary dressing	Every 3–4 d
Polymeric membrane	PolyMem	Ferris	Where cleansing required		Depending on exudate levels
Bordered dressings	Mepilex Border/Border Lite Alleyvn Gentle Border	Mölnlycke Healthcare Smith & Nephew	Isolated wounds Dominant dystrophic and mild dystrophic EB	May require removal with Silicone Medical Adhesive Remover to avoid skin stripping	3–4 d depending on personal choice

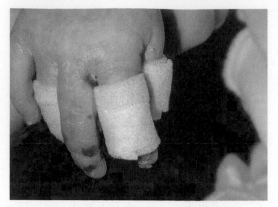

Fig. 1. Dress digits individually to avoid fusion.

difficult to prevent damage to the naked infant. For this reason dressings should be changed on a limb by limb basis rather than all dressings being removed at one time. If the correct dressing is used the wound should not require cleansing, but if needed gentle irrigation can be done using warmed saline delivered via a syringe.

Nappy area care requires adaptation in those with EB. Cleansing with water can sting open wounds and therefore cleansing with equal parts of liquid and white soft paraffin in the form of an ointment or aerosol spray is advocated (commercially available as Emollin 50/50 emollient spray, CD Medical Ltd). The nappy should be lined with a soft disposable cloth to prevent friction and trauma from the edges of the nappy. Open wounds in the nappy area should be covered with a hydrogel-impregnated gauze (Intrasite Conformable, Smith & Nephew) which is replaced at every nappy change. Avoid the temptation to use a larger size nappy than indicated by the size of the baby or to fasten the nappy loosely, as this will encourage friction when the baby moves inside the nappy.

Regular analgesia is paramount in this age group, as evidence suggests neonates may be highly sensitive to pain,[5] and poor management in the neonatal period can cause heightened sensitivity throughout life. Assessment may be complex in this age group as a lack of vigorous responses to pain may be demonstrated.[6]

DRESSING MANAGEMENT IN EB SIMPLEX

This group of children is difficult to manage, as dressings may cause blistering around the edges and heat from the dressing can result in additional blistering. Probably the most challenging are infants who are severely affected with Dowling-Meara EB simplex. These infants often have large areas of skin loss, but traditional dressing management frequently leads to blistering around the edges of the dressings (Fig. 3).[7] The best tolerated dressing is a Hydrofiber (see Table 1) and this can be used to protect skin from friction from the edges of other dressings. As soon as the wound is healed it is recommended that dressings be removed and the infant dressed in soft, flat, seamed clothing or that clothes with raised seams are worn inside out. The main management is to lance the multiple blisters as soon as they arise (Fig. 4). Simple cornflour applied to the blistered area helps it to dry and reduces friction. Catrix powder (bovine cartilage powder; Cranage Healthcare International) (see Table 1) is a prescribable medically approved alternative, and early work has suggested more rapid resolution of blisters when Catrix is applied. Children often suffer from repeated infections, and the author has had success in reducing the incidence of bacterial overgrowth by using garments containing a silver thread.

Older children with Dowling Meara and those with localized EB simplex encounter a higher

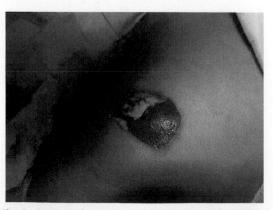

Fig. 2. Damage from attempted insertion of umbilical catheter.

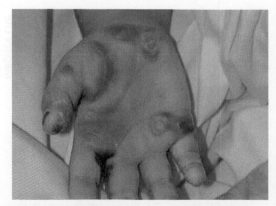

Fig. 3. Blistering from tubular retention bandage.

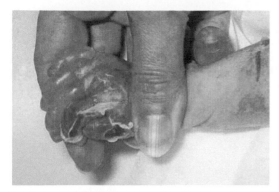

Fig. 4. Lance blisters to prevent enlargement.

incidence of blistering in hot and humid conditions. Dressings are principally required for the feet, and preference varies. Thin silicone-based foams are generally well tolerated. Many like to use sheet hydrogels, as these have a cooling effect that reduces pain.

A large proportion of affected children prefer not to use any dressings at all. Commercial socks containing a silver thread help to reduce heat and bacterial load, and are popular with this group of patients. Dermasilk socks provide an anti friction layer and also reduce the bacterial load.

DRESSING MANAGEMENT FOR THOSE WITH JUNCTIONAL EB
Herlitz Junctional EB

Affected infants often present with minimal skin damage at birth, but there is a marked tendency for chronic wounds to develop early in this group of largely life-limited children. A small number of infants have large, heavily exuding wounds present at birth, and these are very difficult to dress as there is a tendency for the dressings to slip. In these cases the author has found that using a Hydrofiber dressing directly to the wound and covering this with an absorbent dressing provides a stable option.

In general, dressings such as soft silicone and foams that aid healing in other types of EB provide comfort, but do not appear to be effective in those with Herlitz Junctional EB. In the author's experience the best form of management is to use a lipidocolloid dressing to cover open wounds, and use hydrogel-impregnated gauze as a secondary dressing (see **Table 2**) which is then secured with tubular bandage that must be cut shorter than the secondary dressing to avoid blistering from the edges of both the dressing and retention agent. The hydrogel dressings should be changed as soon as they begin to dry out, but the primary dressing can be left in place for several days.

Successful healing has resulted from this method and despite progressive cachexia and dysphasia, infants have maintained largely intact skin throughout life.

Those with non-Herlitz forms of Junctional EB and longer-term survivors with Herlitz Junctional EB benefit from more traditional dressings recommended for dystrophic EB, as the method described here is not always practical in older children.

DRESSING MANAGEMENT FOR THOSE WITH DYSTROPHIC EB
Mild Recessive and Dominant Dystrophic

Children with mild recessive or dominant dystrophic EB generally require dressings for wounds that have developed over bony prominences such as knees, ankles, backs of hands, and digits. Many can tolerate bordered silicone or adhesive dressings (see **Table 3**) although a Silicone Medical Adhesive Remover may be required if skin stripping occurs on removal.[8,9] Children often like these dressings, as they do not need retention bandaging and look like regular sticking plasters as used by their peers.

Severe Generalized Dystrophic EB

Those affected by severe forms of dystrophic EB may require extensive dressings in an attempt to heal wounds, and to offer protection against friction and shearing forces. A range of dressings is suitable for those with dystrophic EB but choice is often limited by size of the dressing. A large proportion will suffer from chronic wounds, which are challenging for all concerned. Atraumatic primary dressings include soft silicone mesh and lipidocolloid dressings. These require a secondary dressing for exudate management and protection. Foam dressings are commonly used, although additional highly absorptive dressings may be required if exudate is excessive.

Infection and critical colonization appear to be a major factor in the persistence of wounds, and use of an antimicrobial applied topically or medicated dressings are recommended (**Table 4**).[10] Silver-impregnated dressings are very effective in reducing the bioburden[11] but as there is a concern about raised plasma silver levels the author currently does not use these in children. Honey dressings or stabilized topical hydrogen peroxide cream is prescribed in preference to silver products. Honey is available in the form of impregnated dressings and ointments, and is effective both in the management of chronic wounds and reduction of the bioburden.[12] Unfortunately, some patients experience stinging and pain in response to the

Table 4
Recommended dressings for infected and critically colonized wounds and where biofilm is present

Type	Brand	Manufacturer	Specific Indication	Contraindication/Comments	Wear Time
Honey			Malodorous wounds Infection/critical colonization	Pain In conditions where insects are rife May need to use over recommended primary dressing to ensure nonadherence	3–7 d depending on patient choice May need to change secondary dressing more frequently due to increase in exudate
	Algivon	Advancis Medical			
	Medihoney Gel Sheet	Medihoney	Sensitive wounds where removal resisted		Replace when no evidence of gel sheet remains
	Mesitran S (ointment)	Aspen Medical	Sensitive wounds		Apply at each dressing change
Silver	Mepilex Ag	Mölnlycke Health care	Where foam dressing required		
	Urgotul Silver/SSD	Urgo	Primary dressing		
	PolyMem Silver	Ferris			
	Aquacel Ag	Convatec	EB simplex with diabetes mellitus		
Other	Suprasorb X+ PHMB	Activa Healthcare Lohmann & Rauscher	Pain Itching		Daily for optimum pain relief and cooling effect
Other	Cutimed Sorbact	BSN			As dictated by strike through on secondary dressing
Other	PolyMem	Ferris			When strike through observed
Other	Crystacide	Derma	Superficial infection		

pH level and the osmotic pull. Cutimed Sorbact (BSN) dressings remove bacteria by the process of hydrophobic interaction; the dressings are coated with a fatty acid derivative that attracts bacteria to the dressing, where they become bound. Initial studies have shown this dressing to be effective in wound healing in those with chronic wounds associated with EB.

Dressings containing Polyhexanide (PHMB) such as Suprasorb X+ PHMB (Activa Healthcare, Lohmann & Rauscher, UK) offer antimicrobial management of critically colonized and infected wounds, and are recommended for long-term use. Polymeric membrane dressing (PolyMem, Ferris, OH, USA) contains a cleanser (surfactant) that also reduces the bioburden and has enabled healing of recalcitrant wounds. Polymeric membrane dressings also have the advantage of being a "stand-alone" dressing without the need for a nonadherent primary dressing or secondary dressing for protection or exudate management. Frequency of dressing changes is determined by personal choice, time available, and level of exudate. Infected or critically colonized wounds require more frequent dressing changes. Use of honey products and polymeric membrane dressings increase exudate initially, so commitment to daily dressing changes must be ascertained before starting these.

Bathing is encouraged for those with severe forms of EB but may not be tolerated due to difficulties resulting from pain management and handling. It has been reported that adding an unspecified large amount of salt to the water reduces pain both while in the bath and while waiting for the wounds to be redressed. The author's experience reflects this. When bathing is not possible and the child also refuses cleansing of the wound, polymeric membrane dressings have proved very effective in reducing the bioburden. Adequate pain relief before use of dressings is essential, and additional sedation may also be required. Need for medication varies from simple analgesia such as paracetamol or ibuprofen to opiates including tramadol and morphine.[13,14]

Dressings impregnated with ibuprofen (Biatain-Ibu) have proved helpful for some wounds, although these are not licensed for children younger than 12 years.[15] Topical morphine in hydrogel is also effective. Other dressings with pain-relieving properties include biosynthetic cellulose such as Suprasorb X, which has an additional cooling effect and is helpful in reducing pain associated with both blisters and wounds. Therapies such as guided imagery and distraction techniques can be taught to families and carers to reduce the distress of procedural pain.

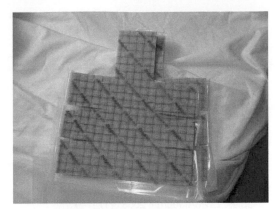
Fig. 5. Template for foot dressing.

TIPS AND HINTS

- Turn off fans before removing dressings to reduce pain from the circulating air.
- Cut templates of dressing shapes to aid carers who are unfamiliar with the wound requirements (**Fig. 5**).
- Cut all dressings anticipated for dressing change before starting.
- Demonstrate new products in advance of their use, FOR EXAMPLE, Silicone Medical Adhesive Removers
- If using new products such as honey based products that have the potential to sting, try it on a small wound first before widespread application.
- Use tubular bandage as retention where possible. Place bandage above or below wound before dressing is applied, so it can be pulled into place quickly before dressing moves.

REFERENCES

1. Haynes L. Clinical practice guidelines for nutrition support in children with epidermolysis bullosa. Autumn 2007. Available at: www.nutricia-clinical-care.co.uk. Accessed January 21, 2010.
2. Denyer J. Management of severe blistering disorders. Semin Neonatol 2000;5(4):321–4.
3. White R. Evidence for atraumatic soft silicone wound dressing use. Wounds UK 2005;1(3):104–9.
4. Blanchet-Bardon C, Bohot S. Using Urgotul dressing for the management of epidermolysis bullosa skin lesions. J Wound Care 2005;14(10):490–1, 494–96.
5. Anand KJS, Hickey PR. Clinical importance of pain and stress in preterm newborn infants. Biol Neonate 1998;73:1–9.
6. Anand KJ, The International Evidence-Based Group for Neonatal Pain. Consensus statement for the

prevention and management of pain in the newborn. Arch Pediatr Adolesc Med 2001;155:173–80.

7. Denyer J. Epidermolysis bullosa. Chapter 10. In: Denyer J, White R, editors. Paediatric skin and wound care. Aberdeen (UK): Wounds UK; 2006. p. 154.

8. Mather C, Denyer J. Removing dressings in epidermolysis bullosa. Nurs Times 2008;104(14):46–8.

9. Cutting K. Silicone and skin adhesives. J Community Nurs 2006;20(11):36–7.

10. White RJ, Cooper R, Kingsley A. Wound colonisation and infection; the role of topical antimicrobials. Br J Nurs 2001;10(9):563–78.

11. Cutting K. Wound healing, bacteria and topical therapies. EWMA Journal 2003;3(1):17–9.

12. Hon J. Using honey to heal a chronic wound in a patient with epidermolysis bullosa. Br J Nurs 2005;14(19):S4–S12 Tissue Viability Supplement.

13. Herod J, Denyer J, Goldman A, et al. Epidermolysis bullosa in children, pathophysiology, anaesthesia and pain management. Paediatr Anaesth 2001; 12(5):388–97.

14. Weiner M. Pain management in epidermolysis bullosa an intractable problem. Ostomy Wound Manage 2004;50(8):13–4.

15. Jorgenson B, Friis GJ, Gottru F. Pain and quality of life for patients with venous leg ulcers; proof of concept of the efficacy of Biatain-Ibu, a new pain reducing dressing. Wound Repair Regen 2006;14:233–9.

Bathing for Individuals with Epidermolysis Bullosa

H. Alan Arbuckle, MD[a,b,*]

KEYWORDS

- Epidermolysis bullosa • Bathing
- Activity of daily living • Pool salt

Whereas bathing is an activity of daily living (AOL) that most of us take for granted, this is certainly not true for individuals with EB. Showering may anecdotally be quite painful for some patients with EB due to the pressure of the water on open wounds. Hence, bathing was recommended, particularly in the era of dressings that would adhere to the wounds, in order to soak them off. With more modern nonstick dressings, some patients prefer to have "dry dressing" changes and spraying of their skin; one advantage of this is that bacteria that might colonize one wound may not spread from wound to wound. In the United Kingdom, the Dystrophic Epidermolysis Bullosa Research Association (DebRA) nurses advocate this method for newborn babies as they believe that it is easier for parents to change one limb at a time and that the newborns are less likely to kick the raw skin off the opposite limb, for example, when they are agitated. There has never been a randomized trial of bathing/showering or dry dressing changes in EB.

Despite the significant pain associated with bathing there is very little in the way of research to document or quantify how this impacts EB patients. Most of the information in the literature addresses overall AOL, or some therapeutic modality to improve pain with associated procedures, wound care, or dressing changes.

In 2004, Fine and colleagues[1] documented, through the United States–based National EB Registry, the percentage of EB children reported to be totally independent versus dependent for major AOL (toileting, feeding, bathing, dressing, grooming, and walking). Each activity was subcategorized based on subtype of EB (simplex, junctional, dominant dystrophic, and recessive dystrophic). With regard to bathing, 100% of dominant dystrophic and 46.7% of recessive dystrophic patients felt that they were totally independent for AOL, whereas 95.8% of simplex and 65.4% of junctional EB patients considered themselves independent. Not surprisingly, those who reported being dependent on others for AOL scored highest for the more severe forms of EB (26.9% and 26.7% for junctional and recessive dystrophic, respectfully), whereas those with the more mild forms were least dependent (2.1% for simplex). Of note, no patients with dominant dystrophic EB reported dependency.

Other reports addressing bathing are mostly related to the safety of sedation or anesthesia. In 1999, Chiu and colleagues[2] documented the safety of midazolam, along with cognitive behavior techniques, 20 minutes before bathing in a 9-year-old male with nonlethal junctional EB. In 2007, Wu[3] showed that propofol and propofol with ketamine was safe and efficacious in 2 patients with "severe dystrophic EB" who required whirlpool baths for wound care.

In their EB center in Denver, Colorado the authors learned from the guest editor of

[a] Epidermolysis Bullosa Center of Excellence and Wound Care Clinic, The Children's Hospital, 13123 East 16th Avenue, B570 Aurora, CO 80045, USA
[b] VA Medical Center, Department of Dermatology, 1055 Clermont Street, Denver, CO 80220, USA
* Epidermolysis Bullosa Center of Excellence and Wound Care Clinic, The Children's Hospital, 13123 East 16th Avenue, B570 Aurora, CO 80045.
E-mail address: Alan.Arbuckle@ucdenver.edu

Dermatol Clin 28 (2010) 265–266
doi:10.1016/j.det.2010.01.003
0733-8635/10/$ – see front matter. Published by Elsevier Inc.

this issue, Professor Murrell, a very simple treatment to decrease the pain associated with bathing. In Australia, it is the standard of care to recommend the addition of salt to bath water. Professor Murrell first learned this several years ago from Anna Kemble-Welch, Director of DeBRA New Zealand (personal communication, 2009). In their Denver clinic the authors recommend adding 1 pound of salt, whereas Professor Murrell has had excellent results with the addition of 1 kg per standard adult bath size, to be isotonic with normal saline in the body. The authors are currently working with Professor Murrell to quantify this change using a validated quality of life survey.

Although there are very few data regarding bathing and EB, the simple addition of pool salt to the bath water can dramatically decrease the pain and anxiety of bathing.

REFERENCES

1. Fine JD, Johnson LB, Weiner M, et al. Assessment of mobility, activities and pain in different subtypes of epidermolysis bullosa. Clin Exp Dermatol 2004;29: 122–7.
2. Chiu YK, Prendiville JS, Bennett SM, et al. Pain management of junctional epidermolysis bullosa in an 11 year old boy. Pediatr Dermatol 1999;16(6):465–8.
3. Wu J. Case report: deep sedation with intravenous infusion of combined propofol and ketamine during dressing changes and whirlpool bath in patients with severe epidermolysis bullosa. Paediatr Anaesth 2007;17:592–6.

Infection and Colonization in Epidermolysis Bullosa

Jemima E. Mellerio, MD, FRCP[a,b,*]

KEYWORDS

- Blister • Genodermatosis • Critical colonization
- Infection • Antimicrobial • Antibiotic

WOUNDS AND BACTERIA: CONTAMINATION, COLONIZATION, AND INFECTION

Ulceration of the skin in epidermolysis bullosa (EB) invariably leads to the presence of bacteria, although the extent to which this happens and its clinical implications vary greatly.[1] It is useful to consider bacterial load in a wound as a continuum (Fig. 1).[2] At one end there is contamination, with bacteria over the wound surface, usually as a result of inoculation from hands, fomites, or airborne contamination: in this situation bacteria do not impede healing of the wound and no treatment is necessary. When bacteria are present in greater numbers, but not impairing healing, the wound can be said to be colonized. If bacterial proliferation increases further, the wound may become "stuck," where it is unable to heal, although not extending in size. At this stage, the term "critical colonization" is used. At the far end of the spectrum, with still greater bioburden, is infection: this is usually considered to occur once there are 10^5 bacteria present per gram of tissue.[3] Wound infection is essentially a clinical diagnosis characterized by increasing size, exudate, odor, and pain, and surrounding erythema, swelling and edema,[4,5] although these signs may be less marked in chronic EB wounds. Systemic upset and fever may also accompany a wound infection. As with all wounds, EB management relies on recognition of colonization or frank infection, and tailoring treatment accordingly.

COLONIZATION AND INFECTION IN EB

There are no good data concerning the incidence of critical colonization or wound infection in EB but, anecdotally, this is a sizeable problem, particularly for patients with more severe and generalized forms who have large numbers of chronic wounds.[1,6] These wounds cause considerable morbidity, including pain, exudate and odor, and may demand many hours of dressing changes on a daily basis; they are also responsible for a significant economic burden, necessitating large quantities of often expensive, specialized dressings.

Sepsis, in the majority of cases arising from cutaneous infection, is an important cause of death of EB patients, particularly neonates and infants with junctional and recessive dystrophic EB. The use of intravenous lines and indwelling ports are also a significant source of septicemia in this group due to chronically colonized or infected surrounding or overlying skin. These

The author acknowledges financial support from the Department of Health via the National Institute for Health Research (NIHR) comprehensive Biomedical Research Centre award to Guy's & St Thomas' NHS Foundation Trust in partnership with King's College London and King's College Hospital NHS Foundation Trust.

[a] St John's Institute of Dermatology, Guy's and St Thomas' NHS Foundation Trust, St Thomas' Hospital, Westminster Bridge Road, London SE1 7EH, UK

[b] Department of Dermatology, Great Ormond Street Hospital for Children NHS Trust, Great Ormond Street, London WC1N 3JH, UK

* Department of Dermatology, Great Ormond Street Hospital for Children NHS Trust, Great Ormond Street, London WC1N 3JH, UK.

E-mail address: jemima.mellerio@kcl.ac.uk

Dermatol Clin 28 (2010) 267–269
doi:10.1016/j.det.2010.01.004
0733-8635/10/$ – see front matter

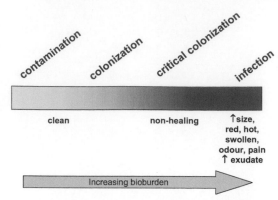

Fig. 1. The bioburden in a wound is a continuum, and reflects a balance between numbers and virulence of bacteria, and the host defenses. Contamination and colonization can be viewed as normal states, although critical colonization (in which the wound fails to heal) and infection (increased wound size and local signs) are abnormal and require treatment to enable healing to occur.

patients may be particularly susceptible to infections due to anemia, poor nutrition, and relative immunosuppression as a result of their systemic disease.

The most common bacteria isolated from EB wounds include gram-positive organisms, particularly *Staphylococcus aureus* and *Streptococci*, as well as gram-negatives and anaerobes such as *Pseudomonas aeruginosa* and *Proteus*. It is common to find a mixed growth of organisms in EB wounds, particularly those that are chronic. The emergence of antibiotic-resistant strains of bacteria is a particular problem: methicillin-resistant *Staphylococcus aureus* and, increasingly, ciprofloxacin-resistant *Pseudomonas*, are frequently isolated from EB wounds. It may be impossible to eradicate these bacteria fully, and it is possibly unfeasible to aim to do so in EB patients. Rather, efforts should be made to restrict treatment to clinically significant infections, and to limit spread within health care settings and the community as much as possible.

INVESTIGATION OF WOUND INFECTIONS IN EB

Although the gold standard for identifying pathogens in an infected wound is a skin biopsy for culture and sensitivity, this is rarely indicated in clinical practice. Instead, a swab should be taken from the wound bed after any necrotic debris or exudate has been cleaned off. If the wound is dry, the swab should first be moistened with sterile saline or transport medium. Light pressure should be applied to the tip of the swab as it is passed across the wound bed in a zig-zag pattern and at the same time rotated through 360° to maximize

contact with the swab tip.[2] The swab is then placed in transport medium and sent to the laboratory for culture and sensitivity. The diagnosis of wound infection should be based on clinical features as listed above: if felt to be infected, appropriate antibiotic treatment should be initiated empirically and altered later if necessary, depending on the swab results when received.

MANAGEMENT OF COLONIZATION AND INFECTION OF EB WOUNDS

Contamination of EB wounds can be considered inevitable and, because it does not generally interfere with healing, no specific treatment is required beyond using an appropriate atraumatic dressing (**Fig. 2**). Once a wound becomes critically colonized and fails to heal, steps should be taken to try and reduce the bioburden, usually with topical antimicrobials or specialized dressings.[6] Frank infection almost always requires systemic antibiotic therapy, often in conjunction with topical measures (**Fig. 3**).

Topical Antimicrobial Agents and Dressings

Simple measures such as bathing will reduce bacteria in EB wounds and should be advocated whenever possible. The use of emollient lotions containing antimicrobials, such as chlorhexidine chloride or benzalkonium chloride (eg, Dermol lotion), may be useful. Similarly, a 0.25% solution of acetic acid (reduced if stinging occurs) or a solution of bleach (5–10 mL in 5 L water, washed off thoroughly after) may be helpful used in the bath or as a compress applied to the wound for 15 to 20 minutes, particularly if there is recurrent infection with *Pseudomonas*. Lipid-stabilized hydrogen peroxide cream (Crystacide) is well tolerated, with

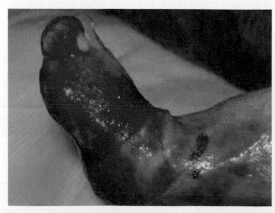

Fig. 2. Extensive ulceration but no clinical signs of infection on the foot of a neonate with recessive dystrophic EB. Atraumatic dressings are needed but there is no need for specific antimicrobial measures.

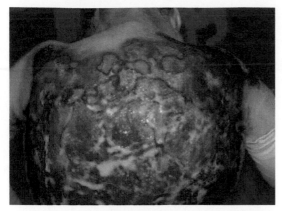

Fig. 3. Nonhealing ulceration of large areas of the back in recessive dystrophic EB with exudate and surrounding erythema. Systemic antibiotic therapy is indicated.

a broad spectrum of action, and can be used directly onto a colonized or infected wound.

Topical antibiotics should be used sparingly and with caution in EB: they may lead to the emergence of antibiotic-resistant bacteria and some, for example, mupirocin, neomycin, and fucidic acid, can to lead to sensitization. If used, they should be rotated every 2 to 6 weeks to minimize these risks.

Silver preparations either as creams (eg, silver sulfadiazine) or incorporated into dressings (eg, Mepilex Ag, Urgotul SSD, Aquacel Ag) may help to reduce bacterial load in wounds. Silver has a very broad antimicrobial spectrum and is therefore useful where there is a mixed growth of organisms in an EB wound. Silver preparations should be used for limited periods of time since the silver may be absorbed, and argyria has been reported in EB patient using silver for prolonged periods.[7,8]

Medical grade honey (γ-irradiated to remove any *Clostridium* spores) in ointments (eg, Mesitran S) or dressings (eg, Activon Tulle) can be used for sloughy or infected wounds, including in EB.[9] Honey is thought to reduce pathogens by virtue of its low pH, high osmolality, and production of low levels of hydrogen peroxide.[10] Honey usually causes a transient increase in wound exudate when first used, so a highly absorbent dressing and possibly a barrier film (eg, Cavilon) should be used to avoid maceration of surrounding skin; it may also be stingy or painful due to its osmotic pull and acidity.

Systemic Treatment of Infections

Where there are overt clinical signs of infection in an EB wound, systemic therapy with an appropriate antibiotic according to swab results is often indicated. Oral antibiotics are normally adequate although they may be needed for reasonably long periods (eg, 14 days) to ensure clearance. If the patient is systemically unwell, or if dictated by bacterial sensitivities, intravenous antibiotics may occasionally be indicated.

The presence of group A β-hemolytic streptococci on skin swabs, even in the absence of overt infection, should always prompt treatment with antibiotics to minimize the risks of worsening soft tissue infections and complications such as post-streptococcal glomerulonephritis.

SUMMARY

Contamination and colonization of EB wounds is extremely common and is not generally a problem requiring treatment unless healing is becoming impaired, suggesting critical colonization. Topical measures are often sufficient to keep colonization down to a level at which exudate and odor are controlled and wound healing is not impaired. The diagnosis of infection of an EB wounds should be made clinically, and usually requires systemic treatment.

REFERENCES

1. Abercrombie EM, Mather CA, Hon J, et al. Recessive dystrophic epidermolysis bullosa. Part 2: care of the adult patient. Br J Nurs 2008;17.36, S8, S10.
2. Kingsley A. The wound infection continuum and its application to clinical practice. Ostomy Wound Manage 2003;49(Suppl 7A):1–7.
3. Robson MC, Heggers JP. Bacterial quantification of open wounds. Mil Med 1969;134:19–24.
4. Cutting KF, White R. Defined and refined: criteria for identifying wound infection revisited. Br J Community Nurs 2004;9:S6–15.
5. Sibbald RG, Woo K, Ayello EA. Increased bacterial burden and infection: the story of NERDS and STONES. Adv Skin Wound Care 2006;19:447–61.
6. Mellerio JE, Weiner M, Denyer JE, et al. Medical management of epidermolysis bullosa: proceedings of the IInd International Symposium on Epidermolysis Bullosa, Santiago, Chile, 2005. Int J Dermatol 2007;46:795–800.
7. Browning JC, Levy ML. Argyria related to silvadene application in a patient with dystrophic epidermolysis bullosa. Dermatol Online J 2008;14:9.
8. Flohr C, Heague J, Leach I, et al. Topical silver sulphadiazine-induced systemic argyria in a patient with severe generalized dystrophic epidermolysis bullosa. Br J Dermatol 2008;159:740–1.
9. Hon J. Using honey to heal a chronic wound in a patient with epidermolysis bullosa. Br J Nurs 2005;14:S4–12.
10. Molan PC. The evidence supporting the use of honey as a wound dressing. Int J Low Extrem Wounds 2006;5:40–54.

Tests to Monitor in Patients with Severe Types of Epidermolysis Bullosa

Anna E. Martinez, MBBS, MRCP, MRCPCH

KEYWORDS

• Epidermolysis bullosa • Tests • Monitor

	Investigation	Comment
Chemical Pathology	Urea and electrolytes: Na, K, Ur, Cr	6 monthly unless abnormal
	Liver function tests: total bilirubin, albumin, alkaline phosphatase, alanine aminotransferase, aspartate aminotransferase	6 monthly
	Bone profile: Ca, P, albumin, alkaline phosphatase, vitamin D)	6 monthly
	Trace elements: zinc, selenium	Annual
	Vitamin B_{12}, vitamin A	Annual
	Total iron-binding capacity (TIBC), serum iron, ferritin	3–6 monthly depending on anemia and if having iron infusions
	Urine dipstick test, protein and blood	At each visit
Hematology	Full blood count	3–6 monthly depending on degree of anemia
	Red cell folate, serum folate	Annually
Radiology	Radiograph: lateral thoracic and lumbar spine	Annually from age 4 years
	Whole spine dual energy radiograph absorptiometry (DEXA) scan	
	Radiograph of left hand	Evaluate bone age if indicated
	Echocardiogram	Annually from age 2 years
	Renal ultrasound	Annually in patients with junctional epidermolysis bullosa (JEB) and JEB-PA
Microbiology	Wound swab	If clinical evidence of infection
	Urine culture	If positive dipstick
Endocrinology for Pubertal Delay	Female patients: follicle-stimulating hormone (FSH), luteinizing hormone (LH), and estradiol	Pelvic ultrasound to assess ovaries and uterus if clinically indicated
	Male patients: FSH, LH, and testosterone	

Department of Paediatric Dermatology, Great Ormond Street Hospital for Children NHS Trust, Great Ormond Street, London WC1N 3JH, UK
E-mail address: martia@gosh.nhs.uk

Dermatol Clin 28 (2010) 271
doi:10.1016/j.det.2010.01.005
0733-8635/10/$ – see front matter © 2010 Elsevier Inc. All rights reserved.

Pain Management in Epidermolysis Bullosa

Kenneth R. Goldschneider, MD[a,b],
Anne W. Lucky, MD[a,c,d],*

KEYWORDS

- Epidermolysis bullosa • Pain management • Pruritus
- Children • Pediatric pain • Pain • Palliative care

Pain is an unfortunate constant in the lives of most patients with epidermolysis bullosa (EB),[1] especially for those with the more severe types of EB. In a survey of 140 patients with all types of EB, the daily level of pain was scored at greater than 5 out of 10 in 14% to 19% of the patients with all types of EB, but present at this level in nearly 50% of those with severe recessive dystrophic epidermolysis bullosa (RDEB). Only 5% of RDEB patients were pain-free.[2] Measurements of pain vary from study to study and methodology can influence the evaluation of degree and quality of pain, although a recent quality of life questionnaire has provided some guidelines for this evaluation.[3] In addition, individuals vary considerably in their pain thresholds and families have different expectations as to what level of pain is tolerable. Prevention and treatment of pain is a major challenge for the clinician caring for patients with EB.[4] The approach to pain management is different in daily life, during intermittent exacerbations or injuries, or when hospitalizations or operative procedures occur. Pediatric pain management in particular has had recent advances and requires a specialized knowledge base, which is becoming more accessible to non–pain care practitioners.[5] An outline of pain management strategies in EB is presented in **Table** 1. This review will focus on the current approaches to the management of pain in patients with EB and especially considers the importance of the delicate balance between comfort and function.

PAIN MANAGEMENT IN THE HOME SETTING
Prevention of Pain

Prevention of pain is far superior to treatment. Most pain in EB is focused on the skin. Pain may exist at rest, during activities, during dressing changes or bathing, or as a result of injury to the skin. Using appropriately protective dressings, wraps and padding, and tailoring activities to the capabilities and safety of the individual can prevent unnecessary trauma to the skin. Promoting physical exercise, using physical therapy, and encouraging active enjoyable physical activities appropriate to the ability of the patient will maximize strength and flexibility, and prevent painful joint contractures and unnecessary injury. Discouraging reliance on devices such as motorized wheelchairs when patients are capable of more independent activity will maximize strength and agility. However, it is always important to weigh the benefits of lifestyle and enjoyment against the risks of skin trauma.

[a] University of Cincinnati College of Medicine, Cincinnati, OH, USA
[b] Division of Pain Management, Department of Anesthesiology, Cincinnati Children's Hospital Medical Center, 3333 Burnet Avenue, Cincinnati, OH 45229, USA
[c] Cincinnati Children's Epidermolysis Bullosa Center, Cincinnati Children's Hospital Medical Center, Cincinnati, OH, USA
[d] Division of Pediatric Dermatology, Cincinnati Children's Hospital Medical Center, 3333 Burnet Avenue, Cincinnati, OH 45229, USA
* Corresponding author. Division of Pediatric Dermatology, Cincinnati Children's Hospital Medical Center, 3333 Burnet Avenue, Cincinnati, OH 45229.
E-mail address: annelucky@fuse.net

Dermatol Clin 28 (2010) 273–282
doi:10.1016/j.det.2010.01.008

Table 1
Outline of pain management

	Daily Activities	Dressings and Baths	Acute Injury	Perioperative
Topical Rx	Occlusive dressings Protective dressings Skin grafts	Occlusive dressings Bath additives (salt, oatmeal) Adhesive removers	Occlusive dressings Skin grafts Topical lidocaine Topical morphine	OR preparation Padding Lubrication
Traditional systemic Rx	Acetominophen Ibuprofen Low-strength opioids	Acetominophen Ibuprofen Combinations Low-strength opioids High-strength opioids	Acetominophen Ibuprofen Combinations Low-strength opioids High-strength opioids	Acetominophen Ibuprofen Combinations Low-strength opioids High-strength opioids Antianxiety Rx Ketamine Nerve blocks Propofol
Nontraditional systemic Rx	Tricyclic antidepressants Anticonvulsants Tetrahydrocannabinol Dronabinol	Tricyclic antidepressants Anticonvulsants Tetrahydrocannabinol Dronabinol	Tricyclic antidepressants Anticonvulsants Tetrahydrocannabinol Dronabinol	
Psychological techniques	Relaxation Visualization Yoga, meditation	Relaxation Visualization Self hypnosis	Relaxation Visualization Self hypnosis	Relaxation Visualization Self hypnosis

Abbreviations: OR, operating room; Rx, prescription.

Sources of Pain

Most EB-related pain arises from 4 major sources: skin, bone/joints, gastrointestinal (GI) tract, and during procedures. Skin pain in EB results from blisters, erosions, and secondary cutaneous infection. Deformities of the joints from scarring and contractures compromise proper joint function and can be painful. Osteoporosis is common, and bone pain is well documented in moderate to severe osteoporosis, sometimes with vertebral compression fractures, and can respond well to treatment with bisphosphonates.[6,7] GI pain starts in the mouth because oral care is difficult, and there is a tendency toward abscesses, gum disease, blisters, erosions, and dental caries. The whole GI tract is often involved, and the complications that contribute to pain from the GI tract include esophageal strictures, gastroesophageal reflux, poorly fitting gastrostomy tubes, constipation, and anal fissures.[8] The procedures that are a painful constant include baths, esophageal dilatations, wound debridement, reconstructive hand surgery, and cancer resection. Noncutaneous pain also can result from a variety of other complications, such as pain on urination that follows urethral blistering,[9] and eye pain often caused by corneal abrasions. These issues and their treatment strategies are discussed in detail elsewhere in this issue (see the article by Almaani and Mellerio elsewhere in this issue for further exploration of this topic.).

Topical Treatment of Pain

Open wounds tend to be most painful when exposed to air or water. Additives to the bathwater such as isotonic salt or oatmeal have anecdotally been said to reduce the pain of entering a bathtub. Occlusive, but not too adherent, dressings can provide pain relief by keeping the wound surface protected from air drying. Semiocclusive dressings, such as ointment-impregnated gauzes, gels, and silicone-based products left in place for 1 to 3 days (depending on the cleanliness of the wounds) can minimize pain.[10] Dressings that stick to the skin are a source of pain and great anxiety in patients with EB. Adhesive removers, especially those with a silicone base, or water/saline soaks, when used before removing adherent dressings, can minimize painful and frightening dressing changes. In some patients, there has been success with the use of biologic semisynthetic grafts that seem to act as "bridges" for more rapid reepithelialization.[11–13] Judicious use of topical lidocaine preparations, or soothing coating products such as sucralfate, may prevent or relieve mouth pain.[14] In some situations, such as perianal pain with defecation or urethral pain with urination, application of topical lidocaine in small amounts can allow for more normal bowel and bladder function. Topical morphine has been an effective adjunct to pain therapy in localized areas for EB and other skin conditions, although data regarding its effect are limited.[15–17] Amniotic membranes can provide instantaneous relief from pain to large surface areas such as in the neonate.[18,19]

Traditional Systemic Treatment of Pain

The type of oral therapy used for pain in EB depends on the severity, chronicity, and location of the discomfort, and also depends on the individual needs, which vary widely. For example, only occasional pain medicine may be needed for daily activities, but bandage changes or baths may require pretreatment with analgesics. When injuries or infections occur, stronger medications are often needed. The role of anticipatory anxiety before dressing changes, baths, or medical procedures cannot be underestimated in this population who experience such frequent pain in their lives that their anxiety can significantly increase the need for analgesia. Conversely, strategies to reduce anxiety (discussed later) can significantly reduce the amount of analgesic used. Pharmacologic approaches to pain and anxiety include traditional and nontraditional agents (Table 2).

For mild pain, acetaminophen (paracetamol) and nonsteroidal anti-inflammatory agents such as ibuprofen often are sufficient. Recognition of potential hepatotoxicity with both of these agents, especially when used chronically or in high doses, needs to be shared with families.[20,21] As pain increases, these medications should be continued, although other medications are added so as to avoid losing whatever analgesic effect the previous medications were contributing.

Opioids are appropriate for managing moderate to severe pain in EB. Low-potency opioids such as hydrocodone or codeine may be given. These 2 agents are limited by their combination with acetaminophen and their unpredictable effect, respectively. Using low doses of more potent opioids is effective, and avoids these limitations. However, there are side effects and concerns about the use of opioids, especially for pruritus and constipation, which are already huge problems in EB. There is also a concern about tolerance to opioids that can lead to escalating doses. However, true addiction is a rare occurrence, and no more than routine caution is warranted.

For severe pain, opioids, such as oxycodone, hydromorphone, and morphine are appropriate.

Table 2
Pharmacologic pain therapies

Class	Generic Names	Routes	Main Uses
Opioids	Morphine Oxycodone Hydromorphone Codeine Fentanyl Others	Oral, IV, intranasal, rectal, subcutaneous, sublingual, percutaneous, others	Pain
Nonsteroidal anti-inflammatory agents	Ibuprofen Ketorolac Celecoxib Naproxen	Oral, rectal, IV	Pain
Tricyclic antidepressants	Amitriptyline Doxepin	Oral	Pain, itch
Anticonvulsants	Gabapentin Pregabalin Valproic acid Oxcarbazepine	Oral	Pain, itch Pain, itch Pain, headache Pain
Anxiolytics	Diazepam Lorazepam Midazolam	Oral, rectal, IV	Muscle spasm, anxiety
Others	Acetaminophen Tramadol Ketamine Dronabinol Clonidine Sucralfate Lidocaine Bisphosphonates Salt, oatmeal	Oral Oral Oral, IV Oral, transpulmonary Oral, IV Oral Topical Oral, IV Topical	Pain Pain Pain, anesthesia Pain, nausea, itch Sleep, anxiety Pain Pain Bone pain (osteopenia) Bath-related pain

Methadone is sometimes useful, but more difficult to use than other opioids, so its use is best managed by those expert in pain treatment. For procedures, transbuccal fentanyl oralets may be helpful.[22] Overall, oral treatment is preferred, but in the very sick or terminal patient, especially in the face of metastatic squamous cell carcinoma, an end-of-life palliative approach is the compassionate one in a home-hospice type of setting. In these children intravenous (IV) infusions, and the use of patient-controlled analgesia pumps wherein the patient can press a button and receive a predetermined dose of analgesic on demand, can improve quality of life. Given that IV access is often difficult to garner and maintain in patients with EB, it is useful to know that subcutaneous opioids have been found to be useful for quite some time[23] when the enteral route is not available. High-concentration morphine and oxycodone (20 mg/ml) are effective as well, and are reasonably absorbed via the sublingual route.[24] In patients

with EB, ankyloglossia may limit this route, and so a physical examination should be done before prescribing this route of administration. Intranasal fentanyl can also be used in end-of-life situations, at least for intermittent dosing.[25,26]

Nontraditional Systemic Treatment of Pain

A variety of medications designed or approved for indications other than pain have proven to be useful in pain management. Anxiety, especially as patients anticipate dressing changes, baths, or medical procedures, can greatly add to the amount of anesthesia needed for a given situation. Anxiolytics such as diazepam, lorazepam, and midazolam may be helpful 15 to 60 minutes before a given dreaded activity. Tricyclic antidepressants such as amitriptyline have been useful for chronic pain of several types,[27–30] although there has been one death from cardiomyopathy supposedly associated with its use in EB.[31] Likewise, some anticonvulsants such as gabapentin, pregabalin, oxcarbazepine, and valproic acid are effective analgesics for several painful conditions,[32–34] and may have a role in EB.

Tetrahydrocannabinol and other cannabinoids, in pill or inhaled form, have been successfully used for pain[35] as well as nausea,[36] anorexia, and pruritis,[37] but tetrahydrocannabinol is illegal even for medical use in some communities and side effects can be limiting. Ketamine has been used when severe chronic pain is difficult to control,[38] and may have a role in the care of patients with EB, especially around baths and dressing changes. The first dose or two of this medication should be administered under medical supervision.

Psychological Approach to Pain Management

The limitations of pharmacologic approaches to pain are well known. The power of psychological approaches is underappreciated, but the use of specific psychological techniques can help patients cope with acute and chronic pain, and are applicable to the population with EB (Table 3). Given that the age, intellectual capacity, disease severity, and family function vary considerably among patients and their families, the wide range of available cognitive-behavioral techniques provides multiple opportunities for intervention. For example, biofeedback is a noninvasive technique by which the patient can learn body self-awareness and relaxation. It has been shown to be useful in several painful conditions[39,40] and is easily learned. However, the authors find that children younger than 6 years and those with difficulty with attention span, or those with a history of

posttraumatic stress disorder (ie, who cannot tolerate the intrusive thoughts that come with deep relaxation) are not optimal candidates for this modality.[41] Coping skills and activity pacing, as well as strategizing approaches to school and other activities, can be excellent uses of a psychologist's skills. There is a large role for parent training, as strategies can be learned by the parents that reduce the focus on pain, and allow for greater functioning of the child with chronic pain.[39] Furthermore, adolescents with chronic pain, who showed little use of coping skills and whose parents used protective approaches, reported more symptoms. This finding suggests a role for coping skills training for the parent and the child.[42] Procedure-centered interventions are useful and include hypnosis, guided imagery, relaxation, and virtual reality. All these techniques have been used successfully for a variety of procedures in the pediatric age group.[43,44]

MANAGEMENT IN THE HOSPITAL

Patients with EB may be hospitalized for a variety of reasons: care in the newborn period, worsening of disease requiring more intensive skin care, operative procedures (including esophageal dilatations, placement of feeding gastrostomy tubes, and hand-release surgeries), or non-EB–related conditions such as appendectomies and pneumonia or end-of-life palliative care in the setting of metastatic squamous cell carcinoma. Each admission requires attention to pain and its prevention. Patients with EB require special care in the hospital with prominent warnings to avoid the application of tape and other adhesives or shearing forces on the skin.

Table 3
Nonpharmacologic pain therapies

Skill	Situation	Patient	Parent[a]	Age Group[b]
Biofeedback	Acute and chronic pain	Yes	No	Older than 6 years
Relaxation, deep breathing	Acute and chronic pain	Yes	Yes	Older than 6 years
Meditation	Chronic pain	Yes	No	Adolescence
Coping skills	Acute and chronic pain	Yes	Yes	All, to varying degree
Yoga, Tai Chi	Chronic pain	Yes	As desired	Older than 6 years
Parent pain assistance skills	Acute and chronic pain	No	Yes	All
Hypnosis, guided imagery	Acute and chronic pain	Yes	No	Older than 6 years

[a] Parents may learn assistive roles in almost all skills, even if not directly using the skills for themselves.
[b] Guidelines only: developmental abilities guide appropriateness more than age.

Management of Dressing Changes

With flares of skin disease, the pain associated with dressing changes may be intolerable with oral pain medications at home (**Fig. 1**). Use of potent oral and IV narcotics as noted earlier is appropriate in this situation on a temporary basis. Anxiety can be significant, so anxiolytics are important. In some cases for which appropriate facilities are available, whirlpool treatment under deep sedation or general anesthesia can promote healing, and reduce bacterial colonization and infection (**Figs. 2 and 3**). Such rapid healing of the skin also reduces the requirement for analgesia. Most dressing changes are done at home, so a plan of care should be devised with the parents. Both monitoring and the ability to rescue the patient are not available in the home, so care should be taken when prescribing sedating medications, especially in combination. Oral medications should be dosed such that adequate time for absorption is allowed, and medications should be added to the regimen one at a time, to allow observation of the effect of each one prior to that of the combination. Intranasal fentanyl has been studied in burn patients and offers another option.[27] A special situation encountered in the newborn nursery is that infants cannot express the sources of their discomfort, and often cry for reasons unrelated to pain. Especially in this situation involving care by personnel unfamiliar with EB, the appearance of the skin can be alarming and there is a tendency to overmedicate infants. It is important to provide balanced treatment, using natural comfort measures such as rocking, swaddling, and holding, and not relying entirely on high-potency analgesics for every bout of crying.

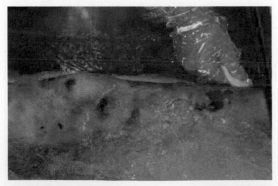

Fig. 1. In the Whirlpool, crusts can be debrided and erosions cleansed without pain under deep sedation, such as in this 18-year-old girl.

Perioperative Pain Management

The perioperative approach to control of pain considers preoperative, intraoperative, and postoperative care,[45] and a detailed discussion is beyond the scope of this article. Education of the entire surgical team is imperative to protect patients during their physical transfers and procedures. Development of written protocols, including warnings to avoid all tape and adhesives, and to provide a padded environment will prevent painful iatrogenic trauma.[46] Any of the standard sedation and general anesthesia techniques can be used. Regional anesthesia (nerve blocks) can be helpful to control the pain of extremity surgeries, as for any such patient, although care must be taken in securing the continuous catheter when one is used (see **Fig. 1**). Otherwise, standard postoperative pain techniques are appropriate. One caveat is that many patients with EB take opioids preoperatively, and dosing postoperatively has to be adjusted upwards to account for the patients' baseline use, to provide adequate analgesia.

Pruritus

Itching is a major negative factor in the quality of life of patients with EB.[1] Although the mechanism is not entirely clear, an inflammatory component, similar to that seen in postburn itching, seems reasonable. The itch-scratch-blister-itch cycle is certainly detrimental to the patients, who generally prefer to be cool, and report that hot weather and sweating make symptoms worse. Certain medications such as opioids can exacerbate pruritus. First-line medications have included antihistamines, although efficacy is mixed as reported anecdotally. Doxepin is a tricyclic antidepressant with a strong antihistaminic effect, so a dose at bedtime may be helpful, although studies are lacking. Gabapentin has been used effectively in patients with postburn itching,[47] so may be worth trying for EB-related itch. Ondansetron has been used with mixed effect in patients with pruritis of uremia and cholestatic jaundice,[48–50] and has been anecdotally helpful in some of these investigators' patients. Other agents that have been reported to be useful in various pruritic conditions and may warrant future investigation include cyclosporine[51] and dronabinol.[52]

Palliative Pain Control

In a sense, many patients with EB spend their entire lives in palliative care. Palliative care no longer is limited to end-of-life care, but represents a continuum of care for patients with diseases producing a compromised quality of life. Palliative

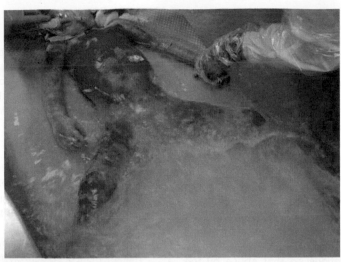

Fig. 2. Whirlpool-based dressing change and wound debridement under general anesthesia in a 4-year-old girl with recessive dystrophic epidermolysis bullosa.

care optimally takes place in conjunction with "traditional" treatment. In this way patients and families obtain full benefit, and when the transition to end-of-life care arrives, it is not seen as "giving up," so much as simply re-weighting the roles of various established care teams. End-of-life care is simply the logical extension of holistic care, and differs little in the patient with EB from that of other dying patients. Quality of life is the focus. End of life is a time when communication becomes

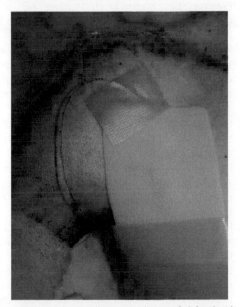

Fig. 3. Regional anesthesia can be useful for both intraoperative and postoperative pain control. The indwelling catheter is secured with silicone-based dressings, here Mepiform (Molnlycke Health Care, Goteborg, Sweden) (*top*) and Mepilex (Molnlycke Health Care, Goteborg, Sweden) (*white square below*).

paramount. It is important to know what the families place in priority, and what their goals and objectives are for the final months, weeks, or days of life. Do they wish to be at home? In the hospital? What are the preferences for feeding and hydration? How do they want wound care to proceed, if at all? There should be no concern for opioid tolerance or addiction at this time, as they are irrelevant consequences of opioid use in dying patients. All too often reluctance to produce addiction can interfere with optimal pain care. However, aggressive pain treatment can reduce alertness and hasten death. The trade-off between these effects and ensuring the comfort of dying patients is a principle of care with long-standing ethical precedent. However, it is one that requires understanding of the patient's goals and family's goals, and education of family and caregivers alike. One should bear in mind that how the patient dies is the memory the family will carry forward. A clear but adaptable plan, good communication, and attention to personal, cultural, and social concerns are crucial.

RISKS OF PAIN THERAPY

When chronic use of pain medications is required, physicians and families often worry about the need for escalating doses. Two main phenomena contribute to the escalation. The first phenomenon is disease progression, with worsening lesions or deformities causing more pain on top of preexisting pain. The second issue is that of tolerance. Patients who take opioid medications for more than a week or two consecutively frequently become tolerant to or become dependent on the opioids. This tolerance is a physiologic phenomenon that differs from addiction, in which opioids are used to the detriment of the patient, and continues despite the patient knowing that harm is being done. Strategies to avoid medication misuse and the fear of addiction include education of patient, family, and care team alike. Clear communication and expectation setting are important. The patient and family need to understand the effects and limits of the medications, their indications, and when to contact the team about problems (including constipation, sedation, lack of efficacy, and change in needs). Goals for pain care should be set together with the patient (when mature enough) and family. Unrealistic or divergent goals can cause conflict and dissent between care providers and patients/families. Ultimately, it is the responsibility of the prescribing physician to make sure that there are appropriate controls on distribution of these medications so that abuse by the patient and, unfortunately, sometimes by the patient's family and friends, does not occur. As patients with EB enter adolescence and young adult life, the availability and the temptation to experiment with alcohol and nonprescription drugs increases. Occasionally, a patient will combine recreational drugs with his or her prescription pain medication. It is imperative that the medical team is aware of which nonprescription drugs or sedating substances (including herbal preparations) are being used so that the addition of prescription medication does not precipitate disastrous consequences such as respiratory arrest or seizures. Periodic urine toxicology screens are a reasonable adjunct to pain care that provide concrete information about which substances are being consumed (expected and unexpected), and can guide discussion, limit-setting, and education. Overall, problems are few, and the overwhelming pain care needs of a large minority of patients with EB mandates appropriate use of potent medications as part of a good pain care plan.

SUMMARY

Patients with EB have a broad spectrum of need for pain treatment, varying with the type of EB, the severity within that type, and the particular physical, emotional, and psychological milieu of each individual. Prevention of situations that precipitate trauma to the skin or exacerbate other pain-inducing complications of this multifaceted disorder is the primary goal of the treating physician. However, inevitably there will be need for pain treatment. Therapy should be geared to the severity of the pain in the home or the hospital setting. Strategies that maximize function without compromising comfort best serve this population.

REFERENCES

1. van Scheppingen C, Lettinga AT, Duipmans JC, et al. Main problems experienced by children with epidermolysis bullosa: a qualitative study with semi-structured interviews. Acta Derm Venereol 2008;88(2):143–50.
2. Fine JD, Johnson LB, Weiner M, et al. Assessment of mobility, activities and pain in different subtypes of epidermolysis bullosa. Clin Exp Dermatol 2004; 29(2):122–7.
3. Frew JW, Martin LK, Nijsten T, et al. Quality of life evaluation in epidermolysis bullosa (EB) through the development of the QOLEB questionnaire: an EB-specific quality of life instrument. Br J Dermatol 2009;161:1323–30. DOI:10.1111/j.1365-2133.2009.09347.x.
4. Mellerio JE, Weiner M, Denyer JE, et al. Medical management of epidermolysis bullosa: proceedings of the IInd international symposium on epidermolysis bullosa, Santiago, Chile, 2005. Int J Dermatol 2007;46(8):795–800.
5. Walco GA, Goldschneider K, editors. Pain in children: a practical guide for primary care. Totowa (NJ): Humana Press; 2008.
6. Fewtrell MS, Allgrove J, Gordon I, et al. Bone mineralization in children with epidermolysis bullosa. Br J Dermatol 2006;154(5):959–62.
7. Perman MJ, Lucky AW, Heubi JE, et al. Severe symptomatic hypocalcemia in a patient with RDEB treated with intravenous zoledronic acid. Arch Dermatol 2009;145(1):95–6.
8. Freeman EB, Koglmeier J, Martinez AE, et al. Gastrointestinal complications of epidermolysis bullosa in children. Br J Dermatol 2008;158(6):1308–14.
9. Fine JD, Johnson LB, Weiner M, et al. Genitourinary complications of inherited epidermolysis bullosa: experience of the national epidermolysis bullosa registry and review of the literature. J Urol 2004; 172(5 Pt 1):2040–4.
10. Ly L, Su JC. Dressings used in epidermolysis bullosa blister wounds: a review. J Wound Care 2008;17(11): 482, 484–486, 488 passim.
11. Falabella AF, Valencia IC, Eaglstein WH, et al. Tissue-engineered skin (Apligraf) in the healing of patients with epidermolysis bullosa wounds. Arch Dermatol 2000;136(10):1225–30.
12. Fivenson DP, Scherschun L, Choucair M, et al. Graftskin therapy in epidermolysis bullosa. J Am Acad Dermatol 2003;48(6):886–92.
13. Sibbald RG, Zuker R, Coutts P, et al. Using a dermal skin substitute in the treatment of chronic wounds secondary to recessive dystrophic epidermolysis bullosa: a case series. Ostomy Wound Manage 2005;51(11):22–46.
14. Marini I, Vecchiet F. Sucralfate: a help during oral management in patients with epidermolysis bullosa. J Periodontol 2001;72(5):691–5.

15. Krajnik M, Zylicz Z, Finlay I, et al. Potential uses of topical opioids in palliative care—report of 6 cases. Pain 1999;80(1–2):121–5.

16. Twillman RK, Long TD, Cathers TA, et al. Treatment of painful skin ulcers with topical opioids. J Pain Symptom Manage 1999;17(4):288–92.

17. Watterson G, Howard R, Goldman A. Peripheral opioids in inflammatory pain. Arch Dis Child 2004; 89(7):679–81.

18. Lucky AW, Palisson F, Mellerio JE. The IVth international symposium on epidermolysis bullosa, Santiago, Chile, 27–29 September 2007. J Dermatol Sci 2008; 49(2):178–84.

19. Martinez Pardo ME, Reyes Frias ML, Ramos Duron LE, et al. Clinical application of amniotic membranes on a patient with epidermolysis bullosa. Ann Transplant 1999;4(3–4):68–73.

20. American Academy of Pediatrics, Committee on Drugs. Acetaminophen toxicity in children. Pediatrics 2001;108(4):1020–4.

21. Amar PJ, Schiff ER. Acetaminophen safety and hepatotoxicity—where do we go from here? Expert Opin Drug Saf 2007;6(4):341–55.

22. Schechter NL, Weisman SJ, Rosenblum M, et al. The use of oral transmucosal fentanyl citrate for painful procedures in children. Pediatrics 1995; 95(3):335–9.

23. Lamacraft G, Cooper MG, Cavalletto BP. Subcutaneous cannulae for morphine boluses in children: assessment of a technique. J Pain Symptom Manage 1997;13(1):43–9.

24. Reisfield GM, Wilson GR. Rational use of sublingual opioids in palliative medicine. J Palliat Med 2007; 10(2):465–75.

25. Manjushree R, Lahiri A, Ghosh BR, et al. Intranasal fentanyl provides adequate postoperative analgesia in pediatric patients. Can J Anaesth 2002; 49(2):190–3.

26. Zeppetella G. An assessment of the safety, efficacy, and acceptability of intranasal fentanyl citrate in the management of cancer-related breakthrough pain: a pilot study. J Pain Symptom Manage 2000;20(4): 253–8.

27. Borland ML, Bergesio R, Pascoe EM, et al. Intranasal fentanyl is an equivalent analgesic to oral morphine in paediatric Bur patients for dressing changes: a randomised double blind crossover study. Bur 2005;31(7):831–7.

28. Holroyd KA, O'Donnell FJ, Stensland M, et al. Management of chronic tension-type headache with tricyclic antidepressant medication, stress management therapy, and their combination: a randomized controlled trial. JAMA 2001;285(17): 2208–15.

29. Kalso E, Tasmuth T, Neuvonen PJ. Amitriptyline effectively relieves neuropathic pain following treatment of breast cancer. Pain 1996;64(2): 293–302.

30. Rintala DH, Holmes SA, Courtade D, et al. Comparison of the effectiveness of amitriptyline and gabapentin on chronic neuropathic pain in persons with spinal cord injury. Arch Phys Med Rehabil 2007; 88(12):1547–60.

31. Taibjee SM, Ramani P, Brown R, et al. Lethal cardiomyopathy in epidermolysis bullosa associated with amitriptyline. Arch Dis Child 2005;90(8):871–2.

32. Magenta P, Arghetti S, Di Palma F, et al. Oxcarbazepine is effective and safe in the treatment of neuropathic pain: pooled analysis of seven clinical studies. Neurol Sci 2005;26(4):218–26.

33. Silberstein SD, Collins SD. Safety of divalproex sodium in migraine prophylaxis: an open-label, long-term study. Long-term safety of depakote in headache prophylaxis study group. Headache 1999;39(9):633–43.

34. Moore RA, Straube S, Wiffen PJ, et al. Pregabalin for acute and chronic pain in adults. Cochrane Database Syst Rev 2009;(3):CD007076.

35. Iskedjian M, Bereza B, Gordon A, et al. Meta-analysis of cannabis based treatments for neuropathic and multiple sclerosis-related pain. Curr Med Res Opin 2007;23(1):17–24.

36. Machado Rocha FC, Stefano SC, De Cassia Haiek R, et al. Therapeutic use of Cannabis sativa on chemotherapy-induced nausea and vomiting among cancer patients: systematic review and meta-analysis. Eur J Cancer Care (Engl) 2008;17(5):431–43.

37. Russo EB. Cannabinoids in the management of difficult to treat pain. Ther Clin Risk Manag 2008;4(1): 245–59.

38. Bell RF. Ketamine for chronic non-cancer pain. Pain 2009;141(3):210–4.

39. Allen KD, Shriver MD. Role of parent-mediated pain behavior management strategies in biofeedback treatment of childhood migraines. Behav Ther 1998;29(3):477–90.

40. Hermann C, Blanchard EB. Biofeedback in the treatment of headache and other childhood pain. Appl Psychophysiol Biofeedback 2002; 27(2):143–62.

41. Kashikar-Zuck S, Am L. Psychological interventions for chronic pain. In: Walco GA, Goldschneider K, editors. Pain in children: a practical guide for primary care. Totowa (NJ): Humana Press; 2008. p. 145–52.

42. Simons LE, Claar RL, Logan DL. Chronic pain in adolescence: parental responses, adolescent coping, and their impact on adolescent's pain behaviors. J Pediatr Psychol 2008;33(8):894–904.

43. Gold JI, Kim SH, Kant AJ, et al. Effectiveness of virtual reality for pediatric pain distraction during i.v. placement. Cyberpsychol Behav 2006;9(2):207–12.

44. Kuttner L. Management of young children's acute pain and anxiety during invasive medical procedures. Pediatrician 1989;16(1–2):39–44.

45. Lin YC, Golianu B. Anesthesia and pain management for pediatric patients with dystrophic epidermolysis bullosa. J Clin Anesth 2006;18(4):268–71.

46. Azizkhan RG, Denyer JE, Mellerio JE, et al. Surgical management of epidermolysis bullosa: proceedings of the IInd international symposium on epidermolysis bullosa, Santiago, Chile, 2005. Int J Dermatol 2007;46(8):801–8.

47. Mendham JE. Gabapentin for the treatment of itching produced by burns and wound healing in children: a pilot study. Burns 2004;30(8):851–3.

48. Jones EA, Molenaar HA, Oosting J. Ondansetron and pruritus in chronic liver disease: a controlled study. Hepatogastroenterology 2007;54(76):1196–9.

49. Muller C, Pongratz S, Pidlich J, et al. Treatment of pruritus in chronic liver disease with the 5-hydroxytryptamine receptor type 3 antagonist ondansetron: a randomized, placebo-controlled, double-blind cross-over trial. Eur J Gastroenterol Hepatol 1998;10(10):865–70.

50. Murphy M, Reaich D, Pai P, et al. A randomized, placebo-controlled, double-blind trial of ondansetron in renal itch. Br J Dermatol 2003;148(2):314–7.

51. Calikoglu E, Anadolu R. Management of generalized pruritus in dominant dystrophic epidermolysis bullosa using low-dose oral cyclosporin. Acta Derm Venereol 2002;82(5):380–2.

52. Neff GW, O'Brien CB, Reddy KR, et al. Preliminary observation with dronabinol in patients with intractable pruritus secondary to cholestatic liver disease. Am J Gastroenterol 2002;97(8):2117–9.

Treatment of Skin Cancers in Epidermolysis Bullosa

Supriya S. Venugopal, BSc, MBBS, MMed,
Dédée F. Murrell, MA, BMBCh, FAAD, MD*

KEYWORDS

- Epidermolysis bullosa • Biopsy • Diagnosis

Squamous cell carcinomas (SCCs) are highly aggressive in patients with epidermolysis bullosa (EB). Non–ultraviolet-related SCCs are the leading cause of death in patients with recessive dystrophic EB, particularly recessive dystrophic EB-generalized severe subtype (RDEB-GS).[1,2] The mechanism of SCC development in patients with RDEB continues to be investigated and several theories have been reported in the literature.[3–9]

REGULAR SKIN CHECKS

Regular skin checks are imperative to assess potential premalignant or malignant lesions. Dermatologists recommend 3-monthly full body detailed skin checks for patients with RDEB to be performed after the age of 12 years. Along with the skin check, patients can also receive multidisciplinary care for the wide array of other medical conditions that patients with RDEB suffer from.

The skin checks often last for 2 hours and begin with the patient removing their dressings with or without a bath. Once the patient is undressed and dressings have been removed, digital photography is performed as a baseline for current wounds, to compare with previous photos, and determine any suspicious areas. Biopsies are generally taken from areas of concern during the same visit. Patients and family members are also encouraged to keep a personal account of ulcers that have become symptomatic or are long standing, associated with either poor or no healing. The skin check is performed by several staff members including the dermatologists and supportive dermatology personnel, nursing staff, and family members.

Some institutions offer home services by an experienced nurse who takes photos; these are then assessed by medical staff. However, this process does not allow the clinician to palpate or directly visualize the suspicious area, or ask questions about individual lesions.

EPIDEMIOLOGY

The cumulative risk of developing SCCs in RDEB patients is 90.1% by the age of 55 years; the most common site of involvement is chronic wounds, followed by long-term cutaneous scars.[1,2] Multiple SCCs are common in patients with a median of 3 to 3.5 tumors.[1,2] The leading cause of death in RDEB-GS patients is metastatic SCCs with a staggering 87.3% cumulative risk of death by the age of 45 years.[1,2]

Patients with RDEB-GS develop SCCs at a much earlier age compared with healthy individuals, often in their adolescence.[2] The trend in onset during adolescence suggests that the skin's mechanism of constant repair may be the culprit for SCC development. In healthy patients, Marjolin ulcers take several years to become malignant ranging between several weeks in burn patients to several years in long-term ulcers.[10–15]

The histologic grading of SCCs does not correlate well with the clinical behavior of these malignancies. SCCs in RDEB patients invariably behave in an anaplastic manner despite histopathology reports confirming well or moderate differentiation. The main predictor of mortality in these

Department of Dermatology, St George Hospital, University of New South Wales, Gray Street, Kogarah, Sydney, NSW 2217, Australia
* Corresponding author.
E-mail address: d.murrell@unsw.edu.au

Dermatol Clin 28 (2010) 283–287
doi:10.1016/j.det.2010.01.009
0733-8635/10/$ – see front matter © 2010 Published by Elsevier Inc.

patients is the extent of SCC at diagnosis. Evidence of local or distant metastasis is associated with a poor outcome because of the aggressive nature of the malignancy. However, early detection of potential SCCs before local tissue invasion coupled with effective treatment results in a more favorable outcome. The earliest report of SCC development in EB is 12 years.[16]

MONITORING

The authors recommend regular skin checks (every 3–6 months) from the age of 10 years and every 3 months from 16 years onwards. Ideally patients remove all dressings first, with or without a bath/shower, as this is most time-efficient routine for the specialist responsible for checking the skin. To assist with this, we have found that comparative digital printed or polaroid photography is useful to detect unhealed potentially premalignant or malignant areas.[17] A thorough history from the patient or carers regarding ulcers that do not heal, are growing larger, becoming increasingly painful, pruritic, or changing in appearance along with serial photography allows dermatologists to detect potential skin cancers early. A body chart for recording the progressive history of SCC in each patient is also useful. A useful chart is available on the DebRA UK Web site (http://www.debra.org.uk/).

PERFORMING THE BIOPSIES

The poor compliance of some patients with monitoring for SCCs stems from a combination of the embarrassment of having to remove all the dressings before being checked and the fear of pain when biopsies are taken from nonhealing ulcerated areas. Ideally, a room attached to a private bathing/shower area that is warm, with plenty of room for the dermatologist, nurse, carer, dressings, and assistants doing the biopsies should be available. In an ambulatory hospital facility, oral midazolam may be given to allay anxiety and provide amnesia for the event. The sites of biopsy should be marked on the printed photographs for ease of identification later.

PREVENTION

Isotretinoin can be used in RDEB patients for chemoprevention up to a dosage of 0.5 mg/kg/d and is tolerated well, however the patient should be monitored for increased skin fragility.[18] In our own experience, several adult RDEB-GS patients have tolerated low dose neotigason well; neotigason has been shown to be more specific for prevention of SCC in the immunosuppressed transplant population.[19–21]

It is possible that neotigason might reduce the incidence of SCC but this would require a long controlled study, which is difficult in such an orphan disease. Now that there is a mouse model of restricted RDEB,[22] it may be possible to trial this in the mice if they live long enough and develop SCC.

BOWEN DISEASE

There are rare reports of in situ SCC in EB. One report used 5-aminolevulinic acid photodynamic therapy for treatment of Bowen disease of the fingers in a patient with RDEB without pseudosyndactyly with no recurrence.[23] We would rather recommend excision of any such areas, given the high mortality rates of SCC in EB and because the biopsy may not have contained all the suspicious area.

TREATMENT
Surgery

Once an SCC has been confirmed on biopsy, the patient should be managed quickly by a team including the dermatologist and a plastic surgeon familiar with EB. Localized magnetic resonance imaging (MRI) can determine if tendons are involved. These SCCs should be widely excised and in cases that are not caught early, amputation of the distal extremity may be required (**Fig. 1**).[24] Although Mohs surgery has been reported, this method may have advantages in terms of the

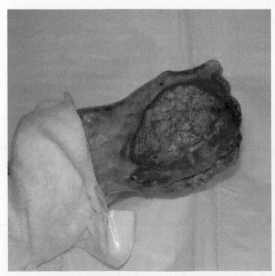

Fig. 1. Right hand of a 20-year-old female presenting with SCC which required amputation.

pathology to be more sure that the SCC is completely excised, but conservative margins may not be wise given the high risk of recurrence.

Staging

Patients should have staging investigations performed including ultrasound and computerized tomography (CT) scans or MRI. Positron emission tomography (PET) scans can also be used to determine extent and presence of hematogenous and lymphatic metastases. Imaging is guided by the extent of the clinician's suspicion for metastases. Because of the aggressive nature of the SCCs, if local invasion has been seen on ultrasound and/or biopsy, CT or MRI, further imaging of the chest, abdomen, and pelvis with or without a PET scan, may be warranted. PET scans are particularly useful for determining the presence of localized metastases difficult to visualize on CT or MRI and can also be used to determine local metastases to lymph nodes. Sentinel lymph node biopsies have also been reported in the literature and postulated to be an additional low morbidity tool in staging and prognostic determination.[25,26]

Surgery

Treatments are largely tailored to the presence or absence of distant metastases and the patient's general health. The surgical treatment of choice for primary SCCs for patients with RDEB or junctional EB is full thickness excision with wide surgical margins.[1,2] For patients with localized involvement, the clinician must carefully assess whether limb-sparing treatments such as wide local excision compared with amputation of the hand/foot/part of the limb is warranted. Longitudinal follow-up of EB registry patients in the United States showed that Mohs surgery did not reduce local recurrence or regional metastases and the value of sentinel lymph node biopsy remains inconclusive.[2,25–27]

SCCs that have invaded the adjacent tendons or soft tissue structures with or without local lymphogenous spread ideally warrant amputation. Amputation is also warranted for recurrent tumors. The problem in proving that amputation is better than local excision in this situation is not being able to detect small distant metastases that may have already occurred and the lack of randomized evidence, but if the tendons have been invaded, wide excision including the invaded tendon would render the hand or foot nonfunctional, which is the reason most patients wish to preserve their hands and feet.

Adjunctive Radiotherapy and/or Chemotherapy

Because of the anaplastic nature of the malignancy, patients requiring localized wide excision can also be offered chemotherapy and/or radiotherapy to the affected areas. Radiotherapy can be useful in debulking large tumors before surgery. Because of the relative dearth of reports in the literature, there is no clear consensus on adjuvant or neoadjuvant treatment regimes for patients with RDEB who are diagnosed with SCCs with local or distant metastases. In the EB registry in the United States, only 5.7% of patient with RDEB had received chemotherapy and only 17% were given radiotherapy when distant metastases were present, with no clinical benefit noted in single or combined use of chemotherapy and radiotherapy.[2] The problem with this evidence is that it is retrospective and reflects old literature reporting concerns about side effects with these modalities, resulting in delays in treatments that are usually given to patients without EB with metastatic or locally advanced SCC. The Australasian EB Registry includes 5 patients with RDEB-GS with SCC which has metastasized to the axilla who underwent fractionated radiotherapy without significant problems to their skin. Any delay in the initiation of radiotherapy allows the tumor to grow exponentially, reducing the likelihood of disease control with radiotherapy. Delays have occurred in different radiotherapy centers because the older literature reports problems with the skin. Another problem has been that generally oncologists do not encounter RDEB-GS patients until the SCC is advanced, and they may perceive that the patient's quality of life is not worth the treatments, whereas those taking care of these patients in the long-term know that these patients generally want to keep living and are used to coping with any skin breakdown that might occur. Hence, it is important for experts in EB to publish case reports of their experience with RDEB-GS and tolerability to radiotherapy.

Palliation

If a patient has extensive disease with distant metastases, the treatments offered are predominantly palliative. The management is largely governed by the wishes of the patient and the family. Limb-sparing operations may be offered in these situations to sustain the patient's quality of life. Adjuvant chemotherapy and radiotherapy can be used; however, there is currently no consensus on the appropriate chemotherapeutic agent and its dosage or duration. Similarly, radiotherapy for EB patients is not routinely recommended because of reports of potential skin breakdown. However, palliative radiotherapy may be particularly useful to treat tumors causing significant impairment to the patient's quality of life such as neuropathy, large fungating, offensive-smelling tumors or tumors with local invasion into blood vessels.

Epidermal Growth Factor Inhibitors

Cetuximab is a monoclonal antibody against epidermal growth factor receptor (EGFR) and has been used to treat locoregionally advanced head and neck cancers, colorectal cancers, and lung and cutaneous SCCs.[28–35] EGFR is over expressed in tumor cells and leads to over stimulation of cell growth and tumorigenesis. Cetuximab binds to EGFR receptors and inhibits the action of EGF via these receptors.

Treatment of locoregionally advanced head and neck cancer with concomitant high-dose radiotherapy plus cetuximab improves locoregional control and reduces mortality, and it has been found that there was no increase in toxic side effects associated with radiotherapy.[35]

Cetuximab can also be used as a single agent in the first-line treatment of patients with unresectable SCCs, and may be considered a therapeutic option.[36] Acneiform rash (in up to 80% of patients) is reported secondary to cetuximab. Other side effects include malaise, nausea, vomiting, diarrhea, constipation, allergic reactions, and susceptibility to infections. Patients should be commenced on pretreatment antihistamines and oral antibiotics, such as minomycin or doxycycline, to prevent an acneiform rash. Cetuximab was well tolerated when given as a weekly intravenous infusion to 1 of our RDEB-GS patients with SCC metastatic to the axilla and chest wall who was taking doxycycline prophylactically.

MULTIDISCIPLINARY MANAGEMENT

Ideally a team of experts should work closely with the patient with RDEB-GS. The team should include a nominated dermatologist, EB nurse, radiologist, plastic surgeon, general surgeon, radiation and medical oncologist, palliative care specialist, and pain specialist. In this way, when an SCC is detected, the team can be mobilized quickly to deliver appropriate care without undue delays.

REFERENCES

1. Fine JD, Johnson LB, Suchindran C, et al. Premature death and inherited epidermolysis bullosa. In: Fine JD, Bauer EA, McGuire J, et al, editors. Epidermolysis bullosa: clinical, epidemiologic, and laboratory advances, and the findings of the National Epidermolysis Bullosa Registry, vol. 1. 1st edition. Baltimore (MD): Johns Hopkins University Press; 1999. p. 206–24.

2. Fine JD, Johnson LB, Weiner M, et al. Epidermolysis bullosa and the risk of life-threatening cancers: The National EB Registry experience, 1986–2006. J Am Acad Dermatol 2009;60(2):203–11.

3. Rodeck U, Uitto J. Recessive dystrophic epidermolysis bullosa-associated squamous-cell carcinoma: an enigmatic entity with complex pathogenesis [comment]. J Invest Dermatol 2007;127(10):2295–6.

4. Rodeck U, Fertala A, Uitto J. Anchorless keratinocyte survival: an emerging pathogenic mechanism for squamous cell carcinoma in recessive dystrophic epidermolysis bullosa [review]. Exp Dermatol 2007; 16(6):465–7.

5. Pourreyron C, Cox G, Mao X, et al. Patients with recessive dystrophic epidermolysis bullosa develop squamous-cell carcinoma regardless of type VII collagen expression [see comment]. J Invest Dermatol 2007;127(10):2438–44.

6. McGrath JA, Schofield OM, Mayou BJ, et al. Epidermolysis bullosa complicated by squamous cell carcinoma: report of 10 cases. J Cutan Pathol 1992;19(2):116–23.

7. Mallipeddi R, Wessagowit V, South AP, et al. Reduced expression of insulin-like growth factor-binding protein-3 (IGFBP-3) in squamous cell carcinoma complicating recessive dystrophic epidermolysis bullosa. J Invest Dermatol 2004; 122(5):1302–9.

8. Arbiser JL, Fine JD, Murrell D, et al. Basic fibroblast growth factor: a missing link between collagen VII, increased collagenase, and squamous cell carcinoma in recessive dystrophic epidermolysis bullosa. Mol Med 1998;4(3):191–5.

9. Arbiser JL, Fan CY, Su X, et al. Involvement of p53 and p16 tumor suppressor genes in recessive dystrophic epidermolysis bullosa-associated squamous cell carcinoma. J Invest Dermatol 2004; 123(4):788–90.

10. Garcia-Morales I, Perez-Gil A, Camacho FM. [Marjolin's ulcer: burn scar carcinoma]. Actas Dermosifiliogr 2006;97(8):529–32 [in Spanish].

11. Copcu E, Sivrioglu N, Baytekin C, et al. Very acute and aggressive form of Marjolin's ulcer caused by single blunt trauma to the burned area. J Burn Care Rehabil 2005;26(5):459–60.

12. Wong A, Johns MM, Teknos TN. Marjolin's ulcer arising in a previously grafted burn of the scalp. Otolaryngol Head Neck Surg 2003;128(6):915–6.

13. Smith J, Mello LF, Nogueira Neto NC, et al. Malignancy in chronic ulcers and scars of the leg (Marjolin's ulcer): a study of 21 patients. Skeletal Radiol 2001;30(6):331–7.

14. Dupree MT, Boyer JD, Cobb MW. Marjolin's ulcer arising in a burn scar. Cutis 1998;62(1):49–51.

15. Fishman JR, Parker MG. Malignancy and chronic wounds: Marjolin's ulcer. J Burn Care Rehabil 1991;12(3):218–23.

16. Kawasaki H, Sawamura D, Iwao F, et al. Squamous cell carcinoma developing in a 12-year-old boy with nonHallopeau-Siemens recessive dystrophic epidermolysis bullosa [review]. Br J Dermatol 2003;148(5):1047–50.

17. Murrell D. Photographic monitoring for squamous cell carcinoma in RDEB. Proceedings of the International EB Professionals Congress. London: Institute for Child Health; 2003.

18. Fine JD, Johnson LB, Weiner M, et al. Chemoprevention of squamous cell carcinoma in recessive dystrophic epidermolysis bullosa: results of a phase 1 trial of systemic isotretinoin. J Am Acad Dermatol 2004;50(4):563–71.

19. Smit JV, de Sevaux RG, Blokx WA, et al. Acitretin treatment in (pre)malignant skin disorders of renal transplant recipients: histologic and immunohistochemical effects. J Am Acad Dermatol 2004;50(2):189–96.

20. Lebwohl M, Tannis C, Carrasco D. Acitretin suppression of squamous cell carcinoma: case report and literature review [review]. J Dermatolog Treat 2003;14(Suppl 2):3–6.

21. George R, Weightman W, Russ GR, et al. Acitretin for chemoprevention of non-melanoma skin cancers in renal transplant recipients. Australas J Dermatol 2002;43(4):269–73.

22. Fritsch A, Loeckermann S, Kern JS, et al. A hypomorphic mouse model of dystrophic epidermolysis bullosa reveals mechanisms of disease and response to fibroblast therapy. J Clin Invest 2008;118:1669–79.

23. Souza CS, Felicio LB, Bentley MV, et al. Topical photodynamic therapy for Bowen's disease of the digit in epidermolysis bullosa [review]. Br J Dermatol 2005;153(3):672–4.

24. Saxena A, Lee JB, Humphreys TR. Mohs micrographic surgery for squamous cell carcinoma associated with epidermolysis bullosa. Dermatol Surg 2006;32(1):128–34.

25. Rokunohe A, Nakano H, Aizu T, et al. Significance of sentinel node biopsy in the management of squamous cell carcinoma arising from recessive dystrophic epidermolysis bullosa. J Dermatol 2008;35(6):336–40.

26. Perez-Naranjo L, Herrera-Saval A, Garcia-Bravo B, et al. Sentinel lymph node biopsy in recessive dystrophic epidermolysis bullosa and squamous cell carcinoma. Arch Dermatol 2005;141(1):110–1.

27. Fine J-D. Possible role of sentinel node biopsy in the management of squamous cell carcinomas in inherited epidermolysis bullosa. Arch Dermatol 2004;140:1012–3.

28. Zhu Z. Targeted cancer therapies based on antibodies directed against epidermal growth factor receptor: status and perspectives [review]. Acta Pharmacol Sin 2007;28(9):1476–93.

29. Suen JK, Bressler L, Shord SS, et al. Cutaneous squamous cell carcinoma responding serially to single-agent cetuximab. Anticancer Drugs 2007;18(7):827–9.

30. Reuter CW, Morgan MA, Eckardt A. Targeting EGF-receptor-signalling in squamous cell carcinomas of the head and neck [review]. Br J Cancer 2007;96(3):408–16.

31. Le Tourneau C, Siu LL. Molecular-targeted therapies in the treatment of squamous cell carcinomas of the head and neck [review]. Curr Opin Oncol 2008;20(3):256–63.

32. Le Tourneau C, Chen EX. Molecularly targeted agents in the treatment of recurrent or metastatic squamous cell carcinomas of the head and neck [review]. Hematol Oncol Clin North Am 2008;22(6):1209–20, ix.

33. Vermorken JB, Trigo J, Hitt R, et al. Open-label, uncontrolled, multicenter phase II study to evaluate the efficacy and toxicity of cetuximab as a single agent in patients with recurrent and/or metastatic squamous cell carcinoma of the head and neck who failed to respond to platinum-based therapy. J Clin Oncol 2007;25(16):2171–7.

34. Bouali S, Chretien AS, Ramacci C, et al. PTEN expression controls cellular response to cetuximab by mediating PI3K/AKT and RAS/RAF/MAPK downstream signaling in KRAS wild-type, hormone refractory prostate cancer cells. Oncol Rep 2009;21(3):731–5.

35. Bonner JA, Harari PM, Giralt J, et al. Radiotherapy plus cetuximab for squamous-cell carcinoma of the head and neck [see comment]. N Engl J Med 2006;354(6):567–78.

36. Maubec E, Petrow P, Duvillard P, et al. Cetuximab as first-line monotherapy in patients with unresectable squamous cell carcinoma of the skin: preliminary results of a phase II multicenter study. J Clin Oncol 2008;26(Suppl) [abstract 9042].

Nutrition for Children with Epidermolysis Bullosa

Lesley Haynes, RD

KEYWORDS

• Epidermolysis Bullosa • Children • Nutrition

Optimization of resistance to infection, growth, sexual maturation, wound healing, and provision of the best possible overall quality of life are important management goals in children with epidermolysis bullosa (EB). However, all these goals rely on the maintenance of optimal nutritional status; and achieving this is extremely challenging in the severe types of EB. Unless a multiplicity of factors, such as inadequate skin care, poor dentition, esophageal stricture, gastroesophageal reflux (GER), painful defecation, and psychological and psychosocial issues are addressed by the collective expertise of the specialist multidisciplinary EB team (MDT), nutritional interventions are destined to founder.

The dearth of published data regarding nutritional support and nutritional requirements in children with EB means that current practice relies on extrapolation from other conditions and expert clinical experience. Strategies to improve nutritional status have the best chance of success when the dietitian or nutritionist works as an integral member of the MDT and is well informed of patients' situations, family dynamics, and prognoses. However, in the more severe forms of EB, the burden of caring for children with such a distressing and life-limiting condition can be immense; and parents have to prioritize numerous aspects of care. Even the best-coordinated dietetic interventions may exert only limited impact.

NUTRITIONAL COMPROMISE

Nutritional compromise corresponds to EB severity, and occurs mainly in generalized forms of recessive dystrophic EB (RDEB) and junctional EB (JEB). In these patients, multiple organ system involvement affects the child physically and psychologically, directly and indirectly. **Fig. 1** illustrates the interactions between causes and effects of inadequate nutritional intake in severe EB. In the Dowling-Meara subtype of EB simplex, infants and younger children often experience difficulties in maintaining satisfactory nutritional status and growth. However, in these EB types, excess weight is commonly gained in the preteenage and teenage years because lesions become mainly confined to feet and enforce a predominantly sedentary lifestyle, whereas factors that had previously caused poor oral intake diminish.[1]

Nutritional compromise is a consequence of
- The hypercatabolic inflammatory state, in which open skin lesions with consequent losses of blood and serous fluid, increased protein turnover, heat loss, and infection all contribute to increased requirements. As in the patient with thermal burns, nutrient needs reflect the severity of lesions[2]
- The degree to which oral, oropharyngeal, esophageal, and other gastrointestinal (GI) complications limit intake or affect absorption. Fecal loading and painful defecation (with or without chronic constipation) are extremely common and frequently cause apathy and secondary anorexia.[1,3]

NUTRITIONAL SUPPORT

Nutritional support generally aims to[1]
- Alleviate the stresses of feeding and minimize nutritional deficiencies

Dietetic Department, Great Ormond Street Hospital for Children NHS Trust, Great Ormond Street, London WC1N 3JH, UK
E-mail address: lesley.haynes@debra.org.uk

Dermatol Clin 28 (2010) 289–301
doi:10.1016/j.det.2010.01.010
0733-8635/10/$ – see front matter © 2010 Elsevier Inc. All rights reserved.

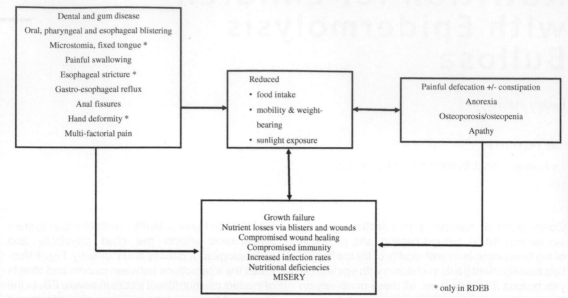

Fig. 1. Causes and effects of nutritional problems in children with severe EB. The asterisk indicates only in RDEB. (*Adapted from* Haynes L. Epidermolysis bullosa. In: Shaw V, Lawson M, editors. Clinical paediatric dietetics. 3rd edition. Oxford: Blackwell Science; 2007; with permission.)

- Optimize bowel function, immune status, and wound healing
- Promote normal body composition and optimize growth
- Promote pubertal development and sexual maturation.

In view of the grave prognosis of Herlitz JEB, these aims must be modified according to the individual patient's situation, with emphasis placed on quality of life.[4] In other severe types of EB, even when nutritional intake is successfully enhanced, few children report significant and consistent improvements in wound healing rates. This fact is disappointing but not surprising, considering the intrinsic flaws in their skin. However, the potential effects of improved nutritional intake in chronic illness are wide ranging.[5] The subtle but positive influence of improved nutritional intake on the complex events surrounding immune status and attempted tissue repair are not fully understood, but it would seem reasonable to optimize intake if deficiency or imbalance is suspected. **Table 1** describes the nutrition-related complications of different EB types and suggests appropriate interventions.

NUTRITIONAL REQUIREMENTS

Nutritional requirements in children with minimal blistering and little or no GI involvement are unlikely to be higher than those of their healthy age- and gender-matched peers, and nationally

recommended daily allowances can be used as a basis for the assessment of nutritional adequacy (bearing in mind that these values are aimed at population groups and do not reflect individual requirements).

In severe EB, however, it is not possible to quantify requirements because of[1]:

- The multisystem, inflammatory, infection-prone nature of the disease
- The variability over time of individual requirements as a reflection of age, extent of skin lesions, presence of infection, need for catch-up growth, and so forth
- The difficulties associated with estimating desirable weight gain when height is compromised because of chronic inflammation, pain, joint contractures, and osteoporosis
- The difficulties associated with conducting clinical trials in such small patient numbers.

Although severe EB lesions bear some similarities to thermal burns, extrapolations from nutrient recommendations in this group should not be applied automatically to severe EB because the megadoses of some nutrients are intended only for the short term. In the absence of specific data in EB, best practice in designing nutrition support currently involves consideration of the following 3 main components.

Component 1. Evaluation of factors affecting nutritional intake using a scoring system such as *THINC* (*Tool to Help Identify Nutritional*

Table 1
Main complications affecting nutritional status and likely nutritional interventions in children with different types of EB

EB Type	Complications	Interventions
Weber-Cockayne EB simplex	Lesions, usually confined to feet and hands, especially in hot weather, often severely limit mobility. Frequently painful defecation ± constipation	Because of reduced mobility and activity, advice on weight maintenance/reduction may be required. Age-appropriate fiber and fluid intakes
Dowling-Meara EB simplex	Generalized blistering tending later to become confined to hands and feet. Feeding problems often severe in infancy, especially GER, but generally resolve before teenage. Often painful defecation ± constipation	As for RDEB in early years, but G-tube placement rarely necessary. Catch-up in weight often occurs preadolescence and if excessive, leads to exacerbation of foot lesions and further reduction in activity and mobility. Age-appropriate fiber and fluid intakes
Herlitz junctional EB	Recurrent moderate to severe lesions. Dental pain caused by abnormal tooth composition. Laryngeal and respiratory complications. Good initial weight gain usually followed by profound failure to thrive; possible PLE. Opioid analgesia often exacerbates constipation. Massive sepsis and respiratory complications. Survivors often profoundly anemic with osteoporosis/osteopenia consequent to immobility and possibly to malabsorption	As for RDEB, but with intention of improving quality of life, rather than quantity. Intervention has no impact on prognosis. G-tube placement not generally advised because it is likely to result in very poor healing around entry site, skin breakdown, and leakage of gastric contents. Specialized formula feeds and exclusion diets have been used experimentally in cases of suspected PLE
Non-Herlitz junctional EB	Recurrent mild to severe lesions. Abnormal tooth composition causes dental pain. Possible PLE. Osteoporosis/ osteopenia when immobility compromised	Global supplementation (as for RDEB) usually required except in mild cases. Specialized formula feeds and exclusion diets have been used experimentally in cases of suspected PLE
Junctional EB with PA	Mild to severe lesions. PA. Usually fatal in infancy, but there are exceptions	As for Herlitz junctional EB
Dominant dystrophic EB	Usually mild lesions. May have oral and esophageal involvement. Anal erosions/fissures cause painful and reluctant defecation ± constipation	Intervention generally not indicated other than age-appropriate fiber and fluid intakes
RDEB	When severe, recurrent moderate to severe lesions heal poorly with generalized scarring and contractures. Internal contractures cause microstomia, dysphagia, and esophageal strictures. Digits fuse in severe generalized type. Anal erosions/fissures cause painful and reluctant defecation ± constipation. Some develop inflammatory bowel disease/colitis. Refractory anemia. Osteoporosis/ osteopenia common	Global supplementation required except in mild cases. Esophageal dilatation ± gastrostomy feeding often indicated. Specialized formula feeds and exclusion diets have been used experimentally with patients with inflammatory bowel disease/colitis

Abbreviations: G tube, gastrostomy tube; PA, pyloric atresia; PLE, protein-losing enteropathy.
Adapted from Haynes L. Epidermolysis bullosa. In: Shaw V, Lawson M, editors. Clinical paediatric dietetics. 3rd edition. Oxford: Blackwell Science; 2007; with permission.

Compromise). *THINC* is meant to aid, not replace, clinical judgment and should be used in conjunction with Clinical Practice Guidelines for Nutrition Support in infants and children with EB (EB CPG).[6] *THINC's* scoring chart rates the 3 key aspects of the child's state: weight and length or height, gastroenterology, and dermatology. The higher the score, the greater is the likelihood of nutritional compromise. **Tables 2** and **3** show the nutritional compromise scoring charts for children younger than and older than 18 months, respectively. According to the total score, algorithms suggesting courses of action can be found in the EB CPG.

Component 2. Comparison of the nutritional intake in children with EB with that of age/height-, age-, and gender-matched unaffected children, with the addition of a factor to allow for increased requirements of certain nutrients. Energy requirements can be calculated using the following formula[7] based on weight for height, age, and additional factors such as blistering, sepsis, and requirement for catch-up growth:

Weight (kg) × (kcal/kg for height age) × [1 + (sum of 3 additional factors)]. Additional factors are

1. Ratio of blisters to body surface area (BSA): 20% BSA = 0.19, 40% BSA = 0.5, 100% BSA = 0.95
2. Sepsis: mild = 0.2, moderate = 0.4, severe = 0.8
3. Catch-up growth: 0.1 to 0.2.

Therefore, for a 6-year old boy; weighing 13 kg; having height for age (25th centile) = 4.7 years, 20% BSA blistered, mild sepsis; and is stunted, the energy requirement calculated by applying the formula is:

$13 \times 90 \times [1 + 0.19 + 0.2 + 0.2] = 1860$ kcal $= 143$ kcal/kg

This calculation may provide twice the child's customary energy intake, so it should be applied with great caution to avoid intolerance of the increased regimen or more seriously, the grave complications of refeeding syndrome. A dietary assessment should also be taken to elucidate the child's usual intake, and the recommended energy intake should initially be based roughly midway between this and the figure achieved from the previously mentioned formula. Carers often overestimate their child's intake, so assessment should be comprehensive and sensitively probed to elicit a representative picture; and the EB CPG[6] includes a proforma for recording intake. In the example discussed earlier, the child currently consuming 1000 kcal should be advised how to increase this to approximately 1300 kcal (100 kcal/kg). This goal can be achieved either with food or with proprietary supplements or both, although many children will be unable to consistently maintain a sufficiently enhanced intake with food alone (see section on alternative feeding routes). The regimen should be individually tailored to the child and family dynamics, introduced slowly, and reviewed regularly to ensure that it remains appropriate and feasible.

Protein requirements are estimated to be approximately 10% to 15% of the energy intake, extrapolated from the recommendation of 9% energy intake for catch-up growth in children with normal skin.[8] Using the earlier example, the child taking 1300 kcal/d would require 33 to 49 g protein/d (2.5–4.0 g/kg). Children with extensive lesions will require an intake at the higher end of the range, especially where there is associated sepsis. Increasing protein intake to this degree will usually require the use of proprietary supplements and, if it is to be maintained, a feeding tube may need to be placed (see section on alternative feeding routes).

Component 3. Evaluation of biochemical and hematological parameters, although the interpretation of results poses great difficulties on account of the effect of the acute-phase inflammatory response in which distribution of minerals is altered. This phenomenon is thought to confer some advantage to the host; for example, sequestration and peripheral uptake of zinc and iron may ensure maximization of their availability for essential metabolic processes.[5] Nevertheless, certain parameters are generally monitored (see the article by Anna E. Martinez elsewhere in this issue for further exploration of this topic). Frequency of sampling depends on disease severity and the need to evaluate the impact of intervention, such as nutrient supplementation or introduction of an alternative feeding method, for example, gastrostomy placement.[1]

Babies

Severe lesions, particularly with sepsis, are likely to increase nutritional requirements (see Component 2 discussed earlier).[9] Extensive blistering may require correspondingly larger feed volumes than the usual 150 to 200 mL/kg, to compensate for additional fluid loss. Breastfeeding should always be encouraged for the many benefits it confers.[10] However, rooting at the breast may cause or exacerbate facial lesions and suckling may lead to blistering of the mouth, tongue, and gums. When possible, babies should be allowed to suckle on demand. Except in mild cases, breast

Table 2
Evaluation of nutritional compromise in children aged less than or equal to 18 months with EB

It is Very Important to Read Guidance Notes in Main Document Before Completing	Nutritional Compromise Rating	Nutritional Compromise Score
(1) Weight and length		
Birth weight centile	>9th = 0 0.4th–9th = 5 <0.4th = 10	
Weight gain/loss in past month	100% expected weight gain = 0 50% expected weight gain = 5 Static weight/weight loss = 10	
Birth length centile	>9th = 0 0.4th–9th = 5 <0.4th = 10	
Length increase in past 2–4 mo	100% expected increase = 0 Unavailable/50% expected increase = 5 Too fragile to measure/No increase = 10	
(2) Feeding and gastroenterological aspects		
Feed in first 4–6 mo	Fully breast fed = 0 Breast milk only (expressed or direct suckling) for first 1–4 weeks = 5 Combined breast milk and formula = 5 No breast milk, fully formula fed = 10	
Mode (past or present)	Oral, regular teat = 5 Oral with Haberman feeder ± NG tube ± G tube = 10 or combination of 2 methods mentioned earlier = 10	
Oral lesions and/or reluctance to feed from breast, bottle or spooned solids and/or GER and/or taking GER medication or medications	No = 0 Occasionally = 5 Usually/always = 10	
Painful defecation and/or constipation and/or diarrhea and/or taking laxatives/stool softeners	No = 0 Occasionally = 5 Usually/always = 10	
(3) Dermatologic aspects		
BSA of denuded/ulcerated skin............% (use grid overleaf)	None = 0 <30% lesions = 5 >30% 10	
Skin infection/sepsis............% (use grid overleaf)	None = 0 1%–30% lesions = 5 >30% 10	
Total score	Maximum possible = 100	

Suggested action for ranges of Nutritional Compromise Scores.

0 to 25: Low risk of nutritional problems; review in 3 to 6 months by relevant professionals.

26 to 50: Moderate risk, address all scores greater than 0, involving relevant professionals, and review in 1 to 3 months.

51 to 75: Significant risk, address all scores greater than 0, involving relevant professionals. May require admission to hospital for more intensive management; review in about 1 month.

76 to 100: Very high risk, admit to hospital and address all scores greater than 0, involving relevant professionals.

Abbreviations: BSA, body surface area; NG tube, nasogastric tube.

From Haynes L. Clinical practice guidelines for nutrition support in infants and children with epidermolysis bullosa (EB). London: Great Ormond Street Hospital for Children NHS Trust; 2007; with permission.

Table 3
Evaluation of nutritional compromise in children older than 18 months with EB

It is Very Important to Read Guidance Notes in Main Document Before Completing	Nutritional Compromise Rating	Nutritional Compromise Score
(1) Weight and height		
Current weight.......... kg, centile	>9th = 0 0.4th–9th = 5 <0.4th = 10	
Current height.......... cm, centile .... Number of centile divisions height centile is greater than weight centile	< 1 = 0 1–2 = 5 >2 = 10	
Approximate weight gain/loss in past 6 months	~75%–100% expected = 0 ~25%–75% expected = 5 >25% or undesirable weight loss = 10 (Score 0 if child overweight)	
(2) Gastroenterological and feeding aspects		
Tethered tongue*	No = 0 Moderate tethering 5 Severe tethering = 10	
Dysphagia and/or pureed diet and/or GER and/or regurgitation of excess mucus/phlegm	Very rarely/never = 0 Occasionally = 5 Frequently/always = 10	
Painful defecation and/or constipation and/or rectal bleeding and/or diarrhea and/or taking laxatives/ stool softeners and/or excessive flatus/bloating and/or taking antireflux medication or medications and/or eliminating dietary component, eg, cows' milk, wheat	Never = 0 Occasionally = 5 Frequently/always = 10	
Gastrostomy/other feeding tube in situ	No = 0 Yes = 5	
(3) Dermatologic aspects		
Body surface area of denuded/ulcerated skin: ....% (use grid overleaf)	1%–10% = 5 11%–30% = 10 31%–50% = 15 >50% = 20	
Skin infection/sepsis: ....% (use grid overleaf)	No = 0 <25% lesions = 5 26%–50% lesions = 10 >50% lesions = 15	
Total score	Maximum possible = 100	

Suggested action for ranges of Nutritional Compromise Scores.

0 to 25: Low risk of nutritional compromise; review in 9 to 12 months by relevant professionals.

30 to 50: Moderate risk, address all scores greater than 0 (except that marked with *), involving relevant professionals, and review in 4 to 6 months.

55 to 75: Significant risk, address all scores greater than 0 (except that marked with *), involving relevant professionals. May require admission to hospital for more intensive management; review in 3 months.

80 to 100: Very high risk, admit to hospital and address all scores greater than 0 (except those marked with *), involving relevant professionals.

From Haynes L. Clinical practice guidelines for nutrition support in infants and children with epidermolysis bullosa (EB). London: Great Ormond Street Hospital for Children NHS Trust; 2007; with permission.

milk alone generally fails to satisfy increased requirements and should be supplemented by a more nutrient-dense feed; this can be achieved in several ways using expressed breast milk (EBM), proprietary infant formulas, and proprietary carbohydrate and fat products.[1] Great care should be taken when modifying feeds to avoid imbalance of macronutrients, and regular review of the infant's weight and feed adequacy is essential. Diarrhea can result with an osmotic load greater than 500 mOsm/kg water; and ready-to-feed nutrient-dense proprietary formulations provide safe alternatives to modifying EBM or formula. A specialized feeder designed for a cleft lip or palate such as the Haberman feeder (Athrodax Healthcare International Ltd, Drybrook, Gloucestershire, UK) is extremely useful. This feeder minimizes trauma to the gum margin, and its internal valve and long shaft allow the carer to control the flow of feed, so that even a weak suck will deliver a satisfactory milk flow. Alternatively, the hole in a conventional teat can be enlarged using a sterile needle. Babies who cannot suck may need to be fed from a spoon or dropper. Nasogastric (NG) tubes are not routinely placed (see section on alternative feeding routes), but their short-term use may be unavoidable.

Vitamin requirements for infants thriving on breast milk or regular infant formulas are unlikely to be greater than normal. However, if in doubt, an age-appropriate multivitamin supplement can be given,[1,3] provided that total intake (particularly of vitamin A) does not exceed the recommended safe upper limits. Although precise requirements have not been determined, the literature and the author's experience suggest that babies who are more severely affected by EB need increased amounts of all vitamins.[3,11] The provision of 150% to 200% of the nationally accepted age-appropriate recommended daily intake should ensure that intakes are within recommended safe limits.

Iron losses from external and internal lesions may necessitate iron supplementation (see section on iron). If so, parents should be warned to look out for signs of constipation and be medically advised regarding an age-appropriate stool softener. In the author's experience, the need for other supplementation (eg, zinc, selenium, calcium) is very unlikely to be indicated in the first year of life.[1]

One gauge of nutritional adequacy is growth, and weight should be documented regularly. Length and head circumference should also be measured. However, downward deviation from the birth weight centile in the first year is common in severe types of EB despite proactive nutritional intervention[1] (see section on body composition and assessing adequacy of growth).

Solid foods can be offered at the same time, and often in the same form, as for an unaffected baby, provided that hard and abrasive foods are omitted. A shallow soft plastic spoon with rounded edges should be used and babies who have an extremely fragile mouth may feed more confidently from the parent's fingertip or from a piece of soft food. Reluctance to try new foods is often a legacy of previously, or ongoing, poorly controlled GER,[12] a very fragile painful mouth, or previous NG tube feeding. Scarring and tongue tethering can cause an uncoordinated swallow with the risk of aspiration.[13] Weaning foods containing soft lumps in a liquid matrix are difficult to control in the mouth, leading to panic and subsequent gagging and choking, thereby compounding negative associations with feeding. Parents should be advised how to increase dietary protein and energy content without increasing bulk.[14] Acceptance of new foods is often extremely slow and parents need ongoing reassurance to allow babies to progress at their own pace. It is crucial to promote confidence and force-feeding is totally counterproductive. The expertise of a pediatric speech and language therapist is invaluable in promoting confidence with different food textures. Some children never progress beyond very soft or smooth foods; this should not be viewed as failure, nor does it jeopardize speech development.

The Over-1s

Over time, the complications associated with severe RDEB in particular, preclude satisfactory nutritional intake. Oral and esophageal problems dictate that even when foods are soft and moist, mealtimes can be protracted and devoid of the pleasures that most of us take for granted. Adequate energy intake may be unachievable without the frequent consumption of fermentable carbohydrate, especially sucrose. Unfortunately, this is highly conducive to the development of dental caries. This apparent conflict of interests between dietitian and dentist can lead to contradictory advice to the child and the carers. However, a compromise is possible, with sweets restricted to the end of mealtimes and continuous sipping of sugary drinks outside mealtimes discouraged.

Liquidized foods can be low in all nutrients, and advice should aim to improve the nutritional value of the child's normal food intake.[15] All modifications should be practical and tailored to family dynamics. The emphasis should be on increased protein and energy intakes, with improvements in vitamin and mineral. Milk often figures prominently in the diets of children with EB, so protein and calcium intakes are generally satisfactory (but see section on calcium and vitamin D). Conversely, the intakes of those who dislike milk and milk products, such as cheese and yogurt, and those who have difficulties chewing and swallowing meat, invariably require supplementation. Realistically, severely affected children need to rely heavily on proprietary multinutrient supplements and energy sources.[1,3]

ALTERNATIVE FEEDING ROUTES

Despite great care, NG tubes can cause internal and external trauma and they should not be placed routinely. NG tubes are difficult to secure, and only nonadhesive dressings or silicone tape that are recommended for fragile skin should be used.[1] Internal friction and scarring by the tube can interfere with oral feeding, and anecdotal evidence suggests that this is associated with later food aversion and possibly an increased tendency to develop esophageal strictures. However, temporary NG feeding may be unavoidable in babies who do not take satisfactory volumes of oral feeds and in those whose mouths become excessively traumatized by suckling. NG feeding may be used as an interim measure in the child, who it is thought would benefit from gastrostomy placement but who needs, or whose carers need, evidence of the effects of improved nutrition before agreeing to surgery. A 6- to 8-week period of NG feeding should be sufficient to show benefit. Whatever the age of the patient, the tube used should be as soft and of as narrow a gauge as possible, and it should not be resited at every feed.

Longer-term NG tube placement is undesirable not only for the reasons cited earlier but also because the tube's unaesthetic appearance attracts further attention to a child who is already a focus for insensitive questions, causing additional distress to carers.[16] When poor oral intake is caused by esophageal stricture or strictures, this can be significantly improved by balloon esophageal dilatation (ED).[17] However, ED does not address the oral and psychological complications that deter eating, and feeding by gastrostomy tube (G tube) should be considered if intake remains poor despite a series of EDs.

There are advantages and disadvantages to G-tube feeding and the decision to place a G tube requires careful consideration (**Table 4**). Although G-tube feeding is not a panacea, parents of many severely affected children recognize that without it, it would be impossible to administer not only the required nutrition but also a large number of medications. A few parents view G-tube placement as condemnation for their failure to nourish their child adequately, and request continued information regarding alternative oral supplements. However, delaying the placement may only add to their stress and frustration, engendering increased feelings of failure. With early intervention, the child is more likely to continue with oral nutrition, albeit in small and varying quantities.[18] This matters socially, when acceptance by, and integration with, peer groups centers so much on eating and drinking.

After G-tube placement, some children are reluctant to continue with oral nutrition, preferring to rely almost entirely on gastrostomy feeds.[1] This preference may reflect previous long-term negativity about eating and relief at having an alternative route for nutrition. However, the large feed volumes required to promote optimal growth may be poorly tolerated, whether they are given overnight, during the day, or a combination of both. To optimize feed tolerance and promote continuing oral intake, it is advisable to begin with small volumes; this may mean as little as 200 to 250 mL of a nutrient-dense feed for a child younger than 5 years, and 300 to 500 mL for an older child. Feeds can be delivered by feeding pump, or gravity bolus, or both, depending on whether they are given in the daytime or overnight. It is more physiologic to be fed during the day and in discrete amounts, and daytime bolus feeds mimic this most closely. However, many children wish to keep daytimes normal, preferring to be fed overnight. A drawback of this timing can be the need to pass urine and sometimes to defecate during the night. It should be possible to address the latter by altering the timing of laxative administration. Some children wear a nappy or incontinence pad, although skin contact with urine or feces during the night is not desirable. In the United Kingdom, carers are advised not to give pureed food via a G tube because of the likelihood of blockage and microbial growth. However, this is not discouraged in all other European countries, and families justify the practice by explaining that the child benefits psychologically from knowing that he or she is eating the same food as other family members.

A jejunal feeding tube may be necessary for a child with impaired gastric emptying, intractable GER, or feed aspiration. Feeding directly into the jejunum limits the rate at which the feed can be delivered and generally requires feeding to be spread over 12 to 18 hours. A proprietary feed that has undergone partial hydrolysis is usually chosen in preference to a whole protein feed based on cow's milk.

Table 4
Factors relating to G-tube feeding in children with EB

Indications for G-Tube Feeding	Benefits of Proactive G-Tube Feeding	General Advantages of G-Tube Feeding	Disadvantages of G-Tube Feeding
Growth rate is less than that expected despite dietetic advice	Undernutrition and growth failure less likely to be established	Discreet device (as opposed to NG tube)	Child dislikes having device changed (experiences pain)
Eating and drinking are aversive/painful	Aversion to eating less likely to be entrenched	Improved compliance with supplements, medications, fiber	Nocturnal enuresis and possibly defecation if overnight feed volumes large
Supplements are refused	Gastrostomy feeds more likely to supplement oral intake (than vice versa). May need only to top-up child on days of poor oral intake	Reduction in painful defecation because of regular laxative/stool softener intake and return to discrete meals	Device leaks feed ± gastric secretions and entry site becomes eroded
Medications are refused	Less awareness of body image and better acceptance of device and lifestyle changes	May be needed for medications only, eg, analgesia, iron, laxatives/softeners	
Mealtimes are increasingly stressful and protracted		Improved quality of life for child and family	
Esophageal dilatation does not alleviate the above issues		Reversible procedure	

BODY COMPOSITION AND ASSESSING ADEQUACY OF GROWTH

Children with severe EB undergo significant changes in body composition (loss of adipose and lean tissues) despite aggressive and proactive nutritional intervention. The picture seen in other children who are critically sick is highly likely to be mirrored in severe EB, because the cascade of events mediated by cytokines and activation of the hypothalamic-pituitary-adrenal axis leads to catabolism and deranged physiology.[5] EB complications generally increase in number and intensity over time, and it is very difficult to judge whether growth and overall nutritional status are optimal. Although serial measurements of weight and height velocity are well-recognized means of evaluating adequacy of growth in sick and well children, comparison of the values of children with severe EB with age- and gender-matched healthy children's growth standards is of limited value. It has been postulated that children with RDEB are significantly lighter at birth than unaffected children, and that the compromise in

growth begins in utero.[19] So any comparison with healthy peers should always be considered in the context of disease severity, and goals should be adjusted accordingly. Painful fixed flexion contractures around joints and osteoporosis in severely affected children make height difficult or impossible to measure. A supine stadiometer or segmental measuring may be more practical.[20] Body mass index (BMI), measured as the weight (in kilograms) divided by height (in meters) squared, gives an indication of relative weight for height; but does not differentiate between lean and fat tissue and is not routinely used (see sections on optimizing growth and mobility, and calcium and vitamin D).

OPTIMIZING GROWTH AND MOBILITY

Determination of optimal growth rates for children with severe EB is difficult and should always be considered in the context of the individual child's disease severity. Nutrition support by gastrostomy feeding (see section on alternative feeding routes) has definite advantages in EB but may be associated with central fat deposition with poor linear growth. The reasons for this are multifactorial and interrelated, and less likely to be caused by gastrostomy feeding per se as to disturbances in growth hormone production mediated by cytokines and increased cortisol production inherent in chronic inflammatory illness.[21] The child whose weight centile deviates upwardly by more than 2 centiles from his height centile may be less mobile and more likely to depend on a wheelchair. It is important to maintain a balance between mobility, growth, and nutritional status because these 3 aspects are interrelated and interdependent. Lack of weight bearing and wheelchair dependency compounds the low bone mass that is frequently seen in children with RDEB and JEB.[22] An increased propensity to bone pain and fractures leads to further immobility. Conversely, undernourished children may fail to attain puberty and to benefit from its associated protective hormonal effect on bone health.

MICRONUTRIENTS

Micronutrients are well recognized as essential intermediaries in metabolism and for their roles in attempted wound healing, cellular immunity, and antioxidant activity. Their importance is widely acknowledged in all children who are critically ill. However, guidelines for their provision are currently empirical whatever the underlying condition.[3] Research in burns and pressure ulcers suggests that it may be beneficial to supplement certain micronutrients in EB.[2] However, in the author's experience single micronutrient supplementation such as zinc is rarely appropriate. Although this is often recommended when biochemical estimation has revealed levels less than the reference range, it is not necessarily the correct course of action (see Component 3 discussed earlier).

Vitamins

If a satisfactory vitamin intake is in doubt (based on Component 1 discussed earlier and dietary assessment), an age-appropriate multivitamin supplement should be recommended, provided that total intake (particularly of vitamin A) does not exceed the nationally recommended safe upper limits. It is likely that severely affected EB children need increased amounts of all vitamins,[6,11] especially vitamin C, whose roles in enhancing iron absorption[23] and in collagen synthesis[24] is recognized. The provision of 150% to 200% of the normal, national recommendations ensures that intakes are still within safe limits. Babies taking increased concentration feeds (see section on babies) automatically receive correspondingly increased amounts of all vitamins, possibly nearing 150% of normal recommendations if large volumes are consumed. However, if a satisfactory intake is in doubt and skin lesions are significant, a comprehensive (ideally liquid) preparation should be prescribed. In the case of vitamin D, even fortified feeds may barely meet the normal requirements and the skin of these babies may be largely covered with dressings, receiving minimal exposure to sunlight (see section on calcium and vitamin D).

Older children consistently consuming significant volumes of multinutrient supplements receive corresponding amounts of vitamins from these, but if, as stated earlier, vitamin intake regularly falls below about 150% of the normal recommendations, a supplement should be prescribed. Although the protective role of antioxidant vitamins (A, C, and E) in the development of malignancy in EB is unproven, it seems prudent to recommend an enhanced intake of these, while keeping within safe upper limits.

Calcium and Vitamin D

Although the low bone mass, abnormal mineralization, and fractures seen in children with the more severe forms of EB may be partly attributable to poor nutrition, additional factors, such as delayed puberty, reduced levels of mobility and weight-bearing exercise, and reduced exposure to sunlight are also implicated.[22] Children consuming significant amounts of milk and milk products, or fortified proprietary feeds consume theoretically adequate levels of calcium and often of vitamin D. However, elevated cytokine concentrations secondary to chronic infection or inflammation may adversely affect bone turnover, and GI complications may interfere with absorption, so combined supplementation may be recommended.

Iron

Iron intake frequently falls short of presumed requirements (based on hematological results and extent of blood loss from internal and external lesions) even when a proprietary feed is consumed. A liquid, rather than tablet form of iron supplement is generally preferable. Iron supplements are often associated with gastric irritation and constipation. Consequently, compliance is poor unless appropriate action is taken (alternative preparations, alternative timing of dosage, stool softeners, and so forth). Debate continues over the merits of daily[25] versus weekly iron administration.[26] The latter view relies on the hypothesis that a mucosal block occurs in intestinal cells, and then these cells cannot absorb therapeutic daily doses of iron until they are renewed by cell turnover at roughly 3-day intervals. In practice, medications given on a less than daily basis are prone to be forgotten, so it is safer to prescribe them on a daily basis as a part of the regular routine. Undesirable side effects may be eased by dividing a daily dose into 2, increasing fiber intake, and prescribing appropriate laxatives or stool softeners.[27] To improve iron absorption, a rich source of vitamin C (eg, blackcurrant or orange juice) can be taken concurrently, provided that this does not irritate the oral mucosa. There is no consensus regarding separate or joint administration of iron and zinc supplements.[28] These 2 micronutrients have the potential to interact, leading to reduced absorption of both. A review article concluded that, although some trials have shown that joint iron and zinc supplementation has less of an effect on biochemical or functional outcomes than does supplementation with either mineral alone, there is no strong evidence to discourage joint supplementation.[29] Whichever regimen is adopted, it is vital to establish compliance. If the scheme proves impractical or the physiologic response is poor, the regimen should be modified accordingly.

Zinc

As an essential cofactor for more than 200 enzymes, zinc plays vital roles in growth, wound healing, immune function, and membrane stability, where its antioxidant properties are crucial.[30] However, the degree of desirable supplementation is unclear,[31] and intakes of more than 200% of the national age-appropriate recommendation are probably unnecessary because improvement in wound healing may only occur in deficiency states, if at all. Excessive intakes have been reported to impair immune responses in adults,[32] and may interfere with copper and iron absorption.[33] Nausea, sometimes accompanied by vomiting, is a common side effect of zinc supplementation and an understandable reason for noncompliance. Flavored zinc lozenges may be better tolerated; these dissolve slowly in the mouth, but their chalky mouth feel is unacceptable to some children and their texture may irritate the fragile oral mucosa. Plasma zinc estimation can be undertaken to provide a baseline, although the interpretation of results is complicated by factors such as low plasma albumin that causes an associated spuriously low zinc result. In such a situation, it is inappropriate to supplement zinc alone; energy and protein intake should also be increased. A liquid zinc supplement is preferable. To optimize absorption and minimize side effects of nausea, the daily dose should be split into 2. It may be prudent to advise giving zinc supplements;

if not on different days from iron supplements, then at least at different times of the day, although no trial has yet shown clearly the merits of either regimen (see section on iron).

Selenium and Carnitine

Selenium and carnitine are considered together as several children who are severely affected by RDEB have developed fatal dilated cardiomyopathy (DCM), which is thought to be associated with deficiencies of selenium and carnitine.[34,35] However, it is equally possible that the extreme, globally malnourished state of these children contributed to the development of DCM. An association has been made between concurrent administration of amitriptyline and cisapride and the development of DCM in EB, because both drugs are potentially cardiotoxic.[36] This study claimed that nutritional deficiency was an unlikely cause of DCM because previously reported cases were under close nutritional supervision. However, such supervision does not automatically equal compliance and efficacy. Indeed, the case described was exceedingly malnourished with all aspects of parental management being extremely poor. Selenium is an essential component of the antioxidant enzyme glutathione peroxidase; and in view of the oxidative stress associated with chronic inflammation and sepsis in severe EB, selenium monitoring should be routinely undertaken.[1] When there is evidence of deficiency, supplementation should be recommended. Selenium supplements that also contain vitamin A should be advised only if intake of vitamin A from other sources is not significant. In the author's experience, biochemical evidence of carnitine deficiency is rarely seen in the under-2s who have been receiving age-appropriate fully fortified proprietary formulas. If supplementation is indicated, this is usually given as L-carnitine.[1]

Specialized and Immune-Enhanced Formulas

These proprietary preparations containing nutrients, such as arginine, glutamine, and essential fatty acids are marketed for adults to promote healing, optimize immune status, and exert a beneficial effect on inflammatory conditions.[37] Although these would be highly advantageous in EB, their efficacy has not yet been robustly tested. More work is required to identify the clinical conditions and the doses of individual micronutrients that actively promote or accelerate healing.[38,39]

OPTIMIZATION OF BOWEL FUNCTION, DIETARY FIBER, PREBIOTICS, AND PROBIOTICS

Chronic constipation (or more accurately, fecal loading) with painful defecation is one of the most frequent, yet underestimated, complications of all types of EB.[3,27] Constipation should be treated without delay if the vicious cycle of pain, conscious ignoring of the gastrocolonic reflex, and secondary anorexia (see **Fig. 1**) is to be avoided. In babies, extra fluid should be offered in the form of water, or if this is refused, 1 teaspoon of fresh fruit juice diluted in 100 mL water or ready-to-feed baby juice diluted with an equal volume of water should be offered. A stool softener may need to be medically prescribed. A fiber-containing proprietary feed, should be introduced at 6 to 9 months and, whether the infant is constipated or not, it is prudent to introduce a fiber source at about 12 months of age, because constipation is such a likely complication of all types of EB.

In the older child, overflow incontinence can be mistaken for diarrhea, and carers often reduce or stop the prescribed laxative therapy, inadvertently exacerbating the situation. When oral lesions, dysphagia, and requirement for a low-bulk nutrient-dense intake prevent the consumption of a conventional high-fiber diet, either a fiber-containing proprietary feed or a pure fiber source should be introduced. Dietary fiber is now a routine component of many proprietary, nutritionally balanced enteral feeds, and its efficacy has been shown in alleviating constipation in children with EB.[27]

Desirable fiber intake can be estimated using the formula of age (in years) + 5 to 10 g daily.[40] Thus, a 3-year old child will require 8 to 13 g fiber per day; adequate fluid intake should be advised concurrently. Before introducing additional fiber, the degree of fecal loading should be assessed and addressed medically. If this is not done, abdominal pain invariably ensues compromising compliance.

Pre- and probiotics have been shown to enhance immune function, improve colonic integrity, reduce incidence and duration of intestinal infections, downregulate the allergic response, and improve digestion and defecation.[41] These effects are all very desirable for children with EB, and in the author's view proprietary feeds containing prebiotics should be chosen over those without, unless medically contraindicated. Although probiotics have been shown to favorably influence immune status and improve GI tolerance to antibiotic therapy, they have also been associated with adverse effects, such as bacteremia, sepsis, and endocarditis.[42] So it would be prudent to advise their use only in selected and carefully monitored EB patients and not in those who are severely debilitated or immunocompromised.

EXCLUSION DIETS

It has been postulated that diarrhea, colitis, and protein-losing enteropathy in some cases of RDEB and JEB arise secondarily to antigenic exposure in the gut lumen as a result of mucosal fragility[43]; and that exclusion of dietary components, such as milk, egg, wheat, and soya may alleviate symptoms. More work is required to establish whether the benefits of imposing such rigid regimes outweigh the significant difficulties that families experience in implementing them.

REFERENCES

1. Haynes L. Epidermolysis bullosa. In: Shaw V, Lawson M, editors. Clinical paediatric dietetics. 3rd edition. Oxford: Blackwell Science; 2007. p. 482–96.
2. Gamelli RL. Nutritional problems of the acute and chronic burn patient. Relevance to epidermolysis bullosa. Arch Dermatol 1988;124:756–9.
3. Allman S, Haynes L, MacKinnon P, et al. Nutrition in dystrophic epidermolysis bullosa. Pediatr Dermatol 1992;9:231–8.
4. Yan EG, Paris JJ, Ahluwalia J, et al. State-of-the-art. Treatment decision-making for patients with the Herlitz subtype of junctional epidermolysis bullosa. J Perinatol 2007;27:307–11.
5. Prelack K. Enteral nutrition support in the critically ill pediatric patient. In: Rolandelli R, Bankhead R, Boullata JI, et al, editors. Clinical nutrition enteral and tube feeding. 4th edition. Philadelphia: Elsevier Saunders; 2005. p. 317–31.
6. Haynes L. Clinical practice guidelines for nutrition support in children with epidermolysis bullosa including THINC (Tool to Help Identify Nutritional Compromise in EB). Great Ormond Street Hospital. 2007. Available at: http://www.nutricia-clinical-care. co.uk.
7. Birge K. Nutrition management of patients with epidermolysis bullosa. J Am Diet Assoc 1995;95:575–9.
8. Smith Z. Faltering growth. In: Shaw V, Lawson M, editors. Clinical paediatric dietetics. 3rd edition. Oxford: Blackwell Science; 2007. p. 556–65.
9. Lechner-Gruskay D, Honig PJ, Pereira G, et al. Nutritional and metabolic profile of children with epidermolysis bullosa. Pediatr Dermatol 1988;5:22–7.
10. Department of Health and Social Security. Report on health and social subjects No. 32: present day practice in infant feeding. London: The Stationery Office; 1988.

11. Fine JD, Tamura T, Johnson L. Blood vitamin and trace metal levels in epidermolysis bullosa. Arch Dermatol 1989;125:374–9.

12. Mathisen B, Worral L, Masel J, et al. Feeding problems in infants with gastro-oesophageal reflux disease: a controlled study. J Paediatr Child Health 1999;35:163–9.

13. Field D, Garland M, Williams K. Correlates of specific childhood feeding problems. J Paediatr Child Health 2003;39:299–304.

14. Haynes L. Nutrition for babies with epidermolysis bullosa; a booklet for parents, carers and professionals. Dystrophic Epidermolysis Bullosa Research Association (DebRA); 2008.

15. Haynes L. Nutrition in epidermolysis bullosa for children over 1 year of age; a booklet for parents, carers and professionals. Dystrophic Epidermolysis Bullosa Research Association (DebRA); 2008.

16. van Scheppingen C, Lettinga AT, Duipmans JC, et al. Main problems experienced by children with epidermolysis bullosa: a qualitative study with semi-structured interviews. Acta Derm Venereol 2008;88:143–50.

17. Azizkhan R, Stehr W, Cohen AP, et al. Esophageal strictures in children with recessive dystrophic epidermolysis bullosa: an 11-year experience with fluoroscopically guided balloon dilatation. J Pediatr Surg 2006;41:55–60.

18. Haynes L, Atherton DJ, Ade-Ajayi N, et al. Gastrostomy and growth in dystrophic epidermolysis bullosa. Br J Dermatol 1996;134:872–9.

19. Fox AT, Alderdice F, Atherton DJ. Are children with recessive dystrophic epidermolysis bullosa of low birthweight? Pediatr Dermatol 2003;20:303–6.

20. Stewart L, McKaig N, Dunlop C, et al. Dietetic assessment and monitoring of children with special needs with faltering growth. British Dietetic Association Paediatric Group Professional Consensus Statement 2006.

21. Van den Berghe G. Dynamic neurodendocrine responses to critical illness. Front Neuroendocrinol 2002;23:370–91.

22. Fewtrell MS, Allgrove J, Gordon I, et al. Bone mineralization in children with epidermolysis bullosa. Br J Dermatol 2006;154:959–62.

23. Seshadri A, Shah A, Bhade S. Haematological response of anaemic pre-school children to ascorbic acid supplementation. Hum Nutr Appl Nutr 1985;39A:151–4.

24. Levene CI, Bates CJ. Ascorbic acid and collagen synthesis in cultured fibroblasts. Ann N Y Acad Sci 1975;258:288–305.

25. Hallberg L. Combating iron deficiency: daily administration of iron is far superior to weekly administration. Am J Clin Nutr 1998;68:213–7.

26. Beard JL. Weekly iron intervention: the case for intermittent iron supplementation. Am J Clin Nutr 1998; 68:209–12.

27. Haynes L, Atherton DJ, Clayden G. Constipation in epidermolysis bullosa: successful treatment with a liquid-fiber-containing formula. Pediatr Dermatol 1997;5:393–6.

28. Whittaker P. Iron and zinc interactions in humans. Am J Clin Nutr 1998;68(Suppl):442S–6S.

29. Walker CF, Kordas K, Stoltzfus RJ, et al. Interactive effects of iron and zinc on biochemical and functional outcomes in supplementation trials. Am J Clin Nutr 2005;82:5–12.

30. Halstead JA. Zinc deficiency in man, the Shiraz experiment. Am J Med 1972;53:277–84.

31. Shankar AH, Prasad AS. Zinc and immune function: the biological basis of altered resistance to infection. Am J Clin Nutr 1998;68(Suppl): 447S–63S.

32. Chandra RK. Excessive intake of zinc impairs immune responses. JAMA 1984;252:1443–6.

33. Walpir RA. Copper absorption and bioavailability. Am J Clin Nutr 1998;67(Suppl):1054S–60S.

34. Melville C, Atherton D, Burch M, et al. Fatal cardiomyopathy in dystrophic epidermolysis bullosa. Br J Dermatol 1996;135:603–6.

35. Sidwell RU, Yates R, Atherton D. Dilated cardiomyopathy in dystrophic epidermolysis bullosa. Arch Dis Child 2000;83:59–63.

36. Taibjee SM, Ramani P, Brown R, et al. Lethal cardiomyopathy in epidermolysis bullosa associated with amitryptiline. Arch Dis Child 2005;90: 871–2.

37. Soriano LF, Lage Vazquez MA, Maristany CP, et al. The effectiveness of oral nutritional supplementation in the healing of pressure ulcers. J Wound Care 2004;13:319–22.

38. Thompson C, Furhman MP. Nutrients and wound healing: still searching for the magic bullet. Nutr Clin Pract 2005;20:331–47.

39. Shenkin A. The key role of micronutrients. Clin Nutr 2006;25:1–13.

40. Williams CL, Bollela M, Wynder EL. A new recommendation for dietary fiber in childhood. Pediatrics 1995;96:985–8.

41. Douglas LC, Sanders ME. Probiotics and prebiotics in dietetics practice. J Am Diet Assoc 2008;108: 510–21.

42. Land MH, Rouster-Stevens K, Woods CR, et al. Experience and reason-briefly recorded. Lactobacillus sepsis associated with probiotic therapy. Pediatrics 2005;115:178–81.

43. Freeman E, Koglmeier J, Martinez A, et al. Gastrointestinal complications of epidermolysis bullosa in children. Br J Dermatol 2008;158(6):1308–14.

Oral Care and Dental Management for Patients with Epidermolysis Bullosa

Susanne M. Krämer, DDS, MSc SND[a,b,c,*]

KEYWORDS

- Epidermolysis bullosa • Dental • Oral
- Treatment • Management

The approach to dental treatment of patients with epidermolysis bullosa (EB), in particular for those with the more severe types, has changed dramatically during the last 30 years. Crawford and colleagues[1] in 1976 stated that extractions were the treatment of choice for patients with recessive dystrophic EB (RDEB). Two decades later, in 1999, Wright[2] declared that it was possible to manage dental abnormalities successfully with a combination of anesthetic and restorative techniques. Recently Skogedal and colleagues[3] showed that caries can be successfully prevented in patients with RDEB by continuous follow-up aimed at dietary advice, oral hygiene habits, frequent professional cleaning, and fluoride therapy. Thus, a preventive protocol is today's dental management approach of choice.[3,4]

Dental treatment is an important part of the multidisciplinary care of patients with EB, especially the severe types. Maintaining a functional dentition reduces the potential for oral and esophageal soft-tissue damage through more efficient mastication and favors nutrition.[5]

The only level of evidence available to support most recommendations is case reports and a few case series.

ACCESS TO DENTAL CARE

Access to dental care can be a challenge for some patients. Even although in most developed countries it is guaranteed, it is still a privilege for many patients around the world. There is a lack of familiarity with the disease in the dental profession and dental care can be complicated by the fears of the patient and the dentist.[6]

EARLY REFERRAL

Patients with EB should be referred to a dentist as early as possible to identify any related feature that needs special attention, for example generalized enamel hypoplasia. Whenever possible, patients should be managed by specialized dental services. This strategy enables dentists to start preventive programs and reduces the risk of developing dental diseases. Many case reports have shown that patients visit the dentist only when they already have several carious lesions or pain.[7–9] However, members of the multidisciplinary team should refer patients to the dentists before oral problems present, as early referral and close follow-up are the keys to maintain oral health.

TREATMENT MODIFICATIONS: PRECAUTIONS

Even although patients with milder oral involvement do not require many modifications to the treatment, a careful approach benefits every patient. Patients with the severe generalized RDEB subtype of EB require the most specific precautions during treatment to minimize soft-tissue damage.

[a] Department of Oral Medicine and Special Needs Dentistry, UCL Eastman Dental Institute, 256 Gray's Inn Road, London, WC1X 8LD, UK
[b] Division of Pediatric Dentistry, School of Dentistry, University of Chile, Calle Sergio Livingstone Pohlhammer 943, Independencia, Santiago, Chile
[c] DebRA Chile, Warren Smith 70 of. 101, Las Condes, Santiago, Chile
* Department of Oral Medicine and Special Needs Dentistry Unit, UCL Eastman Dental Institute, 256 Gray's Inn Road, London, WC1X 8LD, UK
E-mail address: s.kramer@eastman.ucl.ac.uk

Dermatol Clin 28 (2010) 303–309
doi:10.1016/j.det.2010.02.021
0733-8635/10/$ – see front matter © 2010 Elsevier Inc. All rights reserved.

EB Simplex

Most investigators agree that routine dental treatment can be provided for patients with EB simplex (EBS).[2,10] Clinicians should, however, assess history of mucosal fragility because manipulation can precipitate lesions in mildly affected patients.[2]

Junctional EB

Because there is minimal scarring, dental management of junctional EB (JEB) has been described as not requiring many modifications.[1] Mucosal and skin fragility, however, vary considerably between subtypes of JEB and patients. The avoidance of adhesive contact with the skin and careful manipulation are always advised. This group of patients require a special dental rehabilitation plan, as they present with generalized enamel hypoplasia (Fig. 1).

Dominant Dystrophic EB

Patients with dominant dystrophic EB (DDEB) can receive routine dental treatment with little or no modifications.[11] A report describes a patient wearing dentures for several years without difficulties.[1]

RDEB

As patients with severe generalized RDEB present with severe mucosal fragility, oral mucosa blistering, ankyloglossia, vestibule obliteration and microstomia; they require several treatment modifications and a careful approach to avoid as much tissue damage as possible. Ideally, the management of these patients requires a well-organized multidisciplinary team approach.[12,13]

- ◦ Lubrication: Lips, buccal mucosal, gloves, and instruments should always be lubricated before any procedure is performed to reduce adherence and formation of bullae and erosions. Vaseline, petroleum jelly, and

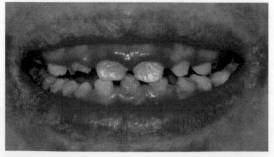

Fig. 1. Generalized enamel hypoplasia in a patient with Junctional EB.

hydrocortisone ointment have been used for this purpose.[2,4,12,14,15]

- ◦ Suction tip: Bullae formation or epithelium sloughing can occur on minimal contact with the suction tip.[4] It is suggested to lean the suction tip on hard tissue (ie, on tooth surface).
- ◦ Bullae: Blood- or fluid-filled bullae that occur during treatment need to be drained with a sterile needle or cut with scissors to avoid spreading.[10]
- ◦ Pressure: Extreme care of the fragile tissue in the patient with RDEB is important. To handle the tissues, a little pressure (compressive force) can be applied, but sliding movements (lateral traction or other shear forces) should be avoided, as these can cause tissue sloughing.[2,9]

Kindler Syndrome

A careful approach to Kindler syndrome is advised as blisters can form after dental treatment such as scaling.[16] The scarce literature available suggests periodontal health as a main area of concern for dental therapy.

ORAL BLISTERS

Only 1 study has been published on a therapeutic approach for oral blisters. Marini and Vecchiet[17] studied the effectiveness of sucralfate powder on the oral mucosa of 5 patients with DEB. They concluded that sucralfate seemed to be a cost-effective treatment to reduce oral blisters and discomfort.

CARIES PREVENTION

Although systemic treatment of EB remains primarily palliative, it is possible to prevent destruction and loss of dentition through appropriate interventions and dental therapy, even in the most severely affected patients with EB.[2] Skogedal and colleagues[3] presented a poster of successful caries prevention in 5 patients with RDEB, among whom after 10 to 13 years of continuous follow-up, only 1 presented with 2 caries and the other 4 were caries free. In 2 of these patients preventive extractions of second and third molars were performed as they were experiencing problems in performing oral hygiene because of reduced mouth opening.

Oral Hygiene

Concern is expressed by some patients, parents, and dentists regarding the use of tooth brushes and potential damage to the oral mucosa. Dentists have described that "preventive techniques, such as regular brushing, are too traumatic for these patients"[13] and several patients do not brush their teeth at all because of bullae formation.[18] However, tooth brushing is possible in all patients with EB, even in patients with the severe generalized RDEB subtype (Fig. 2). The following suggestions may help to find the appropriate tooth brush for each patient:

- Small head.[2,5,9]
- Soft bristles,[2,5,9,14] which can be further softened by soaking in warm water.[6]
- Short bristles may be needed in severe microstomia. For this purpose bristles can be cut.
- Special adaptations of the toothbrush handle can help patients with mitten deformities.
- Parents are advised to assist children to improve plaque removal and reduce tissue damage.

Adjuvant Therapies

Fluoride and chlorhexidine have been widely advised for oral disease prevention in patients with EB.[2,6,8,9,19] A variety of application methods have been used, including mouth washes, swabs, sprays, gels, and topical varnish. The gel has been said to have a better taste than mouth wash (and is therefore preferred).[9] Topical application of high-dose fluoride varnish each visit is preferred by some investigators.[2,19] For children living in non-fluoridated communities, daily fluoride supplements have been suggested.[6] The main concern in EB is that patients with oral lesions can be sensitive to flavoring agents, acids, and alcohol in dental preparations. Neutral, nonflavored, and alcohol-free formulations are advised.[5,6,9]

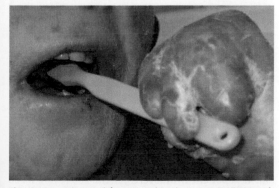

Fig. 2. A patient with generalized severe RDEB tooth brushing despite tissue fragility, microstomia, and mitten deformities on the hands.

Diet

The patients' diet can be an important factor in their increased risk of caries, as they usually choose soft, pureed, or liquid food to avoid mucosal damage,[1,4,8,14] and consume it in small amounts throughout the day.[20] They have a prolonged oral clearance time[6,19] and may be taking medicines that contain sugar.[14] A thoughtful dietary caries prevention program is important and should begin at an early age.[8,14] Suggestions to reduce prolonged oral clearance include increased fluid intake while eating[19] and rinsing with warm water during the day, especially after meals.[6] It is important that dentists and nutritionists work together on thoughtful programs for each patient, instead of giving confusing contradictory advice.

Fissure Sealants and Other Aids

Sealing fissures and fossae has been recommended, as oral hygiene and other preventive measures can be difficult to perform.[6,10] Fitting preformed stainless steel crowns has also been advised.[10]

DENTAL MANAGEMENT
Dental Radiograph

Panoramic radiographs can be taken in all cases. Periapical radiographs can also be taken, but care must be taken not to damage the mucosa.[9] In patients with severe generalized RDEB this technique has been proven to be difficult because of microstomia, ankyloglossia, and scarring of the sublingual area. Although lubrication of the film packet has been advised to avoid tissue damage, orthopantomography is probably the investigation of choice for most patients.

Restorations/Fillings

There are no contraindications to the use of any conventional dental material.[2] The only additional precaution is that all restorations and dentures should be carefully adapted and highly polished.[14] Restorative treatment can be difficult to perform in patients with RDEB because of the high incidence of microstomia, soft-tissue fragility, and complex anesthetic management.[21] Iatrogenic blisters can develop after treatment even if all precautions are in place.[10] Soft-tissue lesions resulting from restorative treatment typically heal in 1 to 2 weeks and require no specific treatment.

Endodontics/Root Canal Treatment

Nowak stated in 1988 that complex endodontic procedures were contraindicated because of the long operative time required and poor access to the mouth.[6] However, there are no reports in the literature of adverse events arising during or after endodontic therapy. In the author's experience 45 endodontic procedures in 9 patients with severe generalized RDEB have been uneventful, suggesting that there are no contraindications for these procedures, unless there is insufficient access because of limited mouth opening.

ORAL REHABILITATION
Removable Dentures

Tolerance to dentures depends on the degree of mucosal fragility of each patient and their EB subtype. Reports of successful tolerance of dentures include patients with EBS, JEB, DDEB, and pretibial RDEB.[1,10,22] For patients with other subtypes, however, removable prostheses may not be acceptable.[4] Overdentures have been described as a practical, economic, nonsurgical treatment option for patients with JEB and generalized hypoplastic enamel who present with failure of eruption.[22]

Fixed Rehabilitation

The use of stainless steel crowns has been reported as a successful approach in children with RDEB and JEB (**Fig. 3**).[1,2,10,18] Successful rehabilitation with fixed bridges has been reported in several patients with severe generalized RDEB.[9,14] Positive outcomes include aesthetic appearance improvement, behavioral changes, and improving feeding ability.[14] In cases with generalized enamel hypoplasia restoration of the entire dentition with full crowns may be necessary. This treatment needs to be planned and discussed with the parents and the patient, as it might consist of several stages until full permanent dentition has been established and restored.[23] Dental implants have been reported in

several patients with EB in recent years, and are an area of increasing interest.

Dental Implants

Successful rehabilitation using dental implants—root shaped titanium screws supporting dental restorations—has been reported in patients with generalized RDEB, non-Herlitz JEB, and RDEB inversa.[2,15] The most extensive report encompasses 38 dental implants with a success rate of 97.9% with a follow-up of 1 to 9 years (average 5.5 years). Peri-implant mucosa remained in good condition in all patients.[15] It has been reported that after rehabilitation patients improved their ability to chew and swallow, and had enhanced quality of life (**Fig. 4**).[15,24]

The results are encouraging and dental implants seemed to be a possible solution for edentulous patients with EB. Patients with RDEB and JEB have been shown to have lower bone mineral density scores than controls.[25] When planning this type of rehabilitation, advice from the medical team should be sought, as extensive surgery might need to be delayed or discouraged because of concomitant disease, such as severe anemia or poor prognosis squamous cell carcinoma.

IMPRESSION TAKING

Although there are no reports of any adverse events (ie, mucosal damage), impressions should be taken with special care. Microstomia can be a real challenge. As an alternative to stock

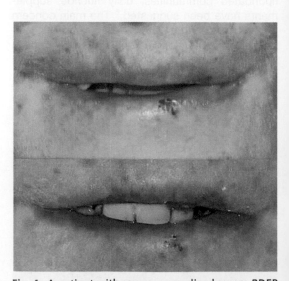

Fig. 4. A patient with severe generalized severe RDEB before and after rehabilitation with fixed crowns. This improved his esthetic appearance, but most of all his ability to eat.

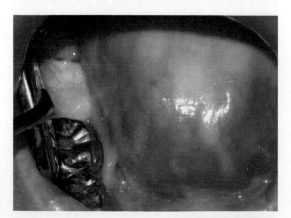

Fig. 3. Stainless steel crowns in a child with RDEB.

impression trays, specially cut topical gel application trays and custom-made acrylic trays have been proposed.[14]

PERIODONTAL TREATMENT

A gentle and careful scale and polish technique can be used in all patients with EB, including RDEB.[9] Lesions might develop, as they can occur after any dental procedure.

ANESTHETIC MANAGEMENT

Dental treatment of patients with EB can be provided under local anesthesia, conscious sedation, or general anesthesia. For patients with mild forms of EB and for small, atraumatic procedures, local anesthesia is the technique of choice. On the other hand, general anesthesia might be indicated for some extensive procedures in patients with severe forms of EB, but the support of an experienced team is crucial.

Local Anesthesia

Some investigators prefer local anesthesia, as it maintains airway patency and provides prolonged postoperative pain relief. Disadvantages are the development of iatrogenic blisters following local anesthesia injection.[9,10,14,26] To avoid blister formation, the anesthetic solution needs to be injected deeply into the tissues and at a slow rate, to avoid the liquid causing a mechanical separation of the tissue.[2,15] Examples of successful treatments provided under local anesthesia include multiple extractions, implants, endodontics, and restorations.[8,26]

General Anesthesia

Treatment under general anesthesia allows the provision of extensive reconstructive dental treatment and multiple extractions regardless of the severity of soft-tissue fragility and microstomia present.[2] When planning a procedure under general anesthesia, the patients' physician/general practitioner needs to be consulted and the availability of an anesthetic team with experience in EB is crucial. The patient's being asleep does not mean that the procedure is easy to perform. Patients with severe fragility still develop intraoperative generalized mucosal sloughing.[4] Oral surgery procedures can be combined with other surgical procedures, such as esophageal dilatation.[4]

SURGICAL EXTRACTIONS

When planning surgical extractions, especially if multiple extractions are needed, it is advised to consult the patient's physician as profound anemia could complicate the dental surgery.[13] An atraumatic technique should be used, making firm and safe mucosal incisions to prevent bullae formation.[6] Hemostasis can be obtained with gentle pressure with gauze packs.[18] There is no agreement in the literature about the use of sutures. Whereas some investigators have decided not to use them to prevent additional blister formation and mucosal tearing,[18] other investigators have used them without reporting any problems.[12] In this author's experience there are no problems related to the use of sutures.

Perioperative Complications

Despite attempts to use as gentle manipulation as possible and all the special precautions, mucosal sloughing and blister formation have been reported after almost every surgical extraction in patients with severe RDEB.[4,10,13,18] Blisters can be found at the angles of the mouth, lips, vestibule, tongue, and any sites of manipulation, some measuring up to 3 cm by 4 cm.[4,13]

Postoperative Complications

Despite the extensive mucosal damage during surgery, no postoperative complications have been reported in most cases of DEB and JEB.[13,27] Healing of the oral tissues occurs gradually after 1 to 2 weeks.[8,18] Healing of the alveolar sockets seems to be uneventful.[26] Postoperative antibiotics are not routinely required for these procedures as individuals with EB have a normal immune system.

ORTHODONTICS

Most patients with EB might be able to tolerate orthodontic treatment with only minor modifications designed to reduce soft-tissue irritation.[2] In patients with generalized severe RDEB, however, the regime more often reported in the literature is the use of serial extractions during the appropriate stage of dental development.[2,5] In severe dentoalveolar disproportions the removal of up to 8 teeth in the premolar area has resulted in reasonably good spontaneous alignment of teeth.[28]

REVIEW APPOINTMENTS

Frequent recall visits have shown to be useful in maintaining dental health in patients with EB.[7,26] There are examples of patients who previously had extensive carious teeth who remained caries free when attending frequent review appointments.[26] On the other hand, case reports have shown that patients who failed to attend the return visits developed several caries within 2 years, despite being given preventive programs.[8,9]

The review sessions should focus on caries prevention, professional plaque removal, topical fluoride application, and dietary advice.[7,10,19] The frequency of dental reviews should be scheduled according to the caries risk, usually every 3 to 6 months.[2,7,10,12]

As patients with RDEB have a higher risk of developing intraoral carcinoma (SSC), which increases with age, cancer screening is an important aspect of the review appointment in these patients.[11,19]

SUMMARY

There is evidence to support the effectiveness of preventive programs in preventing dental caries, even in patients with the most severe subtypes of EB. Oral hygiene, dietary advice, and close follow-up are the key factors. When oral disease does present, restoration of the teeth is important to guarantee function. All patients with EB can receive dental treatment, independent of the EB subtype. For those patients with severe subtypes a multidisciplinary approach is preferred.

REFERENCES

1. Crawford EG Jr, Burkes EJ Jr, Briggaman RA. Hereditary epidermolysis bullosa: oral manifestations and dental therapy. Oral Surg Oral Med Oral Pathol 1976;42(4):490–500.
2. Wright JT. Oral manifestations of epidermolysis bullosa. In: Fine JD, Bauer EA, McGuirre J, et al, editors. Epidermolysis bullosa. Clinical, epidemiologic, and laboratory advances and the findings of the National Epidermolysis Bullosa Registry. Baltimore (MD): The Johns Hopkins University Press; 1999. p. 236–56.
3. Skogedal N, Saltnes S, Storhaug K. Recessive dystrophic epidermolysis bullosa (RDEB) caries prevention and preventive extractions of molars. Clinical presentation of 3 cases. 3rd Scandinavian Conference on Epidermolysis Bullosa. Helsinki, Finland, April 24–25, 2008.
4. Stavropoulos F, Abramowicz S. Management of the oral surgery patient diagnosed with epidermolysis bullosa: report of 3 cases and review of the literature. J Oral Maxillofac Surg 2008;66(3):554–9.
5. Wright JT, Fine JD, Johnson L. Hereditary epidermolysis bullosa: oral manifestations and dental management. Pediatr Dent 1993;15(4):242–8.

6. Nowak AJ. Oropharyngeal lesions and their management in epidermolysis bullosa. Arch Dermatol 1988;124(5):742–5.
7. Momeni A, Pieper K. Junctional epidermolysis bullosa: a case report. Int J Paediatr Dent 2005;15(2):146–50.
8. Silva LC, Cruz RA, Abou-Id LR, et al. Clinical evaluation of patients with epidermolysis bullosa: review of the literature and case reports. Spec Care Dentist 2004;24(1):22–7.
9. Olsen CB, Bourke LF. Recessive dystrophic epidermolysis bullosa. Two case reports with 20-year follow-up. Aust Dent J 1997;42(1):1–7.
10. Serrano C, Silvestre FJ, Bagan JV, et al. [Hereditary epidermolysis bullosa. Dental management of three cases]. Med Oral 2001;6(1):48–56 [in Spanish].
11. Wright JT, Fine JD, Johnson LB. Oral soft tissues in hereditary epidermolysis bullosa. Oral Surg Oral Med Oral Pathol 1991;71(4):440–6.
12. Harel-Raviv M, Bernier S, Raviv E, et al. Oral epidermolysis bullosa in adults. Spec Care Dentist 1995; 15(4):144–8.
13. Album MM, Gaisin A, Lee KW, et al. Epidermolysis bullosa dystrophica polydysplastica. A case of anesthetic management in oral surgery. Oral Surg Oral Med Oral Pathol 1977;43(6):859–72.
14. Siqueira MA, de Souza SJ, Silva FW, et al. Dental treatment in a patient with epidermolysis bullosa. Spec Care Dentist 2008;28(3):92–5.
15. Penarrocha M, Larrazabal C, Balaguer J, et al. Restoration with implants in patients with recessive dystrophic epidermolysis bullosa and patient satisfaction with the implant-supported superstructure. Int J Oral Maxillofac Implants 2007; 22(4):651–5.
16. Wiebe CB, Silver JG, Larjava HS. Early-onset periodontitis associated with Weary-Kindler syndrome: a case report. J Periodontol 1996;67(10):1004–10.
17. Marini I, Vecchiet F. Sucralfate: a help during oral management in patients with epidermolysis bullosa. J Periodontol 2001;72(5):691–5.
18. Lindemeyer R, Wadenya R, Maxwell L. Dental and anaesthetic management of children with dystrophic epidermolysis bullosa. Int J Paediatr Dent 2009; 19(2):127–34.
19. Wright JT, Fine JD, Johnson L. Dental caries risk in hereditary epidermolysis bullosa. Pediatr Dent 1994;16(6):427–32.
20. Allman S, Haynes L, MacKinnon P, et al. Nutrition in dystrophic epidermolysis bullosa. Pediatr Dermatol 1992;9(3):231–8.
21. Wright JT. Epidermolysis bullosa: dental and anesthetic management of two cases. Oral Surg Oral Med Oral Pathol 1984;57(2):155–7.
22. Brooks JK, Bare LC, Davidson J, et al. Junctional epidermolysis bullosa associated with hypoplastic enamel and pervasive failure of tooth eruption: oral rehabilitation with use of an overdenture. Oral Surg

Oral Med Oral Pathol Oral Radiol Endod 2008; 105(4):e24–8.

23. Winter GB, Brook AH. Enamel hypoplasia and anomalies of the enamel. Dent Clin North Am 1975;19(1):3–24.

24. Lee H, Al Mardini M, Ercoli C, et al. Oral rehabilitation of a completely edentulous epidermolysis bullosa patient with an implant-supported prosthesis: a clinical report. J Prosthet Dent 2007;97(2):65–9.

25. Fewtrell MS, Allgrove J, Gordon I, et al. Bone mineralization in children with epidermolysis bullosa. Br J Dermatol 2006;154(5):959–62.

26. Finke C, Haas N, Czarnetzki BM. [Value of dental treatment in interdisciplinary management of a child with epidermolysis bullosa dystrophica hereditaria (Hallopeau-Siemens)]. Hautarzt 1996;47(4):307–10 [in German].

27. Carroll DL, Stephan MJ, Hays GL. Epidermolysis bullosa–review and report of case. J Am Dent Assoc 1983;107(5):749–51.

28. Shah H, McDonald F, Lucas V, et al. A cephalometric analysis of patients with recessive dystrophic epidermolysis bullosa. Angle Orthod 2002; 72(1):55–60.

Epidermolysis Bullosa: Management of Esophageal Strictures and Enteric Access by Gastrostomy

Alan E. Mortell, FRCSI, MD, Richard G. Azizkhan, MD, PhD*

KEYWORDS
- Epidermolysis bullosa • Nutritional failure
- Perioperative management • Esophageal stricture
- Hydrostatic balloon dilatation
- Percutaneous gastrostomy • Long-term outcomes

Epidermolysis bullosa (EB) is a spectrum of rare, inherited, blistering skin disorders, primarily affecting the skin and pharyngoesophageal mucosa.[1] EB affects approximately 2 to 4 per 100,000 children each year.[2] Blistering and scarring occur in response to even the most minor trauma. Broadly speaking, all forms of EB are affected by increased skin fragility and therefore a basic requirement of these children and young adults is satisfactory skin protection and management of wounds. Optimizing skin care can have a dramatic effect on a patient's quality of life and should be proactively managed by health care workers and the patient's family in conjunction with the patients themselves.

NUTRITIONAL FACTORS

Wound healing is promoted by several factors including adequate nutrition and a good tissue blood supply, which can be impaired by iron-deficiency anemia. The main indication for surgical intervention in children with EB is generally nutritional failure caused either by mechanical issues, such as esophageal strictures, or an inability to take in adequate calories to maintain an anabolic state in the face of increased metabolic demands placed on them by their skin disease and constant wound healing. Every patient with EB is different and their nutritional status can vary greatly depending on the type of EB and the extent of their disease. Nutritional deficits in recessive dystrophic epidermolysis bullosa (RDEB) frequently involve a vitamin and trace metal deficiency that may not always be corrected with enteral caloric supplementation.[3] Most patients have significant growth retardation, which can be improved with supplemental gastrostomy feedings but these patients may still have significant protein deficiency. Up to 77% of children with RDEB are at risk for significant malnutrition with 86% being underweight.[4] In contrast 57% of children with junctional epidermolysis bullosa (JEB) and 22% of those with epidermolysis bullosa simplex (EBS) are at risk for malnutrition. Most patients requiring surgical intervention in our institution have RDEB, with smaller numbers of patients with JEB and EBS presenting to our EB Center.

COMMON SURGICAL ISSUES IN EB

Apart from the devastating cutaneous manifestations of EB, several significant systemic and gastrointestinal complications occur.[5] These include lip and oral mucosal involvement with subsequent microstomia and ankyloglossia, which

Division of Pediatric and Thoracic Surgery, Epidermolysis Bullosa Treatment Center, Cincinnati Children's Hospital Medical Center, University of Cincinnati College of Medicine, MLC 3018, 3333 Burnet Avenue, Cincinnati, OH 45229-3039, USA
* Corresponding author.
E-mail address: Richard.Azizkhan@cchmc.org

Dermatol Clin 28 (2010) 311–318
doi:10.1016/j.det.2010.01.012

can make feeding and nutrition difficult and painful. By 12 years of age, more than 50% of patients with RDEB have significant microstomia and ankyloglossia.[6] These abnormalities must also be appreciated before any anesthetic intervention as their presence can make endotracheal intubation extremely challenging and in some cases a fiberoptic bronchoscopic intubation may be necessary to secure the airway for a general anesthetic.

The rapid cell turnover of the skin with concomitant chronic inflammation, repeated wound healing, and poor oral intake leads to a high metabolic demand on the patient with EB, who may already be in a malnourished state with associated chronic iron-deficiency anemia. This state also contributes to a range of nutritional deficits,[7,8] which must be addressed by the responsible clinicians to prolong and improve the quality of life of these fragile patients. Pharyngoesophageal strictures[9] are a common and very morbid complication occurring most commonly in children with RDEB (discussed in greater detail later in this article). Esophageal strictures result in dysphagia and/or odynaphagia with some extreme cases having difficulty swallowing their own saliva. Anorectal disease results in debilitating and painful strictures, which can worsen constipation, creating a vicious cycle of mucosal injury, inflammation, healing, and scarring. Every effort must be made to alleviate these distressing but manageable problems. These patients require support and appropriate intervention by a multidisciplinary team.[4]

ESOPHAGEAL DILATATION

Intensive nutritional support is often enough to maintain patients with EB in a metabolic status quo, however, esophageal dilatations should be performed when required and will enhance the patients ability to tolerate oral feeds. In our experience up to 80% of patients with RDEB will require esophageal dilatation for symptomatic strictures by age 25 years. In the past, patients who underwent esophageal dilatations for strictures had some form of bouginage performed blindly with tapered mercury-filled rubber Maloney dilators or serial Tucker dilators pulled through a gastrostomy with the aid of a string guide. Some modifications of these techniques involve the passage of an endoscope into the esophagus until the stricture is encountered and serial filiform dilators can then be passed through the tight stricture under direct visualization. These previously described techniques were associated with significant postoperative pain and extensive esophageal mucosal sloughing. In many cases, a prolonged period of recovery (7–10 days) was required before adequate

oral intake resumed. Due to the poor outcomes, these techniques have largely been replaced by hydrostatic balloon dilatation techniques. Endoscopic balloon dilatation of EB strictures is performed in many institutions with good outcomes reported.[10,11] Endoscopic-guided dilatation techniques all transmit some degree of shearing force to the mucosal lining of the esophagus potentially resulting in more mucosal blistering and sloughing with the end result of worsening strictures over time. In an attempt to reduce iatrogenic sheer stress esophageal injuries, the authors adopted nonendoscopic and image-guided hydrostatic balloon dilatation as our technique of choice in EB patients with symptomatic esophageal strictures. Theoretically, the advantages include a more specific anatomic identification of length and severity of the stricture(s), and the ability to use a larger balloon size with a fluoroscopic-guided technique than for balloons placed through endoscopes. Direct comparison of endoscopic and nonendoscopic dilatation techniques has not yet been performed to ascertain any differences in complications and outcomes. Duration of postoperative discomfort and recovery time to full oral diet for both techniques are claimed to be similar within a day or so after dilation.

GASTROSTOMY

Despite satisfactory esophageal dilatation, approximately 25% to 35% of patients will have significant failure to thrive and require supplemental feeding.[12] This can be achieved most effectively using a gastrostomy tube. Several approaches to gastrostomy insertion have been used in the past. The standard open approach with a Stamm gastrostomy is an excellent means of obtaining prompt secure access to enteral feeding and the authors advocate this approach in almost all children with EB up to the age of approximately 18 months. Most children presenting in this younger age group tend to have junctional EB (JEB) and the authors advocate an open gastrostomy for these children through a small upper midline incision. The other techniques commonly used for gastrostomy insertion include percutaneous endoscopic gastrostomy (PEG) or laparoscopic-assisted gastrostomy. Both of these procedures have their potential drawbacks in the context of patients with EB. Although PEG insertions are generally a safe and efficient means of obtaining gastric access in many surgeons' and gastroenterologists' hands, the fact that an endoscope must be used can contribute to inadvertent esophageal trauma. A theoretic negative aspect of laparoscopic-assisted gastrostomy is that peritoneal insufflation with gas distends the abdomen and may over stretch the overlying skin, and may result in severe blistering and widespread abdominal skin loss. The authors have adjusted our practice of gastrostomy insertion to take all of these factors into consideration and now use a nonendoscopic percutaneous gastrostomy (push technique) with excellent results in children greater than 2 years of age.

SURGICAL EXPERIENCE

In this article, the authors outline the potential management options for patients with EB complicated by feeding difficulties secondary to esophageal strictures as well as those with nutritional deficiencies requiring a gastrostomy tube for supplemental feeding (Fig. 1). The surgical experience of the senior author (RGA) is summarized in relation to all patients treated in Cincinnati Children's Hospital Medical Center (CCHMC) and 16 patients treated at Clinic Alemana, Santiago, Chile, with a diagnosis of EB over a 16-year period from 1993 to 2009 with esophageal strictures requiring balloon dilatation and those undergoing nonendoscopic percutaneous gastrostomy placement over a 7-year period from 2002 to 2009. These results represent our current standards of care and best practice, which have been developed and tailored to the specific needs of the EB patient population. The various methods and approaches that may be used to manage the potential complications that may arise during or after these interventions are also discussed. These techniques are easily reproducible but require a repertoire of medical, surgical, and radiological skills and strategies to reduce the risk of long-term adverse sequelae.

FLUOROSCOPICALLY GUIDED BALLOON DILATATION OF ESOPHAGEAL STRICTURES

All EB patients undergo a thorough initial medical and nutritional assessment by our multidisciplinary team of pediatric specialists. Patients presenting with dysphagia, nutritional deficiency, or poor weight gain have a contrast esophagogram performed to assess the status of their esophagus and the presence and number of strictures. Initial dilatations are only performed because of a radiologically confirmed esophageal stricture. It is vital to include the pharyngoesophageal junction in the study, as many patients with RDEB can have a high cervical esophageal stricture that could be missed on a routine esophagogram (Fig. 2). A barium esophagogram will delineate the number, level, and severity of the strictures and will facilitate the approach to planning the dilatation. The study should incorporate frontal and lateral projections and must assess the entire esophagus from the oropharynx to the gastroesophageal junction. The proximal cervical esophagus is a common location for strictures in EB patients and can be

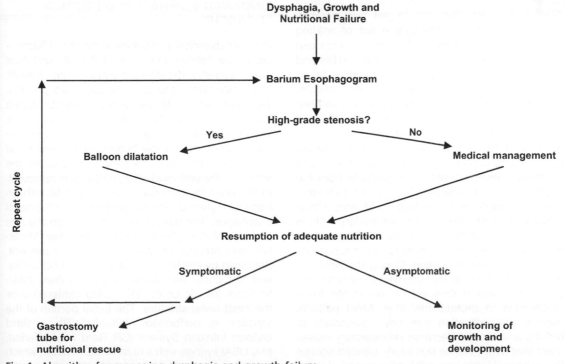

Fig. 1. Algorithm for managing dysphagia and growth failure.

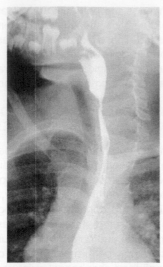

Fig. 2. Barium esophagogram demonstrating a significant esophageal stenosis at C3 and a second stricture at T1.

easily overlooked. An important consideration is the balloon diameter to be used and this can be gauged by the size of the patient's native esophagus and the degree of the stricture to be dilated.

PERIOPERATIVE CARE

The importance of safe anesthesia and airway protection during esophageal dilatation in the EB patient is critical for several reasons.[13] Intensive preoperative planning and diligent perioperative care are essential.[14] The simple act of holding and sealing a facemask on the patients face can cause major skin damage under the mandible and around the mouth and great care must be taken to lubricate all gloves, masks, and instruments, including the laryngoscope blade, with Aquaphor ointment (Beiersdorf Inc, Wilton, CT, USA) or a similar lubricant to prevent skin and mucosal blistering and sloughing. The authors preferentially perform endotracheal intubation for esophageal dilatations when possible. This protects from the potential risk of aspiration as well as providing optimal conditions for balloon dilatation. Other additional challenges to oral intubation include inward angling of the teeth, a scarred tongue, and microstomia. All of these factors may necessitate an oral fiberoptic intubation. During the patients' transition to the operative/interventional radiology suite, they are maintained on egg-crate foam mattresses to protect their skin. Most patients receive premedication with oral midazolam to reduce anxiety and decrease unnecessary movement that might induce skin injury. Limited access to peripheral intravenous (IV) sites can hinder the

induction of anesthesia and therefore patients are usually induced by mask with inhalation anesthetics. If gaining peripheral IV access is difficult, we use ultrasound guidance and interventional radiology to facilitate IV placement. The skin must be protected from tourniquet and blood pressure cuff application by the placement of layers of gauze or Webril (Tyco Healthcare, Mansfield, MA, USA) on the skin initially. IV lines should be secured with an atraumatic soft silicone adhesive dressing, such as Mepitac (Mölnlycke Healthcare, Göteburg, Sweden) and gently wrapped with Webril (Tyco Healthcare, Mansfield, MA, USA) and Coban wrap (3M, St Paul, MN, USA). The endotracheal tube is secured with lubricated cotton tape tied to the tube and placed behind the patients' neck after a protective layer of Mepilex or Mepilex Lite (Mölnlycke Healthcare, Göteburg, Sweden) has been placed on the skin to avoid traction or shearing forces of the tape on the skin. The eyes are lubricated and covered with saline moistened gauze or taped closed with atraumatic Mepitac tape (Mölnlycke Healthcare, Göteburg, Sweden). The adhesive pulse oximeter probe that is commonly used in pediatric anesthesia is exchanged for a clip-type probe, which can be placed on the ear lobe. Alternatively the adhesive can be removed from the probe and it can be secured in place by using the thin malleable metal strip commonly found in the nosepiece of a surgical facemask.

CINCINNATI ESOPHAGEAL DILATATION TECHNIQUE

In the interventional radiology suite, using fluoroscopy, we initially place an 8-French umbilical artery catheter (Boston Scientific Corp, Natick, MA, USA) transorally into the upper esophagus. We then pass a flexible soft-tip Benson (Cook Inc, Bloomington, IN, USA) 0.035-in guidewire into the stomach through the catheter. This procedure is performed under fluoroscopic control and once the guidewire is confirmed to lie within the stomach, the umbilical artery catheter is removed. At this point the high-pressure hydrostatic balloon catheter is placed over the guidewire into the distal esophagus. The balloon size depends on the age and size of the patient as well as the characteristics and number of strictures that are present. We begin by inflating the balloon with a 50% dilution of Optiray 240 water-soluble contrast (Mallinckrodt Inc, St Louis, MO, USA) centered over the most distal stricture. The initial portion of the injection is performed manually with a Bard Balloon Inflation System (CR Bard Inc, Billerica, MA, USA) syringe with a built-in manometer, which is subsequently locked and the handle turned clockwise to apply a gradual increase in balloon pressure up to a pressure of no more than 2 atmospheres at a time. The pressure applied must be kept less than the stated balloon burst pressure at all times. Simultaneous fluoroscopy allows visualization of the stricture/s and their gradual effacement as dilatation progresses (**Fig. 3**). It is important to place the center of the balloon at the midpoint of the stricture to prevent migration of the balloon with resultant shearing forces being applied to the esophageal mucosa. This is also achieved by applying gentle traction to the balloon catheter during balloon inflation. The balloon is left inflated for up to 30 seconds before deflation and repositioning to deal with any other more proximal strictures. If a small amount of contrast is left within the balloon, this can facilitate the identification of further strictures within the esophagus as a waist or narrowing can clearly be seen on pulling the balloon back. We believe it is important to perform this esophageal-mapping maneuver up to and including the pharyngoesophageal junction to avoid missing high strictures commonly found in RDEB, which may not have been picked up on a routine contrast esophagogram. We then replace the balloon catheter with the previously used umbilical artery catheter over the guidewire with the purpose of performing a limited contrast esophagogram. This procedure can help confirm satisfactory patency of the esophageal lumen after dilatation and also rules out esophageal perforation. For this purpose, we use standard Optiray 240 injected through the umbilical artery catheter as it is withdrawn from distal to proximal during fluoroscopy. Any residual contrast is then aspirated from the esophagus to reduce the risk of contrast aspiration postoperatively.

Postoperative Management

Once patients are safely recovered and awake, they are commenced on a clear liquid diet followed by a mechanical soft diet. Patients undergoing dilatation for the first time are usually admitted overnight for observation and discharged home the following day. Those who have previously undergone dilatation at our institution are discharged within 8 hours. Since 2001 we have routinely administered peri- and postoperative steroids in an attempt to potentially delay recurrent stenoses. We administer 0.5 mg/kg of dexamethasone with a maximum dose of 12 mg intravenously at induction followed by a 5-day taper dose of liquid prednisolone starting at 1 mg/kg. We also prescribe a concomitant proton pump inhibitor to reduce the effects of gastroesophageal reflux.

Outcomes

More than 400 hydrostatic balloon dilatations were performed on 126 patients with RDEB over a 16-year period between 1993 and 2009. The mean age at first procedure was 10 ± 8 years (range 1.5–41 years). Seventy-five (60%) patients had a solitary stricture with most (87%) of these found

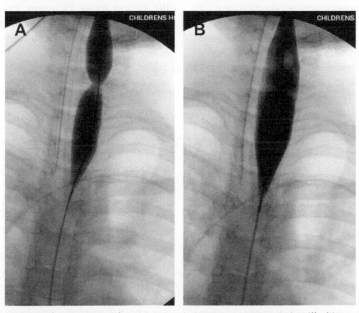

Fig. 3. (*A*) Cervical esophageal stricture with narrow waist seen as contrast is instilled into the balloon port. (*B*) Total effacement of the stricture with full insufflation of the balloon.

in the proximal esophagus. Thirty-five patients (28%) had 2 strictures and the remaining patients had 3 or more strictures each. Balloon diameter varied from 12 to 22 mm, with a median diameter of 18 mm. We performed an average of 4 procedures per patient, however, the number of procedures ranged from 1 to 14. Eight of the patients with high-grade stenoses underwent retrograde esophageal dilatations through their previously placed gastrostomy. Most patients obtained immediate relief of their symptoms with the ability to resume normal diet within 24 hours of the procedure and virtually all had significant weight gain noted at 4 to 6 weeks after dilatation. The mean interval between dilatations was 1 year, with a range of 1.5 months to 6 years. The median follow-up time was 5 years (range 1–13 years). Using this technique, the authors have not seen any dilatation-related esophageal perforations. Two patients, who had concomitant dental procedures performed under the same anesthetic developed aspiration postoperatively requiring antibiotics and intensive respiratory therapy. They both made a satisfactory recovery.

NONENDOSCOPIC PERCUTANEOUS GASTROSTOMY PLACEMENT

All patients undergo a preoperative assessment with a contrast esophagogram and upper gastrointestinal series to look for esophageal strictures along with the size and orientation of the stomach. Those patients who are found to have microgastria or a high-lying stomach are deemed unsuitable for a percutaneous nonendoscopic gastrostomy. In this patient group alternative methods of gastrostomy placement are considered. The anesthetic precautions are the same as previously mentioned with great care taken to avoid any undue trauma to the patient's skin and mucous membranes. To minimize exposure to ionizing radiation, patients and operating staff are shielded and the x-ray beam is collimated to screen only the relevant area of interest. At the same time, only the lowest dose of radiation is used to adequately define the anatomy required for dilatation. This dose is generally less than for most other diagnostic fluoroscopic studies.

PERCUTANEOUS GASTROSTOMY TECHNIQUE

The edges of the liver and spleen are mapped out with ultrasound and lightly marked on the patient's skin with a surgical marker. The transverse and descending colon are outlined by the instillation of 100 to 150 mL of dilute water-soluble contrast via a rectal catheter under fluoroscopic control.

An 8-French umbilical catheter is then passed through the oropharynx into the stomach and 100 to 150 mL of air is insufflated to radiographically delineate the stomach. Before gastric insufflation, 0.1 mg of glucagon is administered intravenously to provoke pylorospasm, thereby reducing the amount of air passing into the duodenum during the procedure. The procedure is facilitated by the availability of anteroposterior and cross-table fluoroscopic guidance for gastrostomy tube placement (**Fig. 4**). Three or 4 needle-mounted T-fasteners are percutaneously passed into the air-filled stomach in a triangular configuration to pull the stomach up against the anterior abdominal wall. The stomach is then percutaneously cannulated with a needle through the midpoint of the T-fasteners. A small amount of water-soluble contrast is injected through the needle to confirm that it is intragastric in position. A guidewire is then inserted through the cannula and the tract is then serially dilated over the wire up to 16- to 20-French depending on the size of the gastrostomy tube to be placed. The 16- to 20-French peel-away introducer sheath is then placed over the guidewire in preparation for the gastrostomy tube. A 14- to 18-French MIC gastrostomy tube with external rubber flange is inserted through the sheath and the balloon is inflated with sterile water. The T-fasteners are then tied down to anchor the gastrostomy tube flange to the abdominal wall after each 3/0 nylon suture (mounted to the T-fastener) has been passed through a layer of Mepilex (Mölnlycke Healthcare, Göteburg, Sweden), dental roll, and the holes in the flange to lie between the patients skin and the flange. This avoids placing skin sutures and anchors the entire gastrostomy system to the abdominal wall. A silk tie is then placed around a groove in the rubber flange to prevent the tube and balloon slipping inwards.

Postoperative Management

Gastrostomy feeds are commenced the following morning after the tube has been left to drain to a Farrell bag reservoir (Corpak Medsystems Inc, Wheeling, IL, USA) overnight. Patients are then discharged after 48 to 72 hours when established on an enteral feeding regimen. The T-fasteners are left in place for 10 to 12 weeks. To remove them, a slight amount of traction is placed on the T-fastener which is then cut flush with the skin. At the same time, the gastrostomy tube is replaced with a low-profile button gastrostomy. The gastrostomy stoma can be dressed with a small piece of cut Mepilex between the button gastrostomy and the patient's skin.

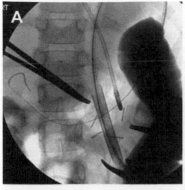
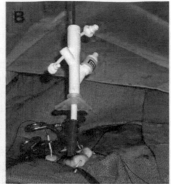
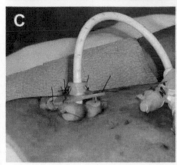
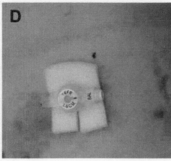

Fig. 4. (*A*) Fluoroscopic image of abdomen during percutaneous gastrostomy placement. Water-soluble contrast is seen within the transverse colon. Four T-fasteners have been positioned to pull the stomach against the abdominal wall. A percutaneously placed guidewire and sheath are seen within the stomach. (*B*) Placement of the 16F gastrostomy tube through the sheath. The T-fasteners on the abdominal wall are anchored through soft dental rolls and Mepilex. (*C*) Gastrostomy in place with flange attached to the T-fasteners and dental rolls. (*D*) Gastrostomy tube is replaced with a low-profile button gastrostomy 10 weeks later.

Outcomes

Eight patients (6 girls and 2 boys, ranging from 6 to 9 years of age) with RDEB and associated nutritional failure were managed with a percutaneous nonendoscopic gastrostomy tube. All of these patients had previously undergone multiple dilatations for esophageal strictures and every effort had been made to optimize their nutritional status with maximal caloric intake. Despite these measures, they had persistent growth failure and a decision was made to proceed to gastrostomy tube placement. All patients tolerated the procedure well and no perioperative complications were encountered. All 8 patients tolerated feeds commenced on postoperative day 1 and all had successful gastrostomy button placement at 10 to 12 weeks postoperatively. Two of the 8 patients (25%) had subsequent retrograde esophageal dilatation performed through the gastrostomy without difficulty. Average follow-up in this series was 24 months (range 3–58 months) and all patients have shown significant gains in weight and height.[12] In addition, parents have noted higher energy and activity levels among the children with less severe blistering and more rapid wound healing than was noted before the gastrostomy.

DISCUSSION

The spectrum of EB treated in our institution broadly reflects the known distribution of the various subtypes, with RDEB comprising most patients presenting to us for management of esophageal strictures. Our experience with fluoroscopically guided balloon dilatation in the challenging condition of EB has shown it to be a safe, gentle, effective, repeatable, and minimally invasive technique with great benefits for the patients and their families. Rapid relief of symptoms with significant improvements in quality of life following esophageal balloon dilatation and after percutaneous nonendoscopic gastrostomy insertion have been reported. This latter technique for providing a secure means of delivering enteral nutrition to EB patients is a safe, effective, and minimally invasive alternative to a commonly performed procedure. Based on our experience, it decreases the potential risk of complications and analgesic requirements compared with the endoscopic approach. Although a PEG is a minimally invasive procedure for many children, the pharyngoesophageal trauma resulting in severe blistering associated with endoscope passage in an EB patient makes it a less than ideal procedure. The degree of discomfort reported after previous endoscopic procedures compared with our current strategy leads us to conclude that the techniques we have described should be used as the first-line treatment option in children with EB. We recommend that endoscopic procedures in this patient population should be avoided or minimized if at all possible. Despite being a versatile instrument, the endoscope has certain limitations, such as the size of the balloons capable of fitting through the scope. Fluoroscopic balloon dilatation achieves a greater diameter of dilatation, thus allowing longer intervals between procedures. The benefits of minimally invasive laparoscopic gastrostomy placement are apparent in patients who do not have EB. However, the consequences of peritoneal insufflation in a child with EB can be devastating with the abdominal skin blistering and sloughing away as a result of distension.

The risks of repeated radiation exposure in patients with EB subjected to frequent dilatations must be balanced against the quality of life achieved from this intervention. This is particularly relevant because of the increased risk of squamous cell skin carcinoma in patients with EB[15] and this prompts us to adhere to strict radiation protection methods at every procedure and to be vigilant for any early sign of malignancy in all patients. A team comprised of pediatric surgeons and pediatric interventional radiologists generally performs the techniques outlined in this article; however, either specialty can safely perform the procedures with adequate training and have the ability to adapt the techniques to each patient's unique anatomy and physiology. Our aim, as clinicians and as an institution, is to provide the best possible care to patients with EB with the ultimate goal of improving their overall quality of life.

REFERENCES

1. Mellerio JE. Molecular pathology of the cutaneous basement membrane zone. Clin Exp Dermatol 1999;24(1):25–32.
2. Wolff K, Goldsmith L, Katz SI, et al. Fitzpatrick's dermatology in general medicine. 7th edition. New York: McGraw-Hill; 2008.
3. Ingen-Housz-Oro S, Blanchet-Bardon C, Vrillat M, et al. Vitamin and trace metal levels in recessive dystrophic epidermolysis bullosa. J Eur Acad Dermatol Venereol 2004;18(6):649–53.
4. Birge K. Nutrition management of patients with epidermolysis bullosa. J Am Diet Assoc 1995;95(5):575–9.
5. Johnston DE, Koehler RE, Balfe DM. Clinical manifestations of epidermolysis bullosa dystrophica. Dig Dis Sci 1981;26(12):1144–9.
6. Fine J-D, Bauer EA, Gedde-Dahl T Jr. Inherited epidermolysis bullosa: definition and historical overview. In: Fine J-D, Bauer EA, McGuire J, et al, editors. Epidermolysis bullosa: clinical, epidemiologic, and laboratory advances and the findings of the National Epidermolysis Bullosa Registry. Baltimore (MD): The Johns Hopkins University Press; 1999. p. 1–19.
7. Allman S, Haynes L, MacKinnon P, et al. Nutrition in dystrophic epidermolysis bullosa. Pediatr Dermatol 1992;9(3):231–8.
8. Mellerio JE, Weiner M, Denyer JE, et al. Medical management of epidermolysis bullosa: Proceedings of the IInd International Symposium on Epidermolysis Bullosa, Santiago, Chile, 2005. Int J Dermatol 2007;46(8):795–800.
9. Pfendner EG, Bruckner A, Conget P, et al. Basic science of epidermolysis bullosa and diagnostic and molecular characterization: Proceedings of the IInd International Symposium on Epidermolysis Bullosa, Santiago, Chile, 2005. Int J Dermatol 2007;46(8):781–94.
10. Castillo RO, Davies YK, Lin YC, et al. Management of esophageal strictures in children with recessive dystrophic epidermolysis bullosa. J Pediatr Gastroenterol Nutr 2002;34(5):535–41.
11. Anderson SH, Meenan J, Williams KN, et al. Efficacy and safety of endoscopic dilation of esophageal strictures in epidermolysis bullosa. Gastrointest Endosc 2004;59(1):28–32.
12. Stehr W, Farrell MK, Lucky AW, et al. Non-endoscopic percutaneous gastrostomy placement in children with recessive dystrophic epidermolysis bullosa. Pediatr Surg Int 2008;24(3):349–54.
13. Iohom G, Lyons B. Anaesthesia for children with epidermolysis bullosa: a review of 20 years' experience. Eur J Anaesthesiol 2001;18(11):745–54.
14. Lin YC, Golianu B. Anesthesia and pain management for pediatric patients with dystrophic epidermolysis bullosa. J Clin Anesth 2006;18(4):268–71.
15. Mallipeddi R. Epidermolysis bullosa and cancer. Clin Exp Dermatol 2002;27(8):616–23.

Anesthesia and Epidermolysis Bullosa

Reema Nandi, MD, FRCA*,
Richard Howard, BSc, MB, ChB, FRCA, FFPMRCA

KEYWORDS

- Epidermolysis bullosa • Anesthesia • Analgesia
- Airway management

Patients with epidermolysis bullosa (EB) may present for anesthesia with an unrelated surgical condition or, more commonly, for diagnostic or therapeutic procedures. Children in particular may require frequent anesthetics. Safe and effective management of anesthesia presents a significant challenge and although there is little rigorous evidence available to aid decision-making, in this article the elements of current good anesthesia care in EB are summarized.

MANAGEMENT OF ANESTHESIA

The primary concerns during anesthesia are maintenance of skin and mucous membrane integrity, safe airway management, prevention of heat and fluid loss, and the provision of effective perioperative analgesia. Several case series have demonstrated that these can be achieved by thorough planning, good communication between clinical teams, and meticulous attention to detail.[1,2] Treatment of patients with EB in specialized units is optimal as it allows accumulation of knowledge and experience by multidisciplinary teams and education of staff, and facilitates implementation of checklists and protocols to guide care. However, if patients require anesthesia outside such centers, whenever possible personnel with the relevant knowledge and experience should be consulted as part of the planning process. The authors recommend that institutions have the necessary policies and protocols in place, however rarely they may expect to manage such patients.

CARE OF THE SKIN AND MUCOUS MEMBRANES

Maintenance of skin and mucosal membrane integrity is of great importance as new bulla formation results in painful wounds, heat and fluid loss, and the risk of secondary infection. Subsequent healing can lead to scarring and deformity resulting in further, sometimes life-threatening, complications. Trauma from friction and shearing forces are largely responsible for new bullae and wound formation, rather than direct pressure, and therefore they should be avoided or reduced as much as possible during anesthesia, surgery, and other procedures.[3] Patients with EB requiring surgical treatment should optimally be admitted to a dermatology ward and their care shared jointly between surgery and dermatology staff. Any special dressings, skin care treatments, and lubricants that are being used should be made available in the operating and procedure room and, as these items are constantly improved and updated, instructions, protocols, and supplies in these areas should be regularly reviewed. Uncertainty about the most reliable and appropriate method for fixation of essential devices such as intravenous, arterial, or central venous lines is best resolved by discussion between teams and planning before surgery. **Table 1** is a checklist of recommended or useful items and

Department of Anesthesia, Great Ormond Street Hospital for Children, London WC1N 3JH, UK
* Corresponding author.
E-mail address: reema.nandi@r2x.com

Dermatol Clin 28 (2010) 319–324
doi:10.1016/j.det.2010.01.011

derm.theclinics.com

Table 1
Checklist of items that are recommended, useful, or to be avoided

Recommended or Useful	To be Avoided
Lubrication of equipment such as laryngoscopes, endotracheal and nasogastric tubes	Friction or any self-adhesives applied directly to the skin
Specialized dressings and tapes that do not cause friction when applied or removed, eg, Mepiform and Mepitel	Regular adhesive tape, except if applied indirectly and never to skin
Petroleum jelly impregnated gauze	Adhesive pulse oximeter probes
Soft cotton gamgee padding	Adhesive ECG electrodes
Clear PVC film wrap	Adhesive electrocautery electrodes
Lubricants: water soluble and petroleum jelly	Adhesive temperature probes
Clip-on pulse oximeter probe	Patslide or other devices causing friction
Eye gelpad	Hard plastic oxygen masks with sharp edges
Gel or soft foam padding for pressure areas	
Bipolar or dry electrocautery electrodes	Rigid nasogastric tubes

Abbreviations: ECG, electrocardiograph; PVC, polyvinyl chloride.

others, frequently encountered in operating rooms, which are to be avoided.

PREOPERATIVE ASSESSMENT

Preoperative assessment forms the basis for perioperative planning. This assessment should take place well in advance of surgery, and is ideally undertaken by the anesthetist who will be present at the procedure. As this is not always possible, thorough protocols for safe and effective management of EB should be in place so that adequate preparation can be made. In the usual way the physical status of the patient, their preferences, and the requirements determined by the procedure to be undertaken are considerations to be synthesized in order to formulate a suitable plan of anesthesia. Some of the most frequent procedures undergone by patients with EB are listed in **Table 2**. Anesthesia risk assessment is often much more complex in this group of patients as

Table 2
Frequent procedures in EB

Change of dressing
Skin biopsy
Dental surgery: dental extraction and conservation
Ophthalmic surgery
Plastic surgery: repair of pseudosyndactyly, surgery to contractures, excision squamous cell carcinoma, skin grafting
General surgery: esophagoscopy and dilatation, gastrostomy, fundoplication

the consequences of anesthesia procedures commonly considered to be "routine," such as endotracheal intubation or regional anesthesia, may carry greater or unknown additional risks.

Management of the airway and assessment of potential airway compromise during anesthesia or sedation are a central component of preoperative assessment. Personal experience, good communication between clinical teams, and a flexible and pragmatic approach to decision-making are likely to be important determinants of the outcome. Possible techniques include local or regional anesthesia, with or without sedation or general anesthesia; and inhalation general anesthesia or total intravenous anesthesia, with or without endotracheal intubation or a laryngeal mask airway (LMA). Cooperative adults are much more likely to tolerate awake or minimal sedation techniques, although the use of continuous spinal epidural (CSE) with sedation in a 6-year-old boy with EB has been described.[4]

Postoperative analgesia is also planned at this time and is discussed with the patient and family. Resumption of oral intake may be relatively delayed in comparison with unaffected patients, especially if endotracheal intubation or other oropharyngeal instrumentation has been used so that intravenous analgesia may be needed. There should also be a full and frank discussion with the patient and family regarding any anticipated risks and possible complications of anesthesia.

MEDICAL HISTORY

A history of oropharyngeal bullae should be sought and all previous anesthesia records reviewed; the patient's previous experiences of anesthesia are especially helpful. EB subtype is important and relevant to airway management: Endotracheal intubation can be performed in patients with the recessive dystrophic type of EB without laryngeal bullae formation, postoperative stridor, or airway obstruction. However, the safety of endotracheal tube placement is not so well documented in patients with junctional EB (JEB), in which the respiratory columnar epithelium can be significantly involved. Infants and children with JEB are known to have a cumulative risk of 39.8% of tracheolaryngeal stenosis or stricture, and require routine surveillance by a pediatric otolaryngologist. The presence of gastroesophageal reflux, renal, and cardiac complications must also be considered (Table 3). Muscular dystrophy is rare but associated with EB simplex;, a history of progressive muscle weakness is suggestive.[5] Intercurrent drug therapy must also be sought, as a recent course of steroids may have perioperative implications.

PHYSICAL EXAMINATION AND INVESTIGATIONS

Airway assessment must be thorough. Recurrent oral blistering may lead to obliteration of the vestibule, ankyloglossia, and microstomia. Difficult

Table 3
Complications associated with EB relevant to anesthesia

Acute	Chronic
Pain	Pain
Fluid loss	Feeding difficulties and failure to thrive
Heat loss	Anemia
Severe pruritus	Dental decay and periodontal disease
Secondary bacterial infection	Constipation
	Ophthalmic disease
	Scarring and contracture formation
	Difficulties in mobility
	Osteopenia
	Stridor
	Renal dysfunction
	Cardiomyopathy
	Squamous cell carcinoma
	Depression

intubation due to limited mouth opening and jaw movement, poor dentition, and difficulty in positioning for laryngoscopy secondary to contractures can occur. Defective enamel, poor oral clearance of foods, and inability to achieve adequate oral hygiene often leads to periodontal disease and extensive dental decay. Therefore the dentition should be examined and the position, security, and viability of the teeth considered.

Venous access should be assessed; this is not usually difficult as veins are often clearly visible. However, the securing of intravenous devices is made much easier if a suitable site is identified. Investigations to determine the extent of intercurrent anemia and renal or cardiac dysfunction may be necessary.

PREMEDICATION

Sedative premedication using for example, 0.5 mg/kg midazolam 45 minutes before anesthesia, is useful in younger children to reduce restlessness, particularly during inhalational induction of general anesthesia. In adults, sedation before general anesthesia is usually not necessary. Excessive salivation can occur so an oral antisialogogue, such as atropine or glycopyrrolate, is sometimes useful. If there is a history of reflux, regurgitation, or a proven esophageal stricture, antacid prophylaxis, for example, Na citrate, should be used.

Local anesthetic creams such as EMLA (lidocaine-prilocaine) or Ametop (amethocaine) are usually used to provide local anesthesia of the skin before intravenous cannulation in children; they can be applied preoperatively using a polyvinyl chloride (PVC) film covering rather than self-adhesive transparent dressings. If opioids are to be given as part of anesthesia or postoperative analgesia, antiemetic or antipruritic agents can also be given at this time or on induction. Patients on long-term corticosteroid therapy are usually prescribed perioperative hydrocortisone.

MONITORING DURING ANESTHESIA

Monitoring can be difficult because many standard probes and monitor electrodes are self-adhesive or cause friction in use or when removed. As they can potentially damage the skin or not function correctly, compliance with recommended monitoring standards is a significant problem. Oxygen saturation can be measured using a "clip-on" rather than adhesive probe. Self-adhesive probes can be applied to a digit that is protected with PVC film or the cut-off digit of a surgical glove if there is no alternative. Self-adhesive electrocardiograph electrodes should not be applied directly to the skin but can be modified in several ways, for example, the adhesive surface can be placed onto electro-conducting gel defibrillator pads, which are then placed directly onto the skin. The defibrillation pads are not adhesive so if the leads are inadvertently pulled, they simply slide off the pads or the pads lift off the skin; it is important to ensure that such "stray" electrodes do not then stick to skin. Noninvasive blood pressure may be measured by conventional means if friction from inflating and deflating sphygmomanometer cuffs is reduced by covering the underlying skin with, for example, PVC film or cotton padding. The same method may be used if a tourniquet is needed for surgery. Nasopharyngeal and rectal temperature probes should be used with extreme care or avoided.

AIRWAY MANAGEMENT

Airway management can be the most challenging aspect of anesthesia. Difficulties may arise because standard techniques for airway control, for example, firm face mask application, oro- or nasopharyngeal airway insertion, or mandibular thrust, easily cause damage to skin, lips, tongue, and mucous membranes. When endotracheal intubation is indicated the anesthetist should always be prepared for difficult intubation in these patients.[6] One series reported only 7 new bullae after 390 general anesthetics, half of which were associated with difficult intubation. One patient required tracheostomy after awake fiberoptic intubation, which remained blister-free and was used on 3 further occasions. An intubation rate of 64.8% in 54 general anesthetics in 16 children has also been reported, 2 of which were difficult (although possible without the use of the fiber-scope). In another report 48% of 25 patients undergoing 121 procedures were intubated.[2] In 64 cases oral tracheal intubation using direct laryngoscopy was performed without difficulty, and in 3 patients fiberoptic tracheal intubation was required due to limited mouth opening and contractures in the neck.

Blind nasal intubation has been advocated by some groups[1,7] and has not been recommended by others.[8] Although intubation may be difficult, it is usually straightforward in maintaining a clear airway, as the tongue is often small and scarred and does not fall back into the pharynx. Despite this, endotracheal intubation is often the preferred method of airway management as it is secure and avoids excessive manipulation. A cuffed endotracheal tube (ETT) half to one size smaller than predicted by standard formulas should be used: the cuff should be inflated gently and maintained at

low pressure. If unhindered surgical access to the oral cavity is required, a nasoendotracheal tube can be placed. Once in position, the ETT should be secured in a manner that does not cause lip or skin damage. Lips are lined with lubricated gauze where they touch the ETT and also beneath the tie to prevent chafing. At the end of the operation pharyngeal suctioning should only be performed under direct vision, taking care not to apply the tip of the sucker directly on to the mucosa. The pharynx and larynx should be inspected before extubation.

The LMA can also be used in patients with EB. A series reporting only one complication after LMA use[9] advocates using an LMA one size smaller than normal, and lubricating the shaft and cuff with a water-based gel. The investigators suggest that the cuff should be inflated to maintain shape but not to be secured within the pharynx, so that there is always a leak. Vaseline gauze can be wrapped around the shaft at the mouth to minimize trauma to the lips. The LMA should be removed before the patient is awake to minimize trauma to the teeth and airway. The LMA has been found to be a useful adjuvant in the management of these patients with difficult airways. Dexamethasone, 0.25 mg/kg (maximum 8 mg) is sometimes given intravenously to reduce airway problems due to local swelling postoperatively following difficult intubation.

INDUCTION OF ANESTHESIA

Patients with EB often undergo frequent anesthetics and may have strong opinions about the type of induction or agents used; whenever possible, these preferences should be accommodated.

Anesthesia and surgery are expected to take longer than usual, due to the extra precautions required to protect the skin, so additional time should be allocated from the outset. Ideally patients should be scheduled at the beginning of surgical lists to minimize the possibility of delays and cancellations.

Handling and transfer of patients from one surface to another should be minimized. In the United Kingdom and many other countries it is conventional to use induction rooms and subsequently transfer anesthetized patients to the operating table. This technique is only suitable if a "nonfriction" method of transfer can be used. As intravenous access and monitoring devices may be less securely fixed than is usual, they are also more likely to become dislodged during such maneuvers. Adults should be anesthetized on the operating table to reduce the number of transfers required. Before induction, children should be placed on a smooth surface on which they can be lifted if necessary without any trauma. Use of rolling or sliding devices to aid transfer is not recommended.

Intravenous induction is generally preferred if there is intravenous access or if veins look easy to cannulate. Shearing forces must be avoided when applying pressure to facilitate cannulation. Intravenous cannulas can be secured with a nonadhesive dressing, for example, Mepiform. Central venous and arterial cannulas are best sutured in place. The intravenous induction agents propofol, thiopentone, and ketamine have all been used successfully in several series.[2,7,10] Ketamine enables easy maintenance of spontaneous respiration, a degree of preservation of protective airway reflexes, and the provision of analgesia, but postoperative restlessness is a disadvantage.

Inhalational induction is also suitable, the rates varying from 21% to 73.4% in published reports. Sevoflurane is the agent of choice.[2,10] The anesthetic face mask should be lubricated at points of contact with the face, for example, by covering with paraffin gauze. The patient's lower mandible should also be protected from friction with paraffin gauze or a suitable dressing. If rapid sequence induction is indicated, for example, in the presence of a full stomach or severe gastroesophageal reflux, the cricoid cartilage should also be protected. Gloves, laryngoscope blades, oral and nasal airways, and intubating forceps should all be well lubricated. These measures reduce shearing and friction forces on the skin but can make equipment and instruments difficult to handle.

Suxamethonium, a short-acting depolarizing muscle relaxant, can be used before intubation. Suxamethonium causes uncontrolled muscle fasciculations immediately after use, which has raised concerns about skin damage and hyperkalemia. Nevertheless, it has been used without complications in several series.[1,2,10] Theoretically, medium-duration, nondepolarizing muscle relaxants, such as atracurium and vecuronium, may have a prolonged duration of action, secondary to changes in volume of distribution as a result of hypoalbuminemia. However, this has not been observed in several series and these drugs have been frequently used without encountering difficulties.[1,2,10]

MAINTENANCE OF ANESTHESIA

Balanced anesthesia, with or without regional anesthesia (RA), is often suitable, despite early reservations concerning the use of central and regional blockade. A 13-year-old girl with dystrophic EB (DEB) undergoing splenectomy and cholecystectomy under general anesthesia and continuous epidural blockade has been described.[11] The epidural catheter was tunneled under the skin and then sutured in place. No bullae, skin lesions, or infections occurred at the insertion point of the epidural catheter or around the subcutaneous tunnel. The presence of uninfected bullae is not a contraindication to RA.[9] The skin can be disinfected by pouring an appropriate antiseptic solution or by using an aerosol; it should not be applied by rubbing. Local anesthetic infiltration of the skin may produce bullae, so the volume of this should be kept to an absolute minimum. Infiltration of the ligaments and muscles is safe. Mepitac or Mepiform dressings can be safely used to secure an epidural catheter.

There are reports of surgical procedures performed under RA alone, including cesarean section in a woman with DEB under spinal anesthesia[12] and a Mitrofanof procedure in a 6-year-old boy with EB using a CSE and sedation.[4]

The eyes are vulnerable during anesthesia and must be carefully protected. To prevent corneal abrasions the eyes should be closed and covered. Adhesive tape, which is often used to keep the eyes closed during anesthesia, is contraindicated. Eye ointment is also best avoided, as this may provoke eye rubbing on waking. If a nasogastric tube is required, one that is suitable for long-term use is preferred and should be secured with Mepiform.

POSTOPERATIVE RECOVERY AND POSTOPERATIVE ANALGESIA

Postanesthesia recovery unit (PACU) staff must be educated regarding safe and suitable monitoring and handling techniques. Touching the skin should be avoided, and children must never be picked up by supporting them under the arms. A notice on the patient's bed to this effect can be a useful reminder for all staff. As in the operating room, plastic oxygen masks with sharp edges, adhesives, and all kinds of friction should be avoided. Temperature can be measured using a tympanic membrane temperature probe if required.

Good postoperative analgesia is essential, particularly during emergence from anesthesia and in the PACU. A patient in pain is likely to be unsettled, and may pull at dressings and be more prone to new skin damage. This situation is particularly problematic in children. Pain management in EB is described in detail elsewhere in this issue; however, there are some important special considerations during the immediate postoperative period. The usual routes for analgesia administration may not be available just after surgery, and resumption of oral intake may be relatively delayed in patients with EB. Postoperative swelling and blistering of lips and oropharynx can contribute to this. The rectal route is also less suitable, as there is a risk of perianal trauma and blistering. Continuous regional analgesia has been used effectively, but is limited by the nature of the surgery. Multimodal analgesia using paracetamol, nonsteroidal anti-inflammatory drugs, and opioids by the intravenous route is the most convenient and effective, and therefore often preferred method.[7]

MANAGEMENT OF PROCEDURAL PAIN

Children with EB undergo many painful procedures that do not require general anesthesia. Guidelines on good practice in procedural pain management have been produced by several professional bodies, including the Association of Paediatric Anaesthetists of Great Britain and Ireland.[13] Pain management should include both pharmacologic and nonpharmacologic strategies whenever possible. Reduction in anticipatory and procedural anxiety by suitable preparatory measures is important. Families, play therapists, nursing staff, and other team members play key roles in this.

Several analgesic strategies are suitable with or without sedation. Staff who administer sedatives should receive adequate instruction in airway management, monitoring, and resuscitation, as determined by local circumstances. Special techniques such as analgesia-sedation with ENTONOX (Nitrous oxide/oxygen) by supervised self-administration can be considered in those older than 6 years. A combination of midazolam and oral morphine can be used for minor procedures in hospital or by families at home with suitable support.

SUMMARY

The management of anesthesia in patients with EB can present a considerable challenge to the perioperative team, and is best conduced in centers with experience and suitable support. Careful planning, good communication between clinical teams, and thorough preprocedure preparation including education of operating room or procedure room staff will reduce skin damage, bullae, and skin wounds. Airway management, monitoring during anesthesia, and postprocedure analgesia

require special consideration as the risk-benefit balance is significantly altered in this patient group.

REFERENCES

1. Ames WA, Mayou BJ, Williams KN. Anaesthetic management of epidermolysis bullosa. Br J Anaesth 1999;82:746–51.
2. Lin AN, Lateef F, Kelly R, et al. Anesthetic management in epidermolysis bullosa: review of 129 anesthetic episodes in 32 patients. J Am Acad Dermatol 1994;30:412–6.
3. Chevaleraud E, Ragot JM, Glicenstein J. [Anesthesia for hand surgery in patients with bullous epidermolysis]. Ann Chir Main Memb Super 1995;14:296–303 [in French].
4. Nasr AA, Almathami A, Alhathal N, et al. Combined spinal and epidural anesthesia in a child with epidermolysis bullosa. Paediatr Anaesth 2008;18:1278–9.
5. Niemi KM, Sommer H, Kero M, et al. Epidermolysis bullosa simplex associated with muscular dystrophy with recessive inheritance. Arch Dermatol 1988;124:551–4.
6. James I, Wark H. Airway management during anesthesia in patients with epidermolysis bullosa dystrophica. Anesthesiology 1982;56:323–6.
7. Griffin RP, Mayou BJ. The anaesthetic management of patients with dystrophic epidermolysis bullosa. A review of 44 patients over a 10 year period. Anaesthesia 1993;48:810–5.
8. Herod J, Denyer J, Goldman A, et al. Epidermolysis bullosa in children: pathophysiology, anaesthesia and pain management. Paediatr Anaesth 2002;12:388–97.
9. Hagen R, Langenberg C. Anaesthetic management in patients with epidermolysis bullosa dystrophica. Anaesthesia 1988;43:482–5.
10. Iohom G, Lyons B. Anaesthesia for children with epidermolysis bullosa: a review of 20 years' experience. Eur J Anaesthesiol 2001;18:745–54.
11. Doi S, Horimoto Y. Subcutaneous tunnelling of an epidural catheter in a child with epidermolysis bullosa. Acta Anaesthesiol Scand 2006;50:394–5.
12. Baloch MS, Fitzwilliams B, Mellerio J, et al. Anaesthetic management of two different modes of delivery in patients with dystrophic epidermolysis bullosa. Int J Obstet Anesth 2008;17:153–8.
13. Howard R, Carter B, Curry J, et al. Good practice in postoperative and procedural pain management: medical procedures. Association of Paediatric Anaesthetists of Great Britain and Ireland. Paediatr Anaesth 2008;18(S1):19–35.

Podiatric Management in Epidermolysis Bullosa

M. Tariq Khan, PhD, BSc (Hons), BSc (Pod Med), DFHom (Pod)[a,b,*]

KEYWORDS

- Epidermolysis bullosa • Podiatrist • Orthotics
- Hyperkeratosis

The foot is an engineering miracle combining grace, durability, and sensitivity. The foot is perhaps one of the most neglected parts of the body, generally hidden from sight, and its importance is only fully appreciated when something goes wrong. Healthy feet in good working order give us the joy of movement. Painful unhealthy feet make one feel tired and irritable, and take the pleasure out of life. Foot problems have plagued the human race since time began. Chiropodists or podiatrists, as they are now increasingly known, give 2 reasons for this.

a. Feet have not yet completed the evolutionary development necessary when our ancestors characteristically changed from the crouched position in which they helped themselves along with their hands.
b. Our feet were made for walking on uneven surfaces such as grass, sand, and earth, and are now pounding hot pavement.

The foot has 2 basic functions: to adapt to the surfaces on which we walk or run and to absorb the shock of impact of the body's weight from above and move it forward. Consider the punishment it absorbs in a lifetime, as we move it through three forward phased motions: heel impact, and transitional balance phase as the weight moves forward, and the thrust of the toes as they flex, just as the heel strike occurs on the opposite foot, walking at a comfortable 100 skips a minute pace. Each heel strikes the pavement with the equivalent of 225-pound jolts, 50 times a minute. As we walk an average of 115,000 miles in a lifetime, that means tens of millions of jolts for each foot. But the foot is built to withstand many times the stresses, so long as the health of its complex structures is maintained. The Achilles tendon counteracts much of the shock of the pounding it gets within each step.[1–4]

EPIDERMOLYSIS BULLOSA

Epidermolysis bullosa (EB) results from genetic defects of molecules in the skin concerned with adhesion. The loss of adhesion results in blister formation.[5]

FOOT STRUCTURE AND FUNCTIONS

To understand the affect of EB on the foot, we must understand the foot and its structure (**Fig. 1**). The foot contains 26 bones, comprising the heel bone, known as the calcaneus, above it the talus, the navicular, the cuboid and the first, second, and third cuneiforms, leading to the metatarsals and then the phalanges. These are housed in ligaments, tendons, and muscles. The foot is

Conflicts of interest: Marigold Therapy having been pioneered by my late father Dr M Taufiq Khan, the Company Marigold Footcare Limited is owned by my family. Alhough I do not have any financial interests, I am consulted by the company on medical matters on an honorary basis.
I do not have any financial interests in the companies Cuxson Gerrard or Molnlycke. nor in any shoe supplier or distributor.
[a] Marigold Clinic, Royal London Homeopathic Hospital, NHS Foundation Trust, 60 Great Ormond Street, London WC1N 3HR, UK
[b] EB Department, Great Ormond Street Hospital for Sick Children, London, UK
* Marigold Clinic, Royal London Homeopathic Hospital, NHS Foundation Trust, 60 Great Ormond Street, London WC1N 3HR, UK.
E-mail address: tariq@hompod.com

Dermatol Clin 28 (2010) 325–333
doi:10.1016/j.det.2010.02.006

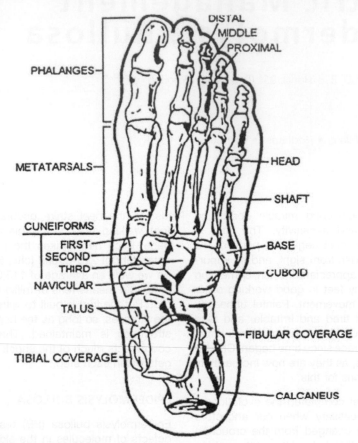

Fig. 1. Diagram of the foot and structure.

divided into 3 parts: the rear foot, the midfoot, and the forefoot.[6]

The rear foot is made up of 2 tarsals, the talus, and the heel bone, which is the largest bone in the foot. The heel bone acts as the shock absorber and balances the foot. The tarsals and metatarsals combine to form arches of the foot, providing a springboard effect to propel the body forward.

The midfoot is made up of 5 small bones, called the tarsals, positioned very closely; they are designed to cope with heavy loads that are transferred down to the feet with every step.

The forefoot includes the toes, which consist of 5 metatarsals and 4 phalanges. The toes are there to take the impact of the body weight and provide balance.[7-9]

The big toe has 2 phalanges whereas the smaller toes have 3. This arrangement gives the feet flexibility and allows them to grip and feel the terrain beneath each step even when wearing shoes. Losing even a single toe in an accident affects balance and gait.[7-9]

Surrounding the bone structures are 5 layers of muscles and fascia, which hold the structure of the foot together. Each compartment of the muscle is either intrinsic or extrinsic. Intrinsic

muscles have their origins and insertions within the foot, whereas extrinsic muscles originate outside the foot and insert in the foot. The muscles work in particular compartments to allow the function of the foot to take place. In general, structures that are on top of the foot coexist with those underneath the foot, working as a counterbalance for movement and function. Encasing this, of course, is the skin, which is considerably thicker than skin in other parts of the body.[10]

The structure of the skin and the sole of the foot consists of the epidermis, dermis, sweat glands, and sensory nerve endings. The key functions of the skin are as follows:

1. A barrier protecting the foot from physical, chemical, or biologic damage
2. Sensory functions enabling us to feel pain, changes in temperature, touch, and vibration
3. Heat regulation
4. Vitamin D production.

If these areas of the skin are not functioning and the skin becomes dry or rough, this generally happens because of the loss of water from the top layer of the skin. Normally cells with high water content are swollen and held tightly together. This arrangement is assisted by a combination of epidermal lipids, which hold the cells together, and the natural moisturizing factors, which keep the skin moist and pliable by attracting and holding water within the cells. However, if the lipid and natural moisturizing factors are reduced, water is lost. The skin then becomes dry, rough, and scaly, which may also result in breaks in the skin called fissures, which can leave the foot vulnerable to infection.[11,12]

The toenails are important because they provide balance for walking. In primitive times the toenails were used for scratching and for picking things up. Nails now have more of an aesthetic value. Toenails, however, do help to protect areas at the end of the toes, which can be vulnerable because of friction and pressure. Nail involvement in EB subtypes is covered by Tosti and Colleagues.[13]

THE WALKING CYCLE (GAIT CYCLE)

The way we walk is termed the gait cycle. The gait cycle begins when the heel of the left foot first comes into contact with the ground (heel strike) and ends with the next heel strike of the same foot.[6,14] Different phases of the gait cycle are as follows.

Heel Strike

Here the heel acts like a rigid lever with the soft tissues contracted over the bones of the feet and the lower limbs brought closely together. This structure enables the force that is generated from striking the ground to be transmitted throughout the body with minimum disruption to the weight-bearing joints throughout the body.[15–20]

Foot Flat and Mid-Stance

As the rest of the foot comes into contact with the ground, the soft tissues expand and the arches lower. These arching soft tissues open up the joints within the foot and lower extremities such as the ankles and the knees. This loosening and lowering enable the lower limb to externally rotate, an action that enables a force generated by the weight of the body to be absorbed as it is transferred vertically over the foot. Such foot functions comprise the mobile adaptor, which is also able to adapt to uneven ground conditions.[15–20]

Push Off or Toe Off

The foot begins its return to the rigid state only after the heel of the foot lifts off the ground. The soft tissues contract and the arches reform externally, rotating the joints in the foot and the lower limb so that they can come closer together. The action is akin to releasing a loaded spring whereby the internal rotation and the shock absorption that has occurred during the mobile stage create the energy. The power provided by this spring release gives strength and stability to the forefoot, allowing it to push off from the ground and propel the body forward.[1–4,19–23]

Foot problems often have their origin in childhood and present at birth, as in EB, either from friction in utero or after heel prick testing at birth. Periodic professional attention and regular foot care can minimize these problems in later life. Neglecting foot health can create problems in other parts of the body such as the legs and back,[24] and can also cause undesirable personality effects. Youngsters with troublesome feet walk awkwardly and usually have poor general posture; as a result, a growing child may become shy and introverted, and avoid athletic and social functions. Consultation between the podiatrist and members of the EB team can help to prevent and resolve some of these related problems.

The toes of young children are often pliable. Abnormal pressure from footwear can easily cause deformity. A child's foot grows rapidly during the first year, reaching almost half the adult foot size. For this reason, foot specialists consider the first year to be the most important in development of the foot.[25] Here are some suggestions to help to show that development can proceed normally[23]:

- Look carefully at the baby's feet, and if you notice something that does not look normal, seek professional care immediately. Deformities do not resolve by themselves.
- Cover babies' feet loosely. Tight covers restrict movements and can retard normal development.
- Provide an opportunity for exercising the feet. Lying on a cover enables the baby to kick and perform other related motions, which will prepare the feet for weight bearing.
- Change babies' positions several times a day; lying too long in one spot, especially on the stomach, can put excess strain on the feet and legs.
- When a child first begins to walk, shoes are not necessarily needed indoors; allowing the youngster to go barefoot or wear just socks helps feet to grow normally and develop muscular joint strength as well as grasping actions of toes. When walking outside or on rough surfaces, babies' feet should be protected in lightweight flexible footwear made of natural materials. Soft cartilage can easily be bent out of shape

in shoes that do not fit, without the parent or child noticing. The layer of puppy fat means that the child will feel no pain while this is happening, and because the baby's foot is so flexible it can easily be squeezed into a badly fitting shoe, storing up trouble for the future. Correct fit prevents this from happening in the first place. Therefore, it is very important that you have your child's foot measured at a reputable High Street shoe shop every 2 to 4 months. As a child's feet continue to develop, it may be necessary to change the shoes and the socks every few months to allow room for the feet to grow.[26,27]

A thorough examination by a podiatrist may detect an underlying defect or condition, which may require immediate treatment or consultation with another specialist.

COMMON FOOT CONDITIONS SEEN IN EB SUFFERERS
Blisters, Vesicles, and Bullas

Some of the most common problems seen with EB sufferers are vesicles and blisters. Blisters are closed, circumscribed, elevated lesions that contain fluid known as "serous fluid." A vesicle is a blister that is 1 cm or less in size whereas a bulla is a blister larger than 1 cm (**Fig. 2**). Friction between a dressing, a shoe, or a boot and skin causes a blister to form. The size of a blister depends on how much friction is placed against the foot. A blister usually develops on the wall of the foot, the back of the heel, or the tops of the toes. A blister is really a protective device. Formation of a blister tells the person that the covering or footwear is rubbing too much against a particular part of the foot.[5]

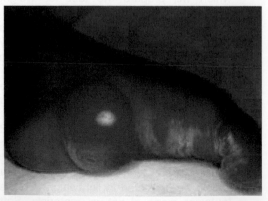

Fig. 2. The most common problems seen with EB sufferers are vesicles and blisters.

Vesicles and bullas cause pain, redness, swelling, and infection if lesions are broken. Treatment of these vesicles and bullas can be tackled in the following way:

1. Open lesions using a sterile needle to drain away fluid. Allow the needle to pierce the blister until it goes through to the other side; this stops the blister from refilling.[5]
2. Place the feet in warm salty water. Salt is a natural cleansing agent that soothes and neutralizes the skin.[5]
3. Dry out the blister using corn flour, which works as an absorbing agent.[5]
4. Use absorbent soft silicone dressing like Mepilex, a soft and highly conformable foam dressing that absorbs exudate and maintains a moist wound environment. Mepilex dressing does not stick to the wound bed yet adheres gently to the surrounding skin, allowing easy application of secondary fixation. In addition, this layer ensures that the dressing can be changed without damaging the wound or surrounding skin or subjecting the patient to additional pain. Mepilex absorbs exudate effectively and ensures a low risk of maceration.[28]
5. Use devices such as removable dressings and insoles to alleviate pressure during walking.[12]
6. Use socks that help with ventilation, such as silver-lined socks (**Fig. 3**). Strands of silver are banded with cotton fibers to make socks, which act by conducting heat away from the feet, thus cooling the feet and stopping the buildup of friction and pressure. These socks also have an additional antibacterial action. It has been reported that the silver fibers present in silver socks can eliminate 99.9% of bacteria in less than 1 hour of exposure, and are static free.[29]

Prevention of Blisters

Blisters can be prevented. The key to success is:

- Make sure that the shoes fit the feet properly;
- Wear socks that fit well, also wearing them inside out to stop the seams from rubbing, and follow the 2-socks method of keeping the feet dry. The 2-socks method is to wear 2 pairs of socks, one on top of the other, which keeps the layer of friction to a minimal amount in the shoe. This method helps to prevent friction between the skin and the shoes, especially when a person is walking or jogging.
- The use of insoles and orthotics is also important (**Figs. 4 and 5**).[12]

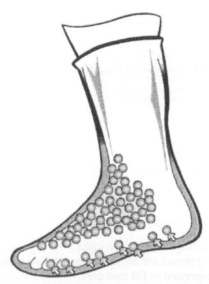

Fig. 3. The use of socks, such as silver-lined socks, conducts heat away from the feet, thereby cooling the feet and stopping the buildup of friction and pressure.

Functional Orthotics

Orthotics are devices that change the way the foot structures work each time a step is taken. Orthotics can be custom-made by the podiatrist or bought ready-made over the counter. Normally they have a posting of up to 4°, which helps to make sure that at the point of heel strike, the subtalar joint (complex of the talus and calcaneus), is in a neutral position and not rotated inwards or outwards, which would lead to uneven pressure to the foot on walking. There are different types of orthotics: rigid and semi-rigid. The rigid orthotic is functional, holding the foot in a corrective position, but can be hard on the surface and can lead to friction on walking. Semi-rigid orthotics are functional and cushioning; they provide support and allow movement, with a cushioning element and reduced friction.[7–10,26,30–34]

These types of orthotics are suitable for most EB foot types, especially EB simplex.

Hyperkeratosis, Corns, and Calluses

Hyperkeratosis, corns, and calluses may be defined as hard, thickened areas of the skin located on the tip of toes or between the toes and soles underneath the metatarsal heads (Fig. 6). The skin is hard and yellow with a nucleus or plug of keratin called a corn. If the skin is reddish the corn is inflamed. The central core of the corn descends into the flesh in a cone-shaped point, killing all the normal cells in its way. A corn grows faster if it keeps rubbing

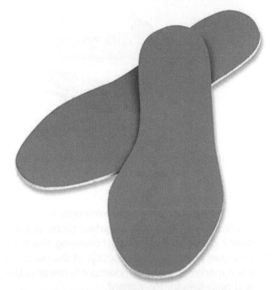

Fig. 4. Poron insoles are not structural devices but are primarily for shock absorbency. These insoles have a unique microporous cellular structure, which allows feet to breathe and rebounds to original thickness step after step, giving the wearer a feeling of walking on sponges. They also allow moisture to move away, leaving the feet feeling cooler. (*Data from* Pawelka S, Kopf A, Zwick E, et al. Comparison of two insole materials using subjective parameters and pedobarography (pedar-system). Clin Biomech (Bristol, Avon) 1997;12(3):S6–7.)

against the shoe because the rubbing provides a constant source of blood to the area. Hyperkeratosis and corns are protective in that they are the body's response to friction and pressure. The hard layers of keratin are trying to protect the skin and the bone beneath the foot from bruises and injury. Corns are consistent with tenderness to pressure, and occur on direct pressure mainly over a prominence, such as the head of a bone, or on direct contact with a hard surface, mainly one single darker area in the middle of a larger yellow area.[11]

1. Management of hyperkeratotic lesions and corns generally involves being seen by a podiatrist to have the overlying hyperkeratosis reduced and corn head enucleated. Chemical ablation with caustics like salicylic acid or monochloroacetic acid is also in regular practice but, because of the delicate EB skin, should not be used by the patient at risk of ulceration and infection. There should be only short-term exposure with the clinician's supervision. Other topical preparations include an extract from a marigold species called "tagetes" that has efficacy in inhibiting the proliferation of excessively proliferating cells, but is self-limiting with no adverse action on healthy

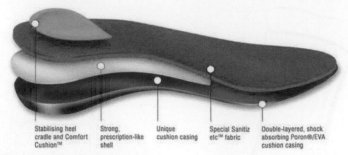

Stabilising heel cradle and Comfort Cushion™   Strong, prescription-like shell   Unique cushion casing   Special Sanitiz etc™ fabric   Double-layered, shock absorbing Poron®/EVA cushion casing

Fig. 5. Functional orthotics are devices that change the way the foot structures work each time a step is taken.

skin.[27] **Fig. 7** shows hyperkeratosis having an application of marigold (tagetes) paste applied over 7 days. After removal of dressing, the color changes and reveals the action of the paste on the hyperkeratosis. Debridement is made easier and pain-free for the patient.

2. The lesion is then dressed with redistributive padding; semi-compressed felt pads would stop friction and pressure returning on to these areas.
3. Patients are given emollients and creams for hydration and reduction of friction and pressure. Urea-based preparations of 20% to 40% are commonly used.
4. Protective padding such as an insole or orthotic device is constructed to help with the mechanical imbalances of the feet, which are the cause of these lesions.[6]

Foot care and shoes are important in that the shoe should be properly fitted with plenty of space so that the foot does not slip or slide during walking.

GENERAL FOOT HEALTH ADVICE

Maintaining foot cleanliness, exercising, and wearing shoes are all good preventative measures and important in EB foot care.

FOOT CLEANLINESS

Practicing good foot hygiene can prevent many, but not all, foot disorders. Proper care of the feet can be achieved by doing the following:

a. Change socks/hosiery and alternate shoes daily. Fresh clean dressing should be applied on a daily basis.
b. Wash feet carefully and dry feet thoroughly, paying particular attention to the area between the toes. In recessive dominant EB, where there are signs of fusion between the toes, the use of digital gel pads to separate the toes is found to be very helpful.
c. Let feet air out sometimes; do not keep them confined in shoes all the time.

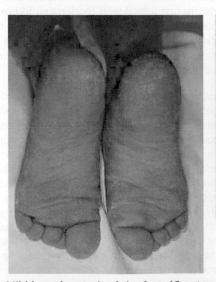
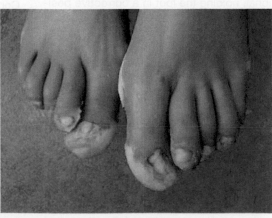

Fig. 6. Mild hyperkeratosis of the feet. (*Courtesy of* Professor Dédée F. Murrell, Sydney, Australia.)

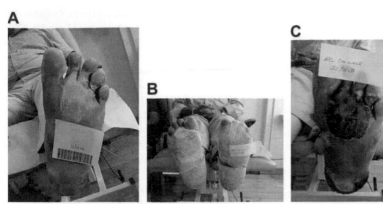

Fig. 7. (*A*) Debrided hyperkeratosis. (*B*) Bandages with marigold paste. (*C*) Marigold action on hyperkeratotic skin. (*D*) After debridement, soft skin and pain free.

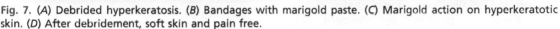

d. Keep toenails trimmed straight across. Soak nails in warm salt water or, after coming out of the bath, file nail surfaces with an emery board. Apply a few drops of baby oil to help stop nail thickening. In junctional EB patients, often the removal of the toenails from their beds is performed via chemical or laser ablation to prevent future problems.
e. Use creams to keep the skin of the feet soft. Also, use powders to absorb excess moisture and to prevent infection and foot odor.[32,35]

FOOT EXERCISE

Exercise the feet to keep them in good health.

a. Walking and running are both good exercises for the feet.
b. A person sitting at a desk or watching television in an easy chair can also perform the following foot exercises.
   1. Lift the feet and rotate them to limber the feet up.
   2. Achilles tendons and calf muscles by tapping the heels and toes on the floor from a sitting position.
   3. Exercise the heel cords by standing and poising the toes on a telephone directory about 2 in thick with the heels of the feet flat on the floor.[35]

SUGGESTIONS FOR SHOES FOR EB

Shoes should ideally have features including:

- Firm, comfortable fit both lengthways and widthways
- Rounded toes
- Plenty of room for the toes
- Flexible, flat soles
- Heel support

- Laces, straps, or equivalent to prevent excessive movement or slipping of the foot inside the shoe
- Material that is not plastic or synthetic; preferably leather because it allows air to circulate.

Shoe Brands

Uggs—Shoes with inner layer of sheepskin; soft and reduce friction on movement, but make feet hot.

Crocs—Molded plastic shoes; provide plenty of room, without causing friction or pressure, but make feet hot if worn constantly.

Climacool—Trainers with mesh lining; allow air to circulate to the feet and additionally have good shock absorption.

Cross-trainers—Multipurpose supporting shoes for comfort and walking.

Ballet pumps—Very thin material shoes with no support; can lead to increased friction to the soles of feet.

Deck shoes/flat-soled trainer—No support for the foot, increased stress and friction to plantar fascia leading to risk of hyperkeratosis and blistering.

Flip flops—No support for the foot, toes become clawed to hold foot to shoe; lead often to blister or callus formation in between first and second toe webbing.

Pedors shoes—Pedors shoes launched their EB shoe program in February of 2000. The program was the result of a request by an adult EB patient to make diabetic shoes for children with EB. The shoes feature an adjustable closure that simplifies fitting and a removable insole for custom orthotics (**Fig. 8**).[35]

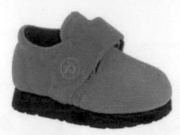

Fig. 8. Pedors shoe.

The evidence about EB sufferers' feet is limited as there are no significant clinical studies in this area. Feedback provided by clinicians and patients has shown several important areas that need to be addressed.

1. The changing shape of the foot structure through aging
2. The type of EB the individual suffers from
3. The type of footwear the individual wears.

With these factors taken into account, management of the EB foot is better controlled. With increasing developments in shoe science and material innovation, the environment within the shoe is more favorable for the feet.

REFERENCES

1. Ball State University. Lab #8: ground reaction forces. Available at: http://www.bsu.edu/web/ykwon/pep294/lab8/grf_laboratory.html. Accessed March 25, 2009.
2. Footmax clinicians corner, for articles. "Critical biomechanical principles", "relevant terminology for the gait cycle" and "bones of the foot. Available at: http://www.footmaxx.com. Accessed March 25, 2009.
3. Sub-talar joint motion—open chain. Available at: http://moon.ouhsc.edu/dthompso/gait/KNMATICS/STJOPEN.HTM. Accessed March 25, 2009.
4. Sub-talar joint motion—closed chain. Available at: http://moon.ouhsc.edu/dthompso/gait/KNMATICS/STJCLOSE.HTM. Accessed March 25, 2009.
5. Atherton DJ, Denyer J. Epidermolysis bullosa an outline for professionals. Berkshire (UK): DebRA; 2003. Available at: www.debra.org.uk. Accessed March 25, 2009.
6. Lorimer D. Neale's common foot disorders—diagnosis and management. 4th edition. London (UK): Churchill Livingston; 1993. ISBN 0-443-04470-8.
7. Pribut SM. Biomechanics of foot and leg problems, Dr. Stephen M. Pribut's sport pages. Available at: http://www.drpribut.com. Accessed March 25, 2009.
8. Prior T. Foot anatomy: bones and joints. Available at: http://www.timeoutdoors.com. Accessed March 25, 2009.
9. Quinn E. Foot anatomy and physiology. Available at: http://www.sportsmedicine.about.com. Accessed March 25, 2009.
10. Tortora GJ, Grabowski SR. Principles of anatomy and physiology. 10th edition. New York: John Wiley and Sons Inc; 2003.
11. Dawber R, Bristow I, Turner W. Text atlas of podiatric dermatology. chapters 1,2,3. London (UK): Matin Dunitz Ltd; 2002. ISBN 1 84184 223 0.
12. Fauli AC, Andres CL, Rosas NP, et al. Physical evaluation of insole materials used to treat the diabetic foot. J Am Podiatr Med Assoc 2008; 98(3):229–38.
13. Tosti A, de Farias DC, Murrell DF. Nail involvement in epidermolysis bullosa. Dermatol Clin 2010;28(1): 153–7.
14. Christensen K. Subluxations: what role do the feet play? Available at: http://www.chiroweb.com. 2003. Accessed March 25, 2009.
15. Austin W. Orthotic therapy: the postural imperative, dynamic chiropractic 1994. Vol 12, Issue 8. Available at: http://www.chiroweb.com/archives/12/08/25.html. Accessed March 25, 2009.
16. Bellinger C. Root cause analysis. Available at: http://www.outsights.com. Accessed March 25, 2009.
17. Bird AR, Payne CB. Foot function and low back pain, the foot, vol. 9. San Diego (CA): Harcourt Publishers Ltd; 1999. p. 75–180.
18. Cash M. Pocket atlas of the moving body. London: Ebury Press; 1999.
19. Charrette M. Shoulder "pronation" and orthotic support. The Chiropractic Journal 2003. Available at: http://www.worldchiropracticalliance.org. Accessed March 25, 2009.
20. Charrette M. Managing an unstable posture. The Chiropractic Journal 2004. Available at: http://www.worldchiropracticalliance.org. Accessed March 25, 2009.
21. Chaitow L. Posture and correct body use, excerpt from osteopathy: a complete health care system. Available at: http://www.healthy.net. Accessed March 25, 2009.
22. Charrette M. The benefits of orthotic therapy. The Chiropractic Journal 2002. Available at: http://www.worldchiropracticalliance.org. Accessed March 25, 2009.
23. Charrette M. Keep an eye on children's feet. The Chiropractic Journal 2004. Available at: http://www.worldchiropracticalliance.org. Accessed March 25, 2009.
24. Fine JD, Johnson LB, Weiner M, et al. Assessment of mobility, activities and pain in different subtypes of epidermolysis bullosa. Clin Exp Dermatol 2004; 29(2):122–7.
25. Watt GF, Goel K. Paediatric podiatry. In: Lorimer D, French G, O'Donnell M, et al, editors. Neale's disorders

of the foot—diagnosis & management. 6th edition. London (UK): Churchill Livingstone; 2001. p. 81–110.

26. Michaud TC. Foot orthoses and other forms of conservative foot care. Philadelphia: Lippincott Williams and Wilkins; 1993.

27. Khan MT, Potter M, Birch I. Podiatric treatment of hyperkeratotic plantar lesions. International Journal of Phytotherapy Research 1996;10:3.

28. Williams C. Mepitel. Br J Nurs 1995;4(1):51–2, 54–5.

29. Sturgis S. Precious meta - foot care takes a shine to silver. Biomechanics, February, 2005.

30. Pratt DJ, Rees PH, Rogers C. Assessment of some shock absorbing insoles. Prosthet Orthot Int 1986; 10(1):43–5.

31. Landsman A, Defronzo D, Anderson J, et al. Scientific assessment of over-the-counter foot orthoses to determine their effects on pain, balance, and foot deformities. J Am Podiatr Med Assoc 2009; 99(3):206–15.

32. Schumann H. Epidermolysis bullosa. An update. Hautarzt 2009;60(8):614–21.

33. Springett K, Otter S, Barry A. A clinical longitudinal evaluation of pre-fabricated, semi rigid foot orthoses prescribed to improve foot function. The Foot 2007; 17:184–9.

34. Van Meerhaeghe T. When and why functional orthotics? Rev Med Brux 2006;27(4):S327–9.

35. Watt G. Children's feet, a practical footcare guide for parents, teachers and children. Foot health information leaflet. London (UK): The Society of Chiropodist and Podiatrists; 2006. Available at: http://www.feetforlife.org/ download/2580/Childrens-Feet-A5-16pp.pdf. Accessed March 26, 2010.

Surgery of the Hand in Recessive Dystrophic Epidermolysis Bullosa

Catina Bernardis, MBBS, BSc, FRCS (Plast)[a,*], Rachel Box, Bsc[b]

KEYWORDS

• Epidermolysis bullosa • Pseudosyndactyly
• Contracture • Skin graft • Surgery • Management

Epidermolysis bullosa (EB) is the name given to a heterogeneous group of rare, inherited skin diseases, characterized by fragility of the epidermis. The underlying genetic abnormalities cause destabilization at the dermo-epidermal junction. Characteristically, therefore, patients with EB are subject to blistering following relatively minor trauma (the Nikolsky sign), and suffer from ulcers and erosions in all areas subject to persistent or repeated friction, such as the hand.[1,2]

More than 20 clinically distinct phenotypes of EB have been described, but there are 3 main subtypes.[3] In epidermolysis bullosa simplex (EBS) the defect causes blister formation within the basal keratinocytes; in junctional epidermolysis bullosa (JEB) the defect causes blister formation within the lamina lucida; and in dystrophic epidermolysis bullosa (DEB) the blistering occurs in the superficial papillary dermis, at the level of the anchoring fibrils. DEB may be transmitted as an autosomal dominant or recessive subtype. The severity of the disease is mainly determined by the particular form of disease from which the patient suffers, but it is useful to broadly categorize the disease into the nonscarring and scarring (dystrophic) types.[2]

EPIDERMOLYSIS BULLOSA AND THE HAND

The typical hand deformities that develop in recessive DEB (RDEB) in particular, where there is reduced or absent collagen VII, include the following: adduction contracture of the thumb; pseudosyndactyly of the digits; flexion contractures of the interphalangeal (IP), metacarpophalangeal (MCP), and wrist joints; and, less frequently, extension contractures of the MCP joints from dorsal scarring. The "mitten" deformity develops when the hand becomes encased in an epidermal cocoon.

All structures in the hand may be affected. Cutaneous involvement results in dermal fibrosis, pseudosyndactyly, contractures, atrophic finger and thumb tips, nail loss (due to subungual blistering) and dermal cocooning. Musculotendinous involvement may result in shortening of the flexor tendons and intrinsic muscle contractures. With time, and lack of use, the IP and MCP joints develop flexion deformities, including contracture and fibrosis of the collateral ligaments. Secondarily, articular involvement produces stiff, subluxed, or even destroyed joints in older patients.[4,5] Generalized osteoporosis and thinned, wedge-shaped distal phalanges may also be found.[5,6]

With each episode of relatively minor trauma to the hand, ulceration produces fibrinous adhesions and scarring; this results in the web spaces being obliterated, progressing to the finger tips and causing pseudosyndactyly. The same process occurs in the first web space, initially causing an adduction contracture. This condition may also progress until the thumb is no longer independent. A grading system may be used to describe adduction deformity of the first web space and pseudosyndactyly.[5,7]

Initially, despite the pain, patients may be able to separate the digits using thread or paper.

ª Department of Plastic Surgery, St Thomas' Hospital, Westminster Bridge Road, London SE1 7EH, UK
ᵇ Department of Hand Therapy, Lambeth Wing, St Thomas' Hospital, Westminster Bridge Road, London SE1 7EH, UK
* Corresponding author.
E-mail address: catina.bernardis@gstt.nhs.uk

Dermatol Clin 28 (2010) 335–341
doi:10.1016/j.det.2010.01.013

However, if left untreated, the resulting pseudo-syndactyly, together with trauma to, and scarring of, the flexion creases produces flexion contractures at the joints (**Fig. 1**). Finally, the whole hand may become encased in an epithelial cocoon, producing the mitten deformity (**Fig. 2**). The term "pseudosyndactyly" is used (as opposed to syndactyly) because the dermis of the adjacent, fused digits remains, with dermis abutting dermis. This abutment is exploited during release of pseudosyndactyly, although a distinct plane may be difficult to find in older children and adults.

Patients with DEB suffer the worst form of the disease, with major implications on all activities of daily living. Those with RDEB have the greatest degree of blistering, ulceration, and deformity. The risk of the hand developing a mitten deformity is 98% in RDEB (generalized severe type) by the age of 20 years.[3]

Finally, it is not uncommon for squamous cell carcinoma to develop in the hand, the limbs and bony prominences being especially susceptible.[8] Consequently, tumors often develop over the dorsum of joints, making surgical excision challenging.

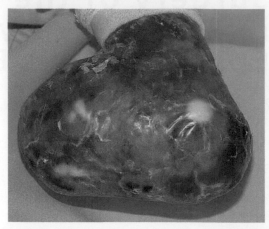

Fig. 2. The whole hand may become encased in an epithelial cocoon, producing the "mitten" deformity.

SURGICAL PLANNING

The aim of surgery is to provide simple pinch grip and grasp, by releasing the first web space and flexion contractures; independent finger movement, by releasing pseudosyndactyly; and improved appearance of the hand. Patients are seen in a multidisciplinary clinic, allowing their condition to be optimized and their admission planned. Wounds are swabbed preoperatively, and active infection treated. Growth of β-hemolytic streptococcus is a contraindication to surgery. The hand therapist spends time with the patient, discussing the nature of the postoperative rehabilitation regime, and emphasizing the need for splintage to delay recurrent contractures for as long as possible.

Surgery is indicated when loss of hand function begins to compromise the patient's independence, but the cosmetic appearance of the hand is also important. Surgery should be performed when the patient's skin, medical, and nutritional condition have been optimized, and at a time when they will be able to attend regular postoperative hand therapy sessions.

Surgery needs careful planning, including: whether to separate the thumb separately from the digits; how to cover the soft tissue defects; whether K-wires will be used; what type of anesthesia is to be used; whether there is an absolute need for postoperative splinting; and close liaison with the hand therapist.

ANESTHESIA

There are multiple anesthetic problems encountered in patients suffering from EB. The reader is referred to the article elsewhere in this issue by Nandi and Howard.

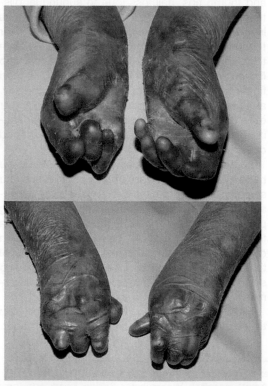

Fig. 1. Patients may be able to separate the digits using thread or paper. However, if left untreated, the resulting pseudosyndactyly, together with trauma to, and scarring of, the flexion creases produces flexion contractures at the joints.

Surgery may be performed under general or regional anesthesia. The latter may be supplemented with an infusion of propofol, particularly if the patient is anxious. Topical local anesthetic cream, or an injection, is used for skin graft harvesting. In children, it is more common to use a general anesthetic. A broad-spectrum antibiotic is given intravenously before surgery begins.

SURGERY

Surgery is usually performed under tourniquet control, although not all surgeons do this.[2,4,5,9] Provided the arm is carefully protected using a layer of Vaseline gauze, followed by cotton wool padding, problems with skin ulceration are avoided. The patient is lifted carefully onto the operating table, which has to be well padded to prevent pressure sores. The authors use the RIK Fluid Operating Table Pad (KCI Medical Ltd, Oxford, UK) and have encountered no problems since its use.

The skin is most safely prepared by using a "dabbing" technique or spraying the skin preparation fluid onto the arm, taking care to prevent fluid from running under the tourniquet, essential if the fluid contains alcohol as it can burn the skin if it seeps under the inflated tourniquet. Sutures are placed through the tips of the digits to act as retractors, preventing unnecessary trauma.

Separation of Digits

Most surgeons release all contractures and affected joints of one hand during the same operation. However, because the thumb contributes 50% to hand function, release of the first web space alone produces significant improvement and can be useful if either the surgeon or the patient prefers to limit the extent of the surgery.[1] The adducted first web space is released by incising the scarred skin from the base of the first metacarpal dorsally, to the thenar muscles volarly. Release of the first dorsal interosseous and the adductor pollicis as well as the overlying fascia may be needed in severe cases, but intraoperative stretching of the muscles may be adequate.[5,10,11] Care must be taken to avoid injury to the neurovascular bundles.

Next, the pseudosyndactyly between the fingers is addressed. Whereas some surgeons "decocoon" the hand to identify the web spaces, the authors have found this not to be necessary, and try to preserve the tissue on the finger tips.[4,12] Starting distally, the interdigital space, lined on each side by dermis, can usually be identified and entered with the tips of scissors. The digits can then be teased apart, down to the web spaces. Sometimes, however, this is not possible, particularly if there has been previous surgery, and sharp dissection with a scalpel may be necessary, exposing subcutaneous tissue.

Division of Flexion Contractures

The flexion contractures are then released. This procedure can be done either using multiple transverse incisions in the IP and MCP joint creases, or with a cruciate incision.[10,13] In children, gentle forced extension of the fingers may sometimes divide any fibrinous adhesions if they alone are causing the flexion contracture. Occasionally, intrinsic muscle contractures need to be released, and shortened flexor tendons may need to be lengthened in selected cases, although this is not common.[5]

K-wires are often used when the IP joints are stiff or subluxed.[1,2,4,5] Like others, the authors prefer not to use wires across the proximal IP joints, unless absolutely necessary, to avoid the complications of prolonged postoperative joint stiffness in extension, potential pin-tract infection, and damage to articular cartilage.[10,13,14] Furthermore, forced extension of the IP joints may cause injury to the neurovascular bundles or subluxation of the joints. As has been noted by others, full release of the distal IP joints may not be possible or useful.[4]

Recurrent flexion deformity of the wrist occurs for several reasons, including the stronger pull of the flexor tendons compared with extensor tendons, the powerful pull of flexor carpi ulnaris, and the complex carpal bone movements that favor ulnar deviation in wrist flexion. In early wrist flexion contractures, which are often ulnarly deviated, simple division of the scarred skin will produce full release of the wrist. In more advanced contractures, division of palmaris longus and flexor carpi radialis may be necessary. If the flexor musculotendinous units are contracted, they may require lengthening in the forearm, though this is not common.[5] Although replacement of joints has been described, this procedure is rare: only 1 adult out of 45 patients required MCP joint replacements in the largest published series.[5]

In the most extreme and neglected cases, the wrist joint is also involved and may need to be fused in a neutral position. In some cases, the potential amount of surgery may be too daunting, and the patient may have learned to function so well that the surgeon is unable to guarantee an improved or predictable outcome (Fig. 3).

Shortening of neurovascular structures is often the limiting factor in release of flexion contractures.

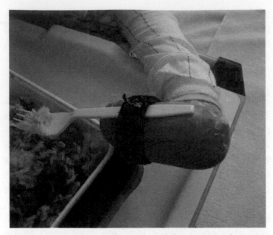

Fig. 3. In some cases, the potential amount of surgery may be too daunting, and the patient may have learned to function so well that the surgeon is unable to guarantee an improved or predictable outcome.

Soft Tissue Cover

Surgeons vary in how they cover the soft tissue defects, and include: no coverage; cultured keratinocytes; using epithelium raised from skin, to split-skin grafts (SSGs) or full-thickness skin grafts (FTSGs); and cellular allograft dermal matrix. Fillet flaps from amputated digits and pedicled flaps from the torso have been described in the past, but are not common practice.[6,15] Those who use no biologic dressing claim that there is no difference in outcome whether grafts are used or not, and the procedure is quicker and simpler.[10,11] Cultured keratinocytes have been used on deepithelialized areas of decocooned hands in 13 patients in an attempt to accelerate healing.[14]

Some surgeons do not cover the lateral defects of the fingers following pseudosyndactyly release, only dermal ones, claiming that the defects reepithelialize in 3 to 4 weeks in children.[4] It is the authors' usual practice in adults to graft these defects, as denuded defects seem to take longer to reepithelialize in adults, and most patients do not tolerate prolonged wounds on their hands.

The first web space and palmar defects are grafted by most surgeons, using FTSGs or SSGs. However, there is little in the literature that proves the superiority of one over the other, and the long-term results may vary little.[9,11] Several factors need to be considered: availability of donor sites and their potential for healing; delaying recurrence of contracture; likelihood of graft take; and patient choice.

FTSGs should delay recurrence of contractures as compared with SSGs, and may be especially useful in the first web space.[9,14,15] However, FTSG take is often poorer than that of SSGs,

potentially resulting in scar formation. The skin stretches less easily than in non-EB skin: therefore, the skin must be harvested with care to fully fit the defect. Furthermore, the donor site will close less readily than in non-EB skin, particularly as the patient ages, limiting the amount of skin graft that can be harvested and increasing the likelihood of scar contracture at the donor site. The epithelium usually separates from the underlying dermis during the procedure.

On the other hand, there is usually an adequate supply of suitable skin for SSG, which the authors harvest freehand with a knife, and this can be meshed 1:1.5 to increase the area of coverage. However, it is not unusual to have delayed donor site healing, particularly if the graft contains significant dermal elements: one of the authors' patients had a donor site still unhealed after 21 years. The authors do not use a dermatome to harvest skin, as the machine can deepithelialize skin adjacent to the planned donor site, increasing morbidity.

Donor site problems can be minimized by harvesting epithelium only, as a "split-off" graft. Not only is healing quicker, but the epithelium can be harvested from wherever there is nonulcerated skin.[16] Recurrent contracture, as early as 6 months, is more common with this technique, but donor site healing is more predictable and usually occurs within 2 weeks.[1,15] The authors have used this technique on several occasions. In one patient, who had an adducted first web space (without significant muscular involvement) it was possible to fully release the contracture with minimal exposure of underlying subcutaneous tissue and cover the defect with harvested epithelium. At 8 months, the first web space remains open and functional, although the patient has unfortunately developed an aggressive squamous cell carcinoma.

Allogeneic composite cultured skin (CCS) allografts have been successfully used on donor sites and between released digits, providing stable donor sites. Biopsies have shown some regeneration of anchoring fibrils, in distinction to when allograft keratinocyte sheets have been used.[17]

Acellular allograft dermal matrix has been used to cover a released first web space contracture in an 11-year old, with application of an ultrathin, unmeshed SSG, stabilized with K-wires.[18] At a 1-year follow-up there had been little blistering in the first web space, but biopsies showed no positive staining for collagen VII. Long-term results are not known.

Graft skin (Apligraf; Organogenesis Inc, Canton, MA, USA and Novartis Pharmaceuticals Corp, East Hanover, NJ, USA), an allogeneic bilayer, has been used with early success in 4 children and in an adult with RDEB.[12] Bulky dressings were applied postoperatively, rather than a splint, and the fingers were dressed individually. A night splint was made at 4 to 6 weeks, when the wounds had healed. No wires were used. However, 3 patients had developed pseudosyndactyly by 18 months, recurrent dorsal erosions were noted in all patients, and recurrent blistering occurred in 3 patients.

The grafts may be held in place with tissue glue (n-butyl cyanoacrylate: Histacryl or Indermil) or absorbable sutures. The grafts are then covered with Vaseline gauze and proflavine impregnated wool; this helps to maintain abduction and extension of the web spaces and digits. The hand is splinted using plaster of Paris, with the wrist extended to 40°, and the fingers and thumb fully extended. Some have advocated the use of suspension frames to aid splinting and positioning of the hand.[2]

Postoperatively, the hand is elevated in a Bradford sling. In adults, the use of patient controlled analgesia (PCA) is discussed with the patient preoperatively, and those who wish to make use of it are given a PCA pump for postoperative pain control. However, regional anesthesia produces long-lasting pain relief. In the authors' experience, most of the pain seems to be due to the joint repositioning.

Patients return to theater for a change of dressing under general or regional anesthesia, or sedation, at 1 and 2 weeks; the wounds or grafts are carefully cleaned and redressed. Microbiological swabs are taken if required. If K-wires have been placed, they are removed at 2 weeks.

HAND THERAPY IN THE MANAGEMENT OF EPIDERMOLYSIS BULLOSA

Postoperatively, once the wounds are manageable with simple dressings, the hand therapist fashions a custom-made splint (Fig. 4). In the authors' practice, this is usually after the second dressing change, in the third week following hand release. The hand is also measured for gloves, range of movement is assessed, exercises are commenced, and wound care advice is given. Close collaboration between the patient and therapist is essential to maintain intraoperative results.

Splints are usually made from perforated thermoplastic.[4,19] This material is ready to wear immediately; it can be remolded; the digits can be supported individually in the positions of achieved extension; and exudate and blood can be cleaned off easily. The perforations reduce overheating, which contributes to skin blistering. Prior to the availability of thermoplastic splinting material,

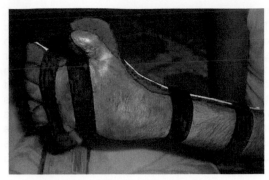

Fig. 4. Postoperatively, once the wounds are manageable with simple dressings, the hand therapist fashions a custom-made splint.

acrylic splints were used. These splints could not be easily adjusted, required an anesthetic to make the impressions, and could damage the skin if the position of digits had altered by the time the splint was ready.[19]

Volar forearm extension splints are used. The wrist is supported in a neutral position, or slight extension; the digits in extension; and the thumb in abduction. Splint fabrication can be difficult as the hands are small and the skin is fragile. While the wounds are healing, the splints are removed only for exercise and dressing changes; once healed, the splints are worn only at night. Uncomfortable splints must be reviewed urgently, as contractures can return within 6 months of surgery if splints are not worn, or adjusted as necessary.[20]

Dynamic splints are used by some clinicians in an attempt to reduce scarring. However, compliance is likely to be poor, especially in adults.[21] These splints are also more time-consuming to make and monitor.

Patients are educated about maintaining their web spaces. Preventative measures that can be taken include the use of bandages or dressings (eg, Vaseline gauze), and wearing rings (Fig. 5) or

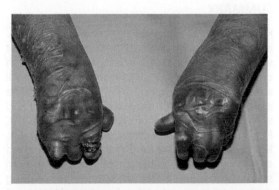

Fig. 5. Measures that can be taken to maintain web spaces include wearing rings.

Interim Gloves (Jobskin Ltd, Nottingham, UK). These gloves are made-to-measure garments: correct fit ensures that they conform to the web spaces. The gloves can be worn 3 weeks after splinting over, or instead of, dressings, and can be cleaned. They are replaced if the position of the digits or web spaces changes. Some patients report finding it easier to complete functional tasks in gloves, as they provide a protective layer. There is little evidence for their efficacy, although it has been suggested that they can deepen the web spaces.[4]

Passive extension and abduction exercises of the digits and thumb are taught, as well as tendon gliding exercises. Functional tasks and heavy activities must not be introduced too quickly to allow grafted areas to heal. Avoidance of microtrauma is essential, and dressings must not adhere to the wound bed or fragile surrounding skin.[22] If they do, painful skin degloving occurs, with the risk of further deformity.[23]

RESULTS

Unfortunately, whatever method of soft tissue cover is used, recurrent contracture is inevitable, although in adulthood the deformities appear to become relatively stable. Long-term results are affected not only by the natural course of the disease but also by failure to use long-term splintage.[4,5] On average, recurrent contracture occurs within 2 to 5 years: the first web space has the poorest outcome, which is partly due to difficulty in splinting this area and the fact that the thumb is used in an adducted position.[5,11,14]

The main complications following surgery are joint stiffness in extension, especially if K-wires have been used; graft failure; and infection. Fortunately, injury to neurovascular structures and osteomyelitis are rare.

SUMMARY

Hand deformities occur in most patients with DEB, and include adduction contractures of the first web space, pseudosyndactyly, and flexion contractures of the IP, MCP, and wrist joints. All structures in the hand may be involved. The severity of the deformity worsens with age, and surgical correction becomes increasingly difficult. Recurrent deformity occurs within 2 to 5 years. Meticulous skin care and the use of well-fitted splints supervised within a multidisciplinary team setting are essential. To date there is no strong evidence base on which to plan surgical treatment of the hand in DEB.

ACKNOWLEDGMENTS

The authors thank Gary Mulcahy, Senior Medical Photographer, for his help with the clinical photos.

REFERENCES

1. Cuono C, Finseth F. Epidermolysis bullosa: current concepts and management of the advanced hand deformity. Plast Reconstr Surg 1978;62:280–5.
2. Greider JL Jr, Flatt AE. Care of the hand in recessive epidermolysis bullosa. Plast Reconstr Surg 1983;72: 222–8.
3. Fine JD, Johnson MW, Stein A, et al. Pseudosyndactyly and musculoskeletal contractures in inherited epidermolysis bullosa: experience of the National Epidermolysis Bullosa Registry, 1986–2002. J Hand Surg 2005;30(1):14–22.
4. Ladd AL, Kibele A, Gibbons S. Surgical treatment and postoperative splinting of recessive dystrophic epidermolysis bullosa. J Hand Surg 1996;21: 888–97.
5. Terrill PJ, Mayou BJ, Pemberton J. Experience in the surgical management of the hand in dystrophic epidermolysis bullosa. Br J Plast Surg 1992;45:435–42.
6. Horner RL, Wiedel JD, Bralliar F. Involvement of the hand in epidermolysis bullosa. J Bone Joint Surg Am 1971;53:1347–56.
7. Colville J. Syndactyly correction. Br J Plast Surg 1989;42:12–6.
8. Mallipeddi R. Epidermolysis bullosa and cancer. Clin Exp Dermatol 2002;27:616–23.
9. Rees TD, Swinyard A. Rehabilitative digital surgery in epidermolysis bullosa. Plast Reconstr Surg 1967;40(2):169–74.
10. Vozdivzhensky SI, Albanova VI. Surgical treatment of contracture and syndactyly of children with epidermolysis bullosa. Br J Plast Surg 1993;46:314–6.
11. Ciccarelli AO, Rothaus KO, Carter DM, et al. Plastic and reconstructive surgery in epidermolysis bullosa: clinical experience with 110 procedures in 25 patients. Ann Plast Surg 1995;35:254–61.
12. Fivenson DP, Scherschun L, Cohen LV. Apligraf in the treatment of severe mitten deformity associated with recessive dystrophic epidermolysis bullosa. Plast Reconstr Surg 2003;112(2):584–8.
13. Cavallo AV, Smith PJ. Surgical treatment of dystrophic epidermolysis bullosa of the hand. Tech Hand Up Extrem Surg 1998;2(3):184–95.
14. Campiglio GL, Pajardi G, Rafanelli G. A new protocol for the treatment of hand deformities in recessive dystrophic epidermolysis bullosa (13 cases). Ann Chir Main 1997;16(2):91–101.
15. Gough MJ, Page RE. Surgical correction of the hand in epidermolysis bullosa dystrophica. Hand 1979; 11(1):55–8.

16. Eastwood DS. Autografting in the treatment of squamous cell carcinoma in epidermolysis bullosa dystrophica. Plast Reconstr Surg 1972;49(1):93–5.

17. Eisenberg M, Llewelyn D. Surgical management of hands in children with recessive dystrophic epidermolysis bullosa: use of allogeneic composite cultured skin grafts. Br J Plast Surg 1998;51:608–13.

18. Witt PD, Cheng CJ, Mallory SB, et al. Surgical treatment of pseudosyndactyly of the hand in epidermolysis bullosa: histological analysis of an acellular allograft dermal matrix. Ann Plast Surg 1999;43: 379–85.

19. Mullett FLH, Smith PJ. Hand splintage following surgery for dystrophic epidermolysis bullosa. Br J Plast Surg 1993;46:192–3.

20. Formsma SA, Maathuis CBG, Robinson PH, et al. Postoperative hand treatment in children with recessive dystrophic epidermolysis bullosa. J Hand Ther 2008;21(1):80–4.

21. Pajardi G, Pivato G, Rafanelli G. Rehabilitation in recessive dystrophic epidermolysis bullosa. Tech Hand Up Extrem Surg 2001;5(3):173–7.

22. Abercrombie E, Mather C, Hon J, et al. Recessive dystrophic epidermolysis bullosa. Part 2: care of the adult patient. Br J Nurs 2008;17(6 Suppl): S6–S20.

23. Schober-Flores C. Epidermolysis bullosa. Wound care pearls for the noninfected and infected wound. Journal of the Dermatology Nurses' Association 2009;1(1):21–8.

Genitourinary Tract Involvement in Epidermolysis Bullosa

Noor Almaani, MRCP[a], Jemima E. Mellerio, MD, FRCP[a,b],*

KEYWORDS

- Blister • Genodermatosis • Urethral stenosis
- Hydronephrosis • Renal failure

GENITOURINARY TRACT OBSTRUCTION IN EPIDERMOLYSIS BULLOSA

Some forms of epidermolysis bullosa (EB) are particularly susceptible to stenosis or obstruction of the genitourinary tract. Patients typically present with a reduced urinary flow, pain on voiding, or recurrent infections, depending on the site and severity of obstruction. Ulceration and scarring of the glans penis and labia may occur and are a particular feature in the inversa form of dystrophic EB (DEB).[1] Urethral meatal stenosis is also well recognized in both sexes, particularly in patients with recessive DEB and junctional EB (JEB), in whom it has been described in 3% to 4% of patients.[2,3] In severe cases, this may lead to bladder distension and subsequently hydroureter and hydronephrosis, with chronic renal failure the ultimate consequence if not treated.[1–3] Partial labial fusion and reflux of urine into the vagina and uterine cavity has been described in one case of DEB.[4] The urethra is also prone to developing strictures (Fig. 1), and these may frequently recur after interventions such as catheterization, urethral dilatation, or electroresection.[1,5–7] If instrumentation of the urogenital tract is necessary, it is probably prudent to use the smallest caliber instruments possible to avoid undue damage,[3] or to avoid surgery if at all possible.[8]

The vesicoureteric junction is another site that is particularly predisposed to stenosis, as well as reflux, particularly in patients with JEB with pyloric atresia.[9–12] Again, this may result in hydroureter and hydronephrosis.[3,9,11,12] Blistering of the bladder mucosa, and thickening and fibrosis of the bladder wall have also been described in patients with EB.[3,5] Expression of proteins implicated in different types of EB, such as laminin 332 and α6β4 integrin, in the urogenital epithelium, particularly in the urethra and at the vesicoureteric junction, presumably leads to fragility at these sites, causing mucosal separation and secondary inflammation and scarring of the underlying structures.

Severe constipation in patients with severe generalized recessive DEB may also result in urinary outflow obstruction with hydroureter and hydronephrosis (Figs. 2 and 3), which may resolve on adequate treatment of the constipation (J.E. Mellerio, personal communication, 2009).

EB-ASSOCIATED RENAL PARENCHYMAL DISEASE

The renal parenchyma itself may be affected in patients with EB, particularly those with the more severe forms, notably severe generalized recessive DEB and JEB with pyloric atresia, although there

Funding: J Mellerio acknowledges financial support from the Department of Health via the National Institute for Health Research (NIHR) comprehensive Biomedical Research Centre award to Guy's & St Thomas' NHS Foundation Trust in partnership with King's College London and King's College Hospital NHS Foundation Trust. N Almaani gratefully acknowledges funding from DebRA UK.
a St John's Institute of Dermatology, Guy's and St Thomas' NHS Foundation Trust, St Thomas' Hospital, Westminster Bridge Road, London, SE1 7EH, UK
b Department of Dermatology, Great Ormond Street Hospital for Children NHS Trust, Great Ormond Street, London WC1N 3JH, UK
* Corresponding author. Department of Dermatology, Great Ormond Street Hospital for Children NHS Trust, Great Ormond Street, London WC1N 3JH, UK.
E-mail address: jemima.mellerio@kcl.ac.uk

Dermatol Clin 28 (2010) 343–346
doi:10.1016/j.det.2010.01.014

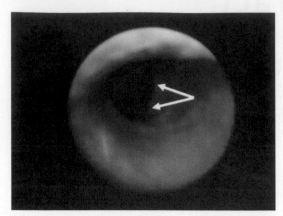

Fig. 1. Urethral stricture (*arrows*) in a boy with non-Herlitz junctional EB who required repeated urethral dilatations and, ultimately, a urethrostomy.

are scant data regarding the frequency with which this complication occurs. Three main patterns of renal parenchymal disease are observed in EB. First, post-infectious glomerulonephritis usually occurs after streptococcal infections of the skin, which are a relatively frequent problem in EB.[7,13] Presentation is usually with hematuria, hypertension, and deteriorating renal function. Second, mesangial IgA nephropathy may occur, and is also postulated to be secondary to repeated mucocutaneous infections.[7,14] Patients usually have hematuria, proteinuria, and hypertension. The third entity seen in EB patients is secondary renal amyloidosis, which usually presents with nephrotic range proteinuria, edema, and hypoalbuminemia.[15–17] Elevated serum amyloid A protein levels may be observed in patients with severe generalized forms of EB without evidence of renal amyloidosis, and the significance of this is therefore unclear.[16] All 3 forms of renal parenchymal disease may progress to chronic renal insufficiency, even if factors amenable to treatment (eg, streptococcal infection) are addressed.

Because infection and inflammation seem to be implicated in the pathogenesis of all 3 patterns of renal parenchymal disease described in EB patients, efforts to reduce bacterial colonization and infection of the skin may be beneficial in reducing the risks of renal impairment. However, the chronicity of skin ulceration in the more severe forms of EB probably means that this is not a realistic option in addition to the measures that are usually taken to primarily improve wound healing.

Hereditary nephritis has also been described in 2 siblings with pretibial DEB,[18] and congenital focal segmental glomerulosclerosis identified in one child with JEB with pyloric atresia.[19] The latter case had homozygous missense mutations in the β4 integrin gene, and reduced β4 integrin expression in the skin and glomerular podocytes, indicating that this protein may have an important role in normal glomerular function.

RENAL INSUFFICIENCY IN EB

Pathology in the kidneys themselves and secondary changes because of outflow obstruction may lead to deteriorating renal function and ultimately end-stage renal failure. Data from the National Epidermolysis Bullosa Registry in the United States found that renal failure was the attributed cause of death in 3.6% patients with severe generalized recessive DEB with a mean age of 24 years (16–38 years), although the cumulative risk of death from renal failure in this type of EB was 12.3% at age 35 years.[20] The risk of mortality from end-stage renal disease in this group comes second only to metastatic squamous cell carcinoma. The cumulative risk of death in other forms of EB was 1.16% by 25 years and older for other types of generalized recessive DEB, and 0.67% by 1 year of age for generalized non-Herlitz JEB. None of the deaths reported in this

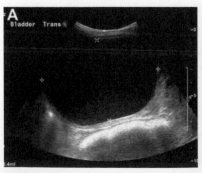
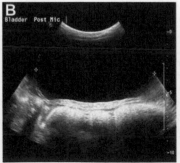
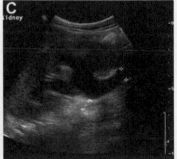

Fig. 2. A 9-year-old girl with severe generalized recessive DEB with severe and chronic constipation causing bladder outflow obstruction. (*A*) Premicturition bladder ultrasound; (*B*) postmicturition bladder ultrasound showing a significant residual volume; (*C*) renal ultrasound showing right hypdronephrosis.

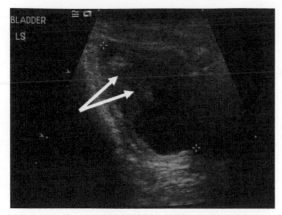

Fig. 3. Polypoid bladder mass (*arrows*) in an 8-year-old boy with junctional EB with pyloric atresia presenting with pain on voiding and hematuria. Biopsy of this lesion showed friable bladder epithelium.

cohort were secondary to renal outflow obstruction.[20]

Hemodialysis[20–22] and peritoneal dialysis[7,20,23] have been reportedly used in 8 and 4 patients with renal failure, respectively, often with reasonable success. However, vascular access may be problematic in EB because of the risks of sepsis from indwelling lines and devices, and the potential for skin breakdown of fistulae. Similarly, it has been suggested that the risk of peritonitis may be greater in EB patients on peritoneal dialysis because of longstanding colonization and infection of skin wounds. Peritoneal access also carries the risks of skin breakdown, catheter obstruction, and adhesions.

MONITORING THE GENITOURINARY TRACT IN EB PATIENTS

Recognizing that genitourinary tract problems may occur in EB, especially in patients with recessive DEB and JEB with pyloric atresia who seem to be at particular risk, is important so that complications can be detected and treated early to minimize the risk of more severe disease occurring. There are currently no published guidelines on how to monitor these patients, although 6-monthly serum urea and electrolytes, blood pressure, and urinalysis should probably be performed in all patients with recessive DEB and JEB. Annual ultrasound imaging in patients with JEB may also be warranted. If any abnormalities are detected, appropriate imaging or functional tests should be performed, and specialist urological or renal opinions sought.

SUMMARY

Genitourinary tract involvement in EB is not uncommon and may be serious, in some cases resulting in end-stage renal failure. Patients with severe generalized recessive DEB and those with JEB, particularly in association with pyloric atresia, are at particular risk. Investigating symptoms suggestive of obstruction, and simple monitoring of renal function, blood pressure, and urinalysis may help detect genitourinary disease earlier in its course and minimize the risks of further complications.

REFERENCES

1. Fine JD, Johnson LB, Weiner M, et al. Genitourinary complications of inherited epidermolysis bullosa (EB): experience of the National EB Registry and review of the literature. J Urol 2004;172:2040–4.
2. Kretkowski RC. Urinary tract involvement in epidermolysis bullosa. Pediatrics 1973;51:938–41.
3. Reitelman C, Burbige KA, Mitchell ME, et al. The urological manifestations of epidermolysis bullosa. J Urol 1986;136:1320–2.
4. Shackelford GD, Bauer EA, Graviss ER, et al. Upper airway and external genital involvement in epidermolysis bullosa dystrophica. Radiology 1982;143: 429–32.
5. Eklof O, Parkkulainen K. Epidermolysis bullosa dystrophica with urinary tract involvement. J Pediatr Surg 1984;19:215–7.
6. Ichiki M, Kasada M, Hachisuka H, et al. Junctional epidermolysis bullosa with urethral stricture. Dermatologica 1987;175:244–8.
7. Chan SM, Dillon MJ, Duffy PG, et al. Nephro-urological complications of epidermolysis bullosa in paediatric patients. Br J Dermatol 2007;156:143–7.
8. Rubin AI, Moran K, Fine JD, et al. Urethral meatal stenosis in junctional epidermolysis bullosa: a rare complication effectively treated with a novel and simple modality. Int J Dermatol 2007;46:1076–7.
9. El Shafie M, Stidham GL, Klippel CH, et al. Pyloric atresia and epidermolysis bullosa letalis: a lethal combination in two premature newborn siblings. J Pediatr Surg 1979;14:446–9.
10. Berger TG, Detliefs RL, Donatucci CF. Junctional epidermolysis bullosa, pyloric atresia, and genitourinary disease. Pediatr Dermatol 1986;3:130–4.
11. Dank JP, Kim S, Parisi MA, et al. Outcome after surgical repair of junctional epidermolysis bullosa-pyloric atresia syndrome. Arch Dermatol 1999;135: 1243–7.
12. Price AP, Hanna M, Katz DS. Epidermolysis bullosa of the bladder. Am J Roentgenol 2001;177:1486–7.
13. Mann JF, Zeier M, Zilow E, et al. The spectrum of renal involvement in epidermolysis bullosa dystrophica hereditaria: report of two cases. Am J Kidney Dis 1988;11:437–41.

14. Nicholls KM, Fairley KF, Dowling JP, et al. The clinical course of mesangial IgA associated nephropathy in adults. Q J Med 1984;53:227–50.

15. Bourke JF, Browne G, Gaffney EF, et al. Fatal systemic amyloidosis (AA type) in two sisters with dystrophic epidermolysis bullosa. J Am Acad Dermatol 1995;33:370–2.

16. Kaneko K, Kakuta M, Ohtomo Y, et al. Renal amyloidosis in recessive dystrophic epidermolysis bullosa. Dermatology 2000;200:209–12.

17. Csikos M, Orosz Z, Bottlik G, et al. Dystrophic epidermolysis bullosa complicated by cutaneous squamous cell carcinoma and pulmonary and renal amyloidosis. Clin Exp Dermatol 2003;28:163–6.

18. Kagan A, Feld S, Chemke J, et al. Occurrence of hereditary nephritis, pretibial epidermolysis bullosa, and beta-thalassemia minor in two siblings with end-stage renal disease. Nephron 1988;49:331–2.

19. Kambham N, Tanji N, Seigle RL, et al. Congenital focal segmental glomerulosclerosis associated with beta4 integrin mutation and epidermolysis bullosa. Am J Kidney Dis 2000;36:190–6.

20. Fine JD, Johnson LB, Weiner M, et al. Inherited epidermolysis bullosa (EB) and the risk of death from renal disease: experience of the National EB Registry. Am J Kidney Dis 2004;44:651–60.

21. Farhi D, Ingen-Housz-Oro S, Ducret F, et al. Recessive dystrophic epidermolysis bullosa (Hallopeau-Siemens) with IgA nephropathy: 4 cases. Ann Dermatol Venereol 2004;131:963–7.

22. Ducret F, Pointet P, Turc-Baron C, et al. Kidney diseases in dystrophic epidermolysis bullosa: case report. Nephrol Ther 2008;4:187–95.

23. Ahmadi J, Antaya R. Successful peritoneal dialysis in a patient with recessive dystrophic epidermolysis bullosa. Pediatr Dermatol 2007;24:589–90.

Dilated Cardiomyopathy in Epidermolysis Bullosa

Irene Lara-Corrales, MD, MSc, Elena Pope, MD, MSc*

KEYWORDS

- Dilated cardiomyopathy • Epidermolysis bullosa
- Carnitine • Selenium

Dilated cardiomyopathy (DC) is a rare disease in the pediatric population, with an incidence of 0.6 to 0.7 per 10,000 children.[1] The World Health Organization defines DC as the progressive dilatation and impaired contractility of the left or both ventricles.[2] A specific cause is determined in only one-third of patients[3] and may involve idiopathic, familial or genetic, viral or autoimmune, and toxic or drug causes. The largest group is idiopathic DC. The term cardiomyopathy is also used for diseases that are associated with specific cardiac or systemic disorders, previously defined as specific heart muscle diseases, such as inflammatory and metabolic cardiomyopathies (micronutrient deficiencies).

The link between epidermolysis bullosa (EB) and DC has recently been described. Current data provided by the National EB Registry of the United States suggest a cumulative risk of DC of 4.51% in recessive dystrophic EB Hallopeau-Siemens type (RDEB-HS) (in or after the age of 20 years), 1.14% in junctional EB (JEB), and 0.4% in non–RDEB-HS.[4] Although the registry provides valuable information, data are based on patients' self-reports, and lack cardiac muscle biopsy specimens and echocardiogram diagnostic confirmation.

The first report of a patient with EB who presented with DC and died was made in 1986 by Sharratt and colleagues,[5] but little information was given about the patient's nutritional status and history. In 1989, Brook and colleagues[6] published a second case of a 17-year-old male patient with RDEB who developed heart failure secondary to DC. Several other case reports and case series have been published since then (Table 1). No clear cause has been identified, but iron overload, low

carnitine, low selenium, concomitant viral illness, chronic anemia, and medications have been proposed as possible contributors to the development of DC in the reported cases.[6–11]

Several observations can be derived from the summary of the published articles. All patients had RDEB and presented with DC at a mean age of 10.0 ± 6.6 years. The ejection fraction was low at diagnosis (9%–37%) with a mean of 20.6% ± 8.5%. The mortality was high (61.5%) and frequently occurred within the first 3 months after diagnosis of DC, suggesting that it may be too late to change the negative outcome if patients are diagnosed when symptomatic. Among the reported cases, low hemoglobin, low selenium, and low carnitine, either alone or in combination with other factors, may have played a role in causing DC.

Similar data were found in the largest retrospective series of patients with EB and DC presented in a poster at the Society of Pediatric Dermatology annual meeting in 2008.[12] Worldwide, a total of 15 patients having EB and with this association were identified. In this report, the mean age at diagnosis of DC was 12.18 ± 4.99 years, and 11 of them were male patients (73%). Eighty-seven percent of these 15 patients had DEB, and 13% had JEB (non-Herlitz subtype). Chronic anemia was diagnosed in 13 of 15 patients (86.7%), all requiring iron supplements. Selenium levels were abnormally low in 55% of patients (n = 11), whereas total carnitine levels were abnormal in 45% of patients at diagnosis (n = 11). Systolic function was moderately impaired, with a mean shortening fraction of 19.38% (standard deviation = 5.04, n = 8). After a mean follow-up period of

The Hospital for Sick Children, 555 University Avenue, Toronto, ON M5G 1X8, Canada
* Corresponding author.
E-mail address: elena.pope@sickkids.ca

Dermatol Clin 28 (2010) 347–351
doi:10.1016/j.det.2010.02.002

Table 1
Reported cases of EB associated with DC

Number of Patients	Age (y)	EF (%)	Outcome	TTD (mo)	Hb (mg/L)	Se	Carnitine	Attributed Cause	References
1	17	10	Alive	—	53	ND	ND	Iron overload	6
2	12.3	?	Dead	0	100	ND	ND	Selenium deficiency	7
	6.7	?	Dead	2	60	Low	Low		
6	12.5	14	Dead	2	88	ND	ND	Carnitine deficiency	8
	6.7	9	Dead	2	100	N	Low		
	5.8	16	Dead	1	67	Low	Low		
	9.9	27	Alive	—	89	N	N		
	8.8	27	Alive	—	94	N	N		
	8.3	28	Alive	—	98	N	N		
1	28	20	Alive	—	78	ND	ND	Viral myocarditis	9
1	5	20	Dead	3	70	N	N	Drugs (TCA)	10
1	2.1	33–37	Dead	11	73	N	N[a]	None	11
1	7	?	Dead	24	ND	ND	ND	None	5

Abbreviations: EF, ejection fraction; Hb, hemoglobin; N, normal; ND, not done; Se, selenium; TCA, tricyclic antidepressants; TTD, time to death; y, year; ?, information not available.
[a] After replacement.

6.3 ± 4.8 years, 6 patients were alive on no medications (40.0%), 2 were alive on medications (13.3%), and 7 had died (46.7%).

Both published and unpublished data raise the potential role of micronutrient deficiencies as predisposing factors to the development of DC in patients with EB.

SELENIUM DEFICIENCY

Selenium is a trace element that is a component of glutathione peroxidase (an enzyme that helps prevent oxidative insults to cells).[13,14] It is still unclear how selenium may contribute to the cardiac changes leading to DC, but it has been shown that selenium supplementation in deficient states, such as Keshan disease, reduces morbidity and mortality and alleviates the clinical course of the disease.[15] Apart from Keshan disease, selenium deficiency has also been associated with peripartum cardiomyopathy[16,17] and in idiopathic DC.[18,19]

In a group of 14 patients with RDEB, 61.5% were identified to have low selenium.[20] Although selenium deficiency may play a role in the development of DC, it is unlikely to be the only causal factor, particularly because some of the EB patients with DC reported in the literature had normal selenium levels.[7,11] In the case series by Sidwell and colleagues,[8] selenium was not found to be significantly lower in the patients with EB and DC when compared with patients having EB and not DC.

CARNITINE DEFICIENCY

Carnitine has also been associated with the development of DC in animals and humans.[21–23] Reports of EB patients with DC and carnitine deficiency have also been published.[7,8,10] The data from the study by Ingen-Housz-Oro and colleagues[24] showed that of the 14 patients reported, 61.5% had low free carnitine (total carnitine was normal in all but 1 patient).

Systemic carnitine deficiency, particularly the enzymatic abnormalities of carnitine palmitoyltransferase, is known to impair fatty acid oxidation that may lead to DC.[25] L-Carnitine is a transmembrane, cotransport molecule that is critical for mitochondrial β-oxidation, and therefore for normal myocardial energy metabolism.[26] Treatment with L-carnitine in patients without EB but with idiopathic DC has sporadically resulted in improvement of left ventricular function and may have a positive impact if DC is truly secondary to carnitine deficiency.[23] However, homozygous primary carnitine deficiency is a rare disorder that presents in infancy, and although heterozygous mutant variants of the carnitine transporter molecule do occur, these variants do not appear to be associated with cardiomyopathy.[27]

Sidwell and colleagues[8] found a statistically significant difference between the total and free carnitine levels of patients with EB and DC and those with EB and not DC ($P = 0.006$), but only 2 of their 6 patients had abnormal levels at diagnosis. Although levels were significantly lower in patients with EB and DC, some of these levels were in the normality range, which makes it difficult to identify patients at risk and also questions the role of carnitine in the pathogenesis of DC. To date, depressed levels of micronutrients, including free carnitine, that appear in isolation in EB are thought not to be significant in the cause of DC.[8,24]

ANEMIA AND IRON OVERLOAD

Many patients with EB and DC have chronic anemia (most likely multifactorial) and respond poorly to supplementation and thus may require repeated transfusion therapy.[12] Iron overload has also been associated with DC in conditions such as β-thalassemia major and other iron storage diseases.[28,29] In one of the first published cases of DC in EB, long-term transfusion therapy was thought to play a role in the development of DC.[6] It would also be important to exclude thalassemia minor in patients with RDEB so that they did not become iron overloaded from iron infusions, as this condition has been missed in the past and could lead to increased risk of cardiomyopathy (DF Murrell, personal communication, May 2009). T2* cardiac magnetic resonance imaging scans have been advocated as a noninvasive screening tool for detecting iron overload in conditions such as β-thalassemia major, and appear to correlate with levels of cardiac impairment.[30] This technique could be used in future cases of EB with DC to assess whether cardiac iron overload is implicated.

VIRAL ETIOLOGIES

Viral-mediated inflammatory cardiomyopathy is a well-recognized cause of DC.[31–33] A clinically apparent prodrome of viral symptoms is not always a constant feature and may be difficult to identify, because it may precede the presentation of DC by several months.[34] Even the analysis of heart tissue may not reveal viral or bacterial RNA or DNA because the microorganisms may no longer persist in myocardial tissue when DC is diagnosed.[35] It is thought that myocarditis and DC may represent the acute and chronic stages of organ-specific autoimmune diseases that can be viral or postinfectious.[33] An influenza-like prodrome was described by Morelli and colleagues[9] in their patient with EB who developed DC. Establishing this relationship in the population with EB as considered by the authors would be a difficult task because symptoms such as breathlessness and fever may go unnoticed in severe cases of EB. Furthermore, the diagnosis of myocarditis, even by endomyocardial biopsy, is challenging.

POSSIBLE GENETIC PREDISPOSITION

To date, there is no evidence that the underlying genetic mutations in type VII collagen or the basement membrane zone proteins in EB have a role in the pathogenesis of DC. Staining of heart tissue from the hearts of 6 children with DC not affected by EB did not show expression of type VII collagen, which makes the direct effect of the mutation in COL7AI an unlikely cause of DC in RDEB.[8] The distribution of collagen VII in a normal heart has not been included in most studies of collagen VII[36] and has been assumed to be negative. This assumption is on the basis that cardiac defects appear to be rare in RDEB, but other normal tissues that are negative for collagen VII, such as the kidney, have been found to stain positive for collagen VII when diseased.[37]

Whether a secondary alteration, which is unrelated to the underlying genetic defect in EB, is involved in DC has not been studied. The role of a secondary autoimmune phenomenon involving proteins present in both the heart and the skin (eg, desmosomal proteins) remains to be determined.

MANAGEMENT

Although limited, the available data highlight the importance of considering the diagnosis of DC as a potential complication of EB, particularly in sicker patients or patients with RDEB or JEB. Mineral deficiencies and chronic anemia are common in patients with EB and have been found to be associated with DC. Therefore, frequent screening and correction of these abnormalities is important. The reported cases also highlight the need for screening for DC in asymptomatic and mildly symptomatic patients. Mild symptoms may be hard to detect in patients with severe EB because of limited mobility and a large surface area being covered by dressings. The authors recommend paying attention to otherwise nonspecific symptoms that reflect a change in the baseline for each individual patient. Early detection allows for medical treatment that delays clinical progression and prolongs survival.

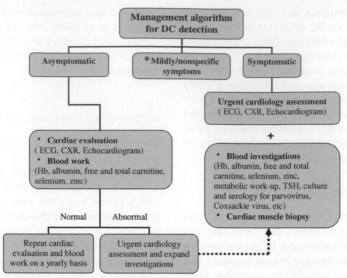

Fig. 1. Management algorithm for DC detection in EB patients. Asterisk indicates changes in exercise tolerance, nonspecific chest pain, poor or excessive weight gain, and poor feeding. CXR, chest radiograph; ECG, electrocardiogram; Hb, hemoglobin; TSH, thyroid-stimulating hormone.

The authors propose that the algorithm shown in **Fig. 1** be implemented for early detection of DC and for screening of DC in patients with EB.

PROGNOSIS

In populations with no EB, the natural history of DC is difficult to predict and is highly variable, ranging from complete recovery to death,[34] the latter occurring within 2 months after presentation.[38] Data from North America in the Pediatric Cardiomyopathy Registry demonstrate that the primary hazard phase for death or cardiac transplantation is in the first 24 months, with a 5-year transplant-free survival rate of approximately 54% in all comers. This phase is influenced by age and echocardiographic severity at presentation and prominently by the cause of DC, with myocarditis being the most favorable category.[39] According to the US Registry, 30% of patients affected with RDEB-HS died of congestive heart failure or cardiomyopathy.[4] Published and unpublished data suggest a higher mortality of 50% and 46.7% respectively.[8,12]

A slightly more favorable outcome of DC in children has been associated with age at presentation (before 2 years of age), a history of prior viral disease (up to 3 months before initial presentation), and improvement of ventricular function in the first 6 months after diagnosis.[3,5,38] Current data suggest that patients are diagnosed at a later age, again emphasizing the need for screening asymptomatic or mildly symptomatic cases.

SUMMARY

DC is a rare but potentially fatal complication of EB. Early detection and correction of potential contributors allows for a better prognosis.

REFERENCES

1. Lipshultz SE, Sleeper LA, Towbin JA, et al. The incidence of pediatric cardiomyopathy in two regions of the United States. N Engl J Med 2003;348(17): 1647–55.
2. Richardson P, McKenna W, Bristow M, et al. Report of the 1995 World Health Organization/International Society and Federation of Cardiology Task Force on the definition and classification of cardiomyopathies. Circulation 1996;93(5):841–2.
3. Gagliardi MG. Dilated cardiomyopathy in children. Acta Paediatr Suppl 2006;95(452):14–6.
4. Fine JD, Hall M, Weiner M, et al. The risk of cardiomyopathy in inherited epidermolysis bullosa. Br J Dermatol 2008;159(3):677–82.
5. Sharratt GP, Lacson AG, Cornel G, et al. Echocardiography of intracardiac filling defects in infants and children. Pediatr Cardiol 1986;7(4):189–94.
6. Brook MM, Weinhouse E, Jarenwattananon M, et al. Dilated cardiomyopathy complicating a case of epidermolysis bullosa dystrophica. Pediatr Dermatol 1989;6(1):21–3.
7. Melville C, Atherton D, Burch M, et al. Fatal cardiomyopathy in dystrophic epidermolysis bullosa. Br J Dermatol 1996;135(4):603–6.

8. Sidwell RU, Yates R, Atherton D. Dilated cardiomy-opathy in dystrophic epidermolysis bullosa. Arch Dis Child 2000;83(1):59–63.

9. Morelli S, Dianzani C, Sgreccia A, et al. Reversible acute global left ventricular dysfunction in a patient with autosomal recessive dystrophic epidermolysis bullosa. Int J Cardiol 2001;79(2–3):321–3.

10. Taibjee SM, Ramani P, Brown R, et al. Lethal cardio-myopathy in epidermolysis bullosa associated with amitriptyline. Arch Dis Child 2005;90(8):871–2.

11. Oh SW, Lee JS, Kim MY, et al. Recessive dystro-phic epidermolysis bullosa associated with dilated cardiomyopathy. Br J Dermatol 2007; 157(3):610–2.

12. Lara-Corrales I, Kantor P, Lucky A, et al. Dilated cardiomyopathy in epidermolysis bullosa, a retro-spective, multicenter study. Presented at the 34th Annual Meeting of the Society for Pediatric Derma-tology. Snowbird (UT), July 10, 2008.

13. Reeves WC, Marcuard SP, Willis SE, et al. Reversible cardiomyopathy due to selenium deficiency. JPEN J Parenter Enteral Nutr 1989;13(6):663–5.

14. Lockitch G. Selenium: clinical significance and analytical concepts. Crit Rev Clin Lab Sci 1989; 27(6):483–541.

15. Cheng TO. Selenium deficiency and cardiomyop-athy. J R Soc Med 2002;95(4):219–20.

16. Cenac A, Toure K, Diarra MB, et al. [Plasma sele-nium and peripartum cardiomyopathy in Bamako, Mali]. Med Trop (Mars) 2004;64(2):151–4 [in French].

17. Phillips SD, Warnes CA. Peripartum cardiomyop-athy: current therapeutic perspectives. Curr Treat Options Cardiovasc Med 2004;6(6):481–8.

18. Vijaya J, Subramanyam G, Sukhaveni V, et al. Sele-nium levels in dilated cardiomyopathy. J Indian Med Assoc 2000;98(4):166–9.

19. Chou HT, Yang HL, Tsou SS, et al. Status of trace elements in patients with idiopathic dilated cardio-myopathy in central Taiwan. Zhonghua Yi Xue Za Zhi (Taipei) 1998;61(4):193–8.

20. Haynes L. Nutritional support for children with epider-molysis bullosa. J Hum Nutr Diet 1998;11(2):163–73.

21. Freeman LM, Rush JE. Nutrition and cardiomyop-athy: lessons from spontaneous animal models. Curr Heart Fail Rep 2007;4(2):84–90.

22. Wang SM, Hou JW, Lin JL. A retrospective epidemi-ological and etiological study of metabolic disorders in children with cardiomyopathies. Acta Paediatr Taiwan 2006;47(2):83–7.

23. Kothari SS, Sharma M. L-carnitine in children with idiopathic dilated cardiomyopathy. Indian Heart J 1998;50(1):59–61.

24. Ingen-Housz-Oro S, Blanchet-Bardon C, Vrillat M, et al. Vitamin and trace metal levels in recessive

dystrophic epidermolysis bullosa. J Eur Acad Der-matol Venereol 2004;18(6):649–53.

25. Gilbert-Barness E. Review: metabolic cardiomyop-athy and conduction system defects in children. Ann Clin Lab Sci 2004;34(1):15–34.

26. El-Aroussy W, Rizk A, Mayhoub G, et al. Plasma carnitine levels as a marker of impaired left ventric-ular functions. Mol Cell Biochem 2000;213(1–2): 37–41.

27. Amat di San Filippo C, Taylor MR, Mestroni L, et al. Cardiomyopathy and carnitine deficiency. Mol Genet Metab 2008;94(2):162–6.

28. Trad O, Hamdan MA, Jamil A, et al. Reversal of iron-induced dilated cardiomyopathy during therapy with deferasirox in beta-thalassemia. Pediatr Blood Cancer 2009;52:426–8.

29. Hahalis G, Alexopoulos D, Kremastinos DT, et al. Heart failure in beta-thalassemia syndromes: a decade of progress. Am J Med 2005;118(9): 957–67.

30. Anderson LJ, Holden S, Davis B, et al. Cardiovas-cular T2-star (T2*) magnetic resonance for the early diagnosis of myocardial iron overload. Eur Heart J 2001;22(23):2171–9.

31. Heymans S. Inflammation and cardiac remodeling during viral myocarditis. Ernst Schering Res Found Workshop 2006;55:197–218.

32. Okazaki T, Honjo T. Pathogenic roles of cardiac auto-antibodies in dilated cardiomyopathy. Trends Mol Med 2005;11(7):322–6.

33. Caforio AL, Mahon NJ, Tona F, et al. Circulating cardiac autoantibodies in dilated cardiomyopathy and myocarditis: pathogenetic and clinical signifi-cance. Eur J Heart Fail 2002;4(4):411–7.

34. Bostan OM, Cil E. Dilated cardiomyopathy in child-hood: prognostic features and outcome. Acta Cardi-ol 2006;61(2):169–74.

35. Maisch B, Richter A, Sandmoller A, et al. Inflamma-tory dilated cardiomyopathy (DCMI). Herz 2005; 30(6):535–44.

36. Wetzels RH, Robben HC, Leigh IM, et al. Distribu-tion patterns of type VII collagen in normal and malignant human tissues. Am J Pathol 1991; 139(2):451–9.

37. Onetti Muda A, Ruzzi L, Bernardini S, et al. Collagen VII expression in glomerular sclerosis. J Pathol 2001; 195(3):383–90.

38. Matitiau A, Perez-Atayde A, Sanders SP, et al. Infan-tile dilated cardiomyopathy. Relation of outcome to left ventricular mechanics, hemodynamics, and histology at the time of presentation. Circulation 1994;90(3):1310–8.

39. Towbin JA, Bowles NE. Dilated cardiomyopathy: a tale of cytoskeletal proteins and beyond. J Cardi-ovasc Electrophysiol 2006;17(8):919–26.

Osteopenia and Osteoporosis in Epidermolysis Bullosa

Anna E. Martinez, MBBS, MRCP, MRCPCH[a],*,
Jemima E. Mellerio, MD, FRCP[a,b]

KEYWORDS

• Osteopenia • Osteoporosis • Vertebral fractures

THE PROBLEM OF POOR BONE HEALTH IN EB

Osteopenia, osteoporosis and fractures may occur in patients with epidermolysis bullosa (EB), particularly in the more severe forms of disease.[1–3] The incidence of vertebral fractures in these patients is unknown but was observed in 13 of 42 children with severe generalized recessive dystrophic EB (RDEB) at Great Ormond Street Hospital (AE Martinez and JE Mellerio, personal communication, 2009) (Fig. 1). Abnormal bone health in patients with EB may not be surprising as it is well documented in association with other chronic inflammatory diseases of childhood such as juvenile idiopathic arthritis (JIA) and inflammatory bowel disease (IBD).[4–6] The combination of inactivity with reduced muscle mass, nutritional compromise with altered nutritional use, chronic inflammation, abnormal growth, and pubertal delay is known to alter bone metabolism.[4–8] These factors hinder the acquisition of peak bone mass during childhood and adolescence, which is an most important determinant of long-term skeletal health.[5]

THE EFFECT OF REDUCED MOBILITY ON BONE HEALTH

Physical activity is critical for skeletal development: mechanical loading promotes increases in lean tissue mass, which is directly related to total bone mineral content. Exercise and mobility have been shown to increase bone mass in healthy children.[9,10] Pain, chronic anemia and contractures all contribute to an often restricted and limited mobility in patients with severe types of EB. In a study of 39 children with different forms of EB (RDEB, junctional EB (JEB), EB simplex Dowling-Meara (EBS-DM)), Fewtrell and colleagues[3] found lower bone mineral density (BMD) in patients with RDEB and JEB compared with patients with EBS-DM and controls, even after correcting for size. The strongest predictor of bone mass was mobility level. Two studies have investigated the effect of vibration therapy in children. Ward and colleagues[11] performed a trial on 20 disabled ambulant children who were randomized to standing on an active or a placebo vibrating device for 10 minutes per day, 5 days a week, for 6 months. Those on treatment had increased tibia and spine trabecular BMD, whereas those on placebo had reduced BMD (measured using a three-dimensional quantitative computed tomography scanner). A second study investigated the effect of 6 months whole-body vibration therapy in a total of 6 immobilized children and reported similar results; vibration therapy improved children's mobility and muscle power, and increased whole-body BMD.[12] Even though there are limited data on the effectiveness of

Funding: Dr Mellerio acknowledges financial support from the Department of Health via the National Institute for Health Research (NIHR) comprehensive Biomedical Research Centre award to Guy's & St Thomas' NHS Foundation Trust in partnership with King's College London and King's College Hospital NHS Foundation Trust.
[a] Department of Paediatric Dermatology (EB Office), Great Ormond Street Hospital for Children NHS Trust, Great Ormond Street, London WC1N 3JH, UK
[b] St John's Institute of Dermatology, Guy's and St Thomas' NHS Foundation Trust, Westminster Bridge Road, London SE1 7EH, UK
* Corresponding author.
E-mail address: martia@gosh.nhs.uk

Dermatol Clin 28 (2010) 353–355
doi:10.1016/j.det.2010.01.006
0733-8635/10/$ – see front matter

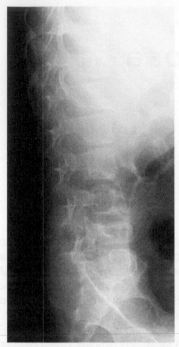

Fig. 1. Lateral spine radiograph showing a wedge vertebral fracture of L4.

vibration therapy in children, platforms are well tolerated in children and seem to have a positive effect on bone status, muscle strength, and mobility. In EB, where skin involvement and contractures often limit or reduce mobility and physical activity, vibrating platforms may be a useful therapeutic approach to consider using in future clinical trials.[13–15]

THE ROLE OF IMPAIRED NUTRITION IN BONE HEALTH

Nutritional compromise in children with severe types of EB is caused by a hypercatabolic inflammatory state with increased metabolic needs, often coupled with a reduced nutritional intake caused by oral and gastrointestinal tract involvement. Low 25-(OH) vitamin D levels may also result from reduced sunlight exposure in EB patients who are more restricted in outdoor activities and who may have extensive bandaging limiting sunlight-induced vitamin D production in the skin. Reyes and colleagues[2] evaluated BMD, vitamin D levels and bone turnover markers in 7 children with RDEB or JEB who were not taking vitamin supplements and found that osteopenia and low 25-(OH) vitamin D levels were present in 4 children. However, in a larger study, children with reduced BMD had normal levels of calcium, phosphate, and alkaline phosphatase, and vitamin

D levels more than 50 nmol/L.[3] Despite gastrostomy feeding and maintaining normal serum bone profile levels, children with severe types of EB still develop osteoporosis and vertebral fractures, highlighting the importance of other factors in contributing to overall poor bone health.

HORMONAL FACTORS AND INFLAMMATION MAY INFLUENCE BONE HEALTH

Delayed onset of puberty and reduced pubertal growth is often reported in patients suffering from chronic inflammatory diseases; the cause is also likely to be multifactorial.[16,17] Abnormalities of growth hormone (GH) and insulin-like growth factor-1 (IGF-1) axis and gonadotrophin secretion have been described in patients with chronic renal failure, cystic fibrosis and Crohn disease.[16] More recently, it has been shown that cytokines produced during chronic diseases such as JIA may affect the GH-IGF-1 axis[4] (see the article by Martinez and colleagues elsewhere in this issue for further exploration of this topic).

An imbalance of proinflammatory cytokines is often seen in patients with inflammatory disease of any cause. These may act individually or in combination to influence growth through systemic effects, and also have a local effect at the level of the growth plate of long bones.[18] Some cytokines have been shown to increase osteoclastic activity; tumor necrosis factor-alpha and interferon-gamma stimulate osteoclast formation both directly and via receptor activator for nuclear factor kappa B ligand (RANKL), having a catabolic effect on bones.[4,5,18,19] Patients with more severe forms of EB are often in a chronic inflammatory state secondary to chronic wounds with recurrent bacterial colonization and infection. This situation is reflected by greatly increased levels of inflammatory markers such as C-reactive protein, erythrocyte sedimentation rate, ferritin and raised platelet counts.

MONITORING AND MANAGEMENT OF BONE HEALTH IN EB PATIENTS

Monitoring BMD and detection of fractures is complicated. We have previously found that in children with EB, BMD Z-scores from anterioposterior lumbar DEXA scans are unlikely to identify individuals at risk of fractures, and may not reliably identify fractures diagnosed on contemporary lateral spine radiographs (A.E. Martinez, personal communication, 2009). However, annual DEXA scans can be useful for detecting osteopenia and osteoporosis. If present, calcium and vitamin D supplementation should be commenced and the serum bone profile monitored. Fractures are best detected with plain lateral radiographs of the thoracic and lumbar spine. We would recommend annual radiographs from age 5 years because of the difficulty in detecting these clinically; pain from other sources such as the skin may effectively mask pain caused by fractures.

Treatment of vertebral fractures remains controversial. Bisphosphonates orally or intravenously have been used to treat osteoporosis and fractures in children with other chronic diseases with variable results.[6] Data are lacking on the effectiveness and safety of bisphosphonate therapy in children with EB. Compared with treatment with intravenous pamidronate, oral risedronate seems to be equally effective in controlling bone pain and shows demonstrable improvement of vertebral fractures and mineralization on subsequent radiographs (A.E. Martinez, J.E. Mellerio, personal communication, 2009).

SUMMARY

Children and adults with EB, as with patients with other chronic inflammatory diseases, may develop osteopenia, osteoporosis and fractures. Recent advances in understanding of the role of inflammation affecting GH and bone growth are promising and may help to design new therapies. However, there remain many other areas that warrant further investigation, both into the cause of poor bone health in EB and the optimal approach to monitoring and management.

REFERENCES

1. Wong WL, Pemberton J. The musculoskeletal manifestations of epidermolysis bullosa: analysis of 19 cases and review of the literature. Br J Radiol 1992;65:480–4.
2. Reyes LM, Cattani A, Gajardo H, et al. Bone metabolism in children with epidermolysis bullosa. J Pediatr 2002;140:467–9.
3. Fewtrell MS, Allgrove J, Gordon I, et al. Bone mineralization in children with epidermolysis bullosa. Br J Dermatol 2006;154:959–62.
4. Pass C, MacRae VE, Ahmed SF, et al. Inflammatory cytokines and the GH-IGF-1 axis: novel actions on bone growth. Cell Biochem Funct 2009;27:119–27.
5. Viswanathan A, Sylvester F. Chronic inflammatory disease: effects on bone. Rev Endocr Metab Disord 2008;9:107–22.
6. Thornton J, Ashcroft DM, Mughal MZ, et al. Systemic review of the effectiveness of bisphosphonates in treatment of low mineral density and fragility fractures in juvenile idiopathic arthritis. Arch Dis Child 2006;91:753–61.
7. Van der Slusi IM, de Munick Keizer-Schrama SM. Osteoporosis in childhood. Bone density of children in health and disease. J Pediatr Endocrinol Metab 2001;14:817–32.
8. Daci E, Van Comphaut S, Bouillon R, et al. Mechanisms influencing bone metabolism in chronic illness. Horm Res 2002;58(Suppl 1):44–5.
9. Inomoto T. Physical activity/sports and bone mineral density. Clin Calcium 2008;18:1339–48.
10. Baxter-Jones AD, Kontulainen SA, Faulkner RA. A longitudinal study of the relationship of physical activity to bone mineral accrual from adolescence to young adulthood. Bone 2008;43:1101–7.
11. Ward K, Alsop C, Caulton J, et al. Low magnitude mechanical loading is osteogenic in children with disabling conditions. J Bone Miner Res 2004;19:360–9.
12. Semler O, Fricke O, Vezyroglou K, et al. Preliminary results on the mobility after whole body vibration in immobilized children and adolescents. J Musculoskelet Neuronal Interact 2007;7:77–01.
13. Torvinen S, Kannus P, Sievanen, et al. Effect of 8-month vertical whole body vibration on bone, muscle performance, and body balance: a randomized controlled study. J Bone Miner Res 2003;18:876–84.
14. Gilsanz V, Wren TA, Sanchez M, et al. Low-level, high-frequency mechanical signals enhance musculoskeletal development of young women with low BMD. J Bone Miner Res 2006;21:1464–74.
15. Roth J, Wust M, Rawer R, et al. Whole body vibration in cystic fibrosis – a pilot study. J Musculoskelet Neuronal Interact 2008;8:179–87.
16. Pozo J, Argente J. Delayed puberty in chronic disease. Best Pract Res Clin Endocrinol Metab 2002;16:73–90.
17. Simon D. Puberty in chronically diseased patients. Horm Res 2002;57:53–6.
18. MacRae VE, Wong SC, Farquharson C, et al. Cytokine actions in growth disorders associated with pediatric chronic inflammatory disease. Int J Mol Med 2006;18:1011–8.
19. Manolagas SC, Jilka RL. Bone marrow cytokines and bone remodeling. Emerging insights into the pathophysiology of osteoporosis. N Engl J Med 1995;332:305–11.

Growth and Pubertal Delay in Patients with Epidermolysis Bullosa

Anna E. Martinez, MBBS, MRCP, MRCPCH[a],*,
Jeremy Allgrove, MA, MD, FRCP, FRCPCH[b,c],
Caroline Brain, MB, BS, MD, MRCP, FRCPCH[c]

KEYWORDS

• Growth • Delayed puberty • Inflammation

Puberty is the acquisition of secondary sexual characteristics, associated with a growth spurt, resulting in the attainment of reproductive function and final adult height.[1] Delayed puberty is defined as the absence of any pubertal development at an age 2 standard deviations more than the mean, which corresponds to an age of approximately 14 years for boys and 13 years for girls. The actual incidence of pubertal delay associated with chronic illness is unknown. Delay is often considered to be acceptable as a consequence of the underlying disease and can be overlooked with other complications of the illness. However, because a larger proportion of patients with chronic disease are surviving longer and beyond the age of normal puberty, correct management of significant delay is increasingly important. Failure to do so may have a detrimental effect on final height, total bone mass and psychological health of the patients.[2]

The degree to which growth and pubertal development are affected in chronic illness depends on the disease itself, as well as factors such as age of onset, duration and severity; the earlier the onset and the more severe the disease, the greater the effect on growth and pubertal development.[2,3] Most children with severe types of EB have abnormal growth and pubertal delay; the possible pathophysiology is discussed.

REGULATION OF GROWTH AND PUBERTAL DEVELOPMENT

The hypothalamo-pituitary-gonadal axis is driven by intermittent discharges of gonadotrophin-releasing hormone (GnRH) generated by hypothalamic neurons known as the GnRH pulse generator.[1] At puberty, increasing levels of GnRH and increased pituitary sensitivity to GnRH result in an increase in luteinizing hormone (LH) and follicle-stimulating hormone (FSH), which in turn stimulates ovarian/testicular activity and is directly responsible for most of the changes seen during puberty.

Leptin, a protein produced by adipocytes, has been proposed as the hormone responsible for the initiation and progression of puberty. Mice and rats deficient in leptin fail to undergo puberty, illustrating the importance of its role in rodents.[4]

The integrity of the growth hormone (GH) insulin-like growth factor-1 (IGF-1) axis is critical for regulating growth during childhood and adolescence. GH is secreted in a pulsatile manner by the pituitary gland and binds to the GH receptor in the liver

[a] Department of Paediatric Dermatology (EB Office), Great Ormond Street Hospital for Children NHS Trust, Great Ormond Street, London, WC1N 3JH, UK
[b] Department of Paediatric Endocrinology, Barts and the London NHS Trust, Royal London Hospital, Whitechapel, London, E1 1BB, UK
[c] Department of Paediatric Endocrinology, Great Ormond Street Hospital for Children NHS Trust, Great Ormond Street, London, WC1N 3JH, UK
* Corresponding author.
E-mail address: martia@gosh.nhs.uk

Dermatol Clin 28 (2010) 357–359
doi:10.1016/j.det.2010.01.007

to generate IGF-1. The latter circulates bound predominately to IGF-binding protein-3 (IGF-BP3), which controls the availability of IGF-1 at tissue level. GH also acts directly on growth plates with amplification of local IGF-1 production.

A family of intracellular proteins known as suppressor of cytokine-inducible signaling (SOCS) are synthesized in response to inflammatory stimuli. They are physiological regulators of cytokine responses, including those that regulate the inflammatory systems.[5] GH and leptin are inhibited by SOCS-2 and SOCS-3, respectively.[6,7] Although at present the role of SOCS proteins in EB is unclear, in such an inflammatory disease it is likely to be important.

CAUSES OF PUBERTAL AND GROWTH DELAY IN PATIENTS WITH EB

Malnutrition is a well-known cause of pubertal delay and this can affect the entire hormonal system (insulin, thyroid hormones, cortisol and GH, and the hypothalamo-pituitary-gonadal axis).[8] The initial process seems to be hypoinsulinemia and an increase in GH secretion, which stimulate lipolysis to provide an alternative energy source.[8] Subsequently modification of the hypothalamic secretion of growth hormone-releasing hormone (GHRH) occurs, resulting in increased serum levels of GH in conjunction with decreased levels of IGF-1 leading to a state of GH resistance and a reduction in growth velocity and skeletal growth.[8] Malnutrition also affects the maturation of the hypothalamo-pituitary-gonadal axis causing delay in the pulsatile secretion of GnRH, the onset of puberty and consequent growth spurt.[2] Patients with severe types of EB and pubertal delay at Great Ormond Street Hospital in London have been found to have hypogonadotrophic hypogonadism; that is, secondary hypogonadism with reduced/low normal serum LH and FSH concentrations (A. Martinez and C. Brain, personal communication, 2010). Although the hormonal system has been poorly evaluated in patients with EB to date, malnutrition or nutritional compromise is likely to play one of the principal roles in delayed growth and puberty in this cohort of patients.

An imbalance of proinflammatory cytokines, notably interleukin-1B (IL-1B), tumor necrosis factor (TNF) and interleukin-6 (IL-6),[9–12] is seen in children with inflammatory diseases. Studies have shown that IL-6 and IL-1 can inhibit steroidogenesis in the ovary and the testis and inhibit secretion of GnRH by direct action on the hypothalamus.[13] In addition, IL-6 inhibits hepatic GH signaling by inducing SOCS-3, as well as increasing proteolysis of IGFBP-3 with impaired

formation of the IGF-1/IGFBP-3/acid labile subunit complex, resulting in a shorter half-life and enhanced clearance of IGF-1.[8] TNF-alpha also lowers IGF-1 by reducing hepatocyte expression of the GH receptors.[14] Although there are no data published on the GH/IGF-1 axis in EB patients, measurement of serum concentrations of IGF-1 and IGF-BP3 have been found to be greatly reduced in children with severe generalized recessive dystrophic EB in a London center (Anna Martinez, personal communication, 2010), supporting the possible effects of the inflammatory cytokines. The combination of nutritional compromise and a chronic inflammatory state are likely therefore to result in abnormalities in the GH/IGF-1 axis with partial GH resistance and effects on the function of the hypothalamo-pituitary-gonadal axis with hypogonadotrophic hypogonadism.

MONITORING AND MANAGEMENT OF GROWTH AND DELAYED PUBERTY

Awareness of the potential for growth and pubertal delay in patients with EB is important, and assessment of height, weight, and secondary sexual characteristic are an important part of the routine physical examination. Charts given to the child/guardian for self-assessment are useful, especially in adolescent boys with EB who are often reticent about any physical examination.

If delay is present, then basal serum levels of LH, FSH together with estradiol (girls) or testosterone (boys) should be obtained. Radiographs of the left hand and wrist to evaluate bone age can assess skeletal maturation[15] and help to confirm a picture of delay. In girls a pelvic ultrasound scan is helpful to assess uterine development and ovarian activity. Annual bone age assessment is recommended for this group of patients as they have multiple risk factors for low bone density.

The attainment of age appropriate secondary sexual characteristics is important not only psychologically for these vulnerable adolescent patients but also to optimize growth and the acquisition of peak bone mineral content. Therefore, carefully planned induction of puberty alongside the children's peer group is recommended but needs to be managed together with a pediatric endocrinologist.

SUMMARY

Proinflammatory cytokines and nutritional compromise have deleterious effects on growth in inflammatory bowel disease and other chronic inflammatory conditions by affecting the hypothalamic-pituitary and GH/IGF-1 axes. A similar mechanism is likely to contribute to growth and pubertal delay commonly encountered in patients with EB. Although supporting poor nutritional status is important, the inability at present to control disease activity and inflammation in patients with EB poses a barrier to the prevention of the impaired growth process most often present in this disease. With a better understanding of the effects of chronic inflammation on growth and pubertal development, it may be possible to develop new therapies in patients with EB.[16]

REFERENCES

1. Traggiai C, Stanhope R. Delayed puberty. Best Pract Res Clin Endocrinol Metab 2002;16:139–51.

2. Pozo J, Argente J. Delayed puberty in chronic illness. Best Pract Res Clin Endocrinol Metab 2002;16:73–90.

3. McKay HA, Bailey DA, Mirwald RL, et al. Peak bone mineral accrual and age at menarche in adolescent girls: a 6-year longitudinal study. J Pediatr 1998;133:682–7.

4. Ahima RS, Prabakaran D, Mantzoros C, et al. Role of leptin in the neuroendocrine response to fasting. Nature 1996;382:250–2.

5. Croker BA, Kiu H, Nicholson SE. SOCS regulation of the JAK/STAT signalling pathway. Semin Cell Dev Biol 2008;19:414–22.

6. Rico-Bautista E, Flores-Morales A, Fernandez-Perez L. Suppressor of cytokine signaling (SOCS) 2, a protein with multiple functions. Cytokine Growth Factor Rev 2006;17:431–9.

7. Yoshimura A, Nishinakamura H, Matsumura Y, et al. Negative regulation of cytokine signaling and immune responses by SOCS proteins. Arthritis Res Ther 2005;7:100–10.

8. Thissen J, Ketelslegers J. Endocrine response to under nutrition: from the experimental model to human physiology. In: Prader A, Rappaport R, editors. Clinical issues in growth disorders: evaluation, diagnosis and therapy. London: Freund Publishing house Ltd; 1994. p. 131–50.

9. Kutukculer N, Caglayan S, Aydogdu F. Study of pro-inflammatory (TNF-alpha, IL-1alpha, IL-6) and T-cell-derived (IL-2, IL-4) cytokines in plasma and synovial fluid of patients with juvenile chronic arthritis: correlations with clinical and laboratory parameters. Clin Rheumatol 1998;17:288–92.

10. Macrae VE, Wong SC, Farquharson C, et al. Cytokine actions in growth disorders associated with pediatric chronic inflammatory diseases [review]. Int J Mol Med 2006;18:1011–8.

11. Rooney M, Varsani H, Martin K, et al. Tumour necrosis factor alpha and its soluble receptors in juvenile chronic arthritis. Rheumatology (Oxford) 2000;39:432–8.

12. Wong SC, Macrae VE, McGrogan P, et al. The role of pro-inflammatory cytokines in inflammatory bowel disease growth retardation. J Pediatr Gastroenterol Nutr 2006;43:144–55.

13. Reichlin S. Neuroendocrine-immune interactions. N Engl J Med 1993;329:1246–53.

14. Barreca A, Ketelslegers JM, Arvigo M, et al. Decreased acid-labile subunit (ALS) levels by endotoxin in vivo and by interleukin-1beta in vitro. Growth Horm IGF Res 1998;8:217–23.

15. Tanner J, Healy H, Goldstein H, et al. Assessment of skeletal maturity and prediction of adult height (TW3 method). 3rd edition. London: WB Saunders; 2001.

16. Pass C, Macrae VE, Ahmed SF, et al. Inflammatory cytokines and the GH/IGF-I axis: novel actions on bone growth. Cell Biochem Funct 2009;27:119–27.

Gene Therapy for Recessive Dystrophic Epidermolysis Bullosa

Matthias Titeux, PhD[a,b], Valérie Pendaries, PhD[a,b],
Alain Hovnanian, MD, PhD[a,c,d],*

KEYWORDS

- Keratinocyte • Fibroblast • Vector
- Type VII collagen

Among the severe genetic disorders of the skin that are suitable for gene and cell therapy, most efforts have been made in the treatment of blistering diseases including dystrophic epidermolysis bullosa (DEB). DEB can be recessively (RDEB, OMIM #226600) or dominantly (DDEB, #131750) inherited, depending on the nature and position of the mutation or mutations in the gene encoding type VII collagen (COL7A1). RDEB is one of the most severe genodermatoses of children and young adults. Individuals with RDEB suffer from lifelong severe skin and mucosal blistering followed by scarring caused by the loss of adhesion between the epidermis and the dermis. Hands and feet in particular are severely affected, and repeated scarring leads to the fusion of digits and their retraction. Aggressive squamous cell carcinomas frequently develop in the areas subjected to repetitive blistering and scarring, and represent the most frequent cause of death in these patients.

The gene encoding type VII collagen, COL7A1, is segmented into 118 exons, spreads over 32 kb on human chromosome 3p21, and encodes a large cDNA of 8.9 kb. Type VII collagen is synthesized as a 290-kDa α1-chain protein precursor that assembles into a homotrimeric-quaternary structure. Homotrimers further assemble into antiparallel dimers in the extracellular matrix to form anchoring fibrils, which are key structures for the dermal-epidermal adherence.

At present, there is no specific treatment for RDEB, and gene and cell therapy approaches hold great promise. The first successful clinical trial of skin gene therapy was performed in a patient suffering from junctional epidermolysis bullosa (JEB).[1] This pioneer work paved the way for future trials aimed at correcting severe genetic skin disorders including RDEB. Meanwhile, novel strategies and technologies based on recent knowledge have been developed, allowing for successful preclinical studies in skin gene therapy trials using different approaches. This article discusses the different gene therapy approaches that have been used for the treatment of RDEB and the new perspectives that they open.

THERAPEUTIC STRATEGIES

The epidermis being a continuously self-renewing tissue, the curative treatment for RDEB must either be repeated throughout the lifetime of the patient or must involve the use or modification of stem cells that are able to permanently reconstitute the tissue. Epidermal stem cells have the capacity to regenerate for a lifetime,[2] and considerable progress has been made in the culture of these human epidermal stem cells. When appropriate culture conditions are used, it is possible to obtain large amounts of cultured epithelia from a small skin specimen, obtained by biopsy, within 3 to 4 weeks.[2,3] Over the past 20 years, cultured

---

[a] Institut National de la santé et de la recherche médicale, U563, F-31400 Toulouse France
[b] University Paul-Sabatier, F-31400 Toulouse, France
[c] Department of Genetics and Dermatology, Necker Hospital for Sick Children, Paris, F-75743 France
[d] University René Descartes, Paris V, F-75270 France
* Corresponding author. Department of Genetics, Necker Hospital for Sick Children, Paris, F-75743 France.
E-mail address: alain.hovnanian@inserm.fr

Dermatol Clin 28 (2010) 361–366
doi:10.1016/j.det.2010.02.003
0733-8635/10/$ – see front matter © 2010 Elsevier Inc. All rights reserved.

epithelial autografts have been successfully used worldwide to treat extensive third-degree burn wounds.[4] Major improvements have also been achieved in in vitro skin-equivalent systems with fibroblast-containing dermal components, tissue engineering, and surgical procedures. These systems have been reported to improve the quality of engrafted skin and wound healing.[5,6] Treatment of RDEB by transplantation of genetically modified skin equivalent could thus benefit from these biotechnological advances.

Strategy at the DNA Level

Genomic locus transfer

The first successful gene transfer applied to RDEB was achieved by microinjecting a PAC vector into a COL7A1-deficient cell line.[7] This genomic approach has several advantages such as the presence of the endogenous regulatory elements for physiologic expression of the transgene, and the maintenance of the genomic environment that can contain additional regions involved in the control of gene transcription. However, the efficiency of transfection methods for large DNA molecules is low, and the pursuit of this type of approach could benefit from systems of high capacity DNA vector such as herpes virus-based vectors.

cDNA transfer

For a long time, gene therapy for RDEB has been hampered because of the inability of the large-sized COL7A1 cDNA (8.9 kb) to transfer. The recent progress in vectorology has permitted vectors to accommodate cDNAs as large as 10 kb, and several groups using different approaches have been able to correct primary human keratinocytes and/or fibroblasts derived from patients with RDEB.

Ex vivo gene transfer The most efficient approach to achieve permanent transgene expression in epidermal stem cells is the ex vivo approach, whereby epidermal stem cells are harvested from the host by a skin biopsy and gene transfer is performed when the cells are growing in tissue culture. Genetically corrected cells are expanded, analyzed, and then grafted back onto the recipient. Several groups have reported successful COL7A1-cDNA transfer into keratinocyte cell lines, primary keratinocytes, or fibroblasts derived from a patient with RDEB using either nonviral gene transfer or virus-mediated gene transfer.

Ortiz-Urda and colleagues[8] have corrected primary keratinocytes from a patient with RDEB using a nonviral gene transfer method. A plasmid encoding the COL7A1 cDNA together with a selectable marker (blasticidin resistance) under the control of the CMV promoter was cotransfected with a plasmid expressing φC31 integrase. This phage-derived integrase mediated the integration of the construct that contained attB sites flanking the expression cassette, at the pseudo-attP sites naturally present in the human genome. Because of the low efficacy of the process, stably modified keratinocytes were selected using blasticidin. Subsequently, the groups of David Woodley and Mei Chen have used a self-inactivating (SIN) lentiviral vector to efficiently transduce immortalized-RDEB keratinocytes[9] or primary-RDEB fibroblasts[10] with the COL7A1 cDNA under the control of a modified retroviral promoter (MND). These investigators have shown functional correction with either keratinocytes or fibroblasts, and have shown that fibroblasts alone can correct the dermal-epidermal adherence defect. Similarly, Goto and colleagues[11] have shown functional correction, by correcting either RDEB keratinocytes or fibroblasts using a classic retroviral vector without selecting the cells with an antibiotic. In parallel, Gache and colleagues[12] have transduced primary-RDEB keratinocytes using a classic retroviral vector expressing COL7A1 cDNA under the control of the viral-LTR (long terminal repeat) and the gene that provides resistance to an antibiotic. The transduced cells were selected with zeocin to enrich the population in corrected cells.

In all cases, demonstration of functional correction was performed using grafting of the genetically corrected cells onto immunodeficient mice to show anchoring fibril formation in vivo in reconstructed human skin. The advantage of the ex vivo gene therapy approach aimed at grafting genetically corrected epithelia or skin equivalents is that it is potentially applicable to every patient with RDEB and that it has already been successful in the treatment of JEB.[1] However, it is a labor-intensive procedure, which is applicable to selected area of the patient's skin, but is more difficult to apply to affected mucosae.

The groups of Paul Khavari[13] and David Woodley[14] have used intradermal injection of ex vivo genetically corrected RDEB fibroblasts in RDEB skin equivalents grafted onto immune deficient mice. In one case, the fibroblasts were transfected with plasmids allowing for the selection of rare recombination events mediated by the φC31 integrase (as discussed earlier). In the second case, cells were transduced using the SIN-lentiviral vector expressing COL7A1 cDNA under the control of the retroviral-MND promoter. Both groups have shown that intradermally injected fibroblasts synthesized and secreted type VII collagen for up to 4 months, leading to anchoring fibril formation at the dermal-epidermal junction and restoration of the dermal-epidermal adherence. This strategy has the potential to treat large body areas of the skin. However, long-term maintenance has not been documented and the feasibility of this approach in patients remains to be assessed.

Collectively, these pioneering studies have established that corrective gene transfer for RDEB is feasible by different means. This research has provided a starting point for further refinement in future preclinical and clinical efforts using safer SIN-viral vectors expressing the *COL7A1* cDNA under the control of human promoters.[15]

In vivo gene transfer Woodley and colleagues[16] have shown functional correction after in vivo injection of a SIN-lentiviral vector expressing type VII collagen into RDEB skin equivalents grafted onto immunodeficient mice. This approach would avoid the need of culturing the cells, could permit treatment of areas not readily accessible, and theoretically would also offer a systemic treatment. However, in vivo injections of such vectors raise major safety concerns. Using this procedure, the possible expression of the transgene in targeted Langerhans cells or dendritic cells could lead to a higher risk of immune response against recombinant type VII collagen. But the main issue of such an approach is that the viral vector that is injected in vivo in a well-vascularized tissue could disseminate into the body and affect other organs, where the effect of ectopic expression of type VII collagen is unknown, or could genetically modify germline cells—an effect which is prohibited by the ethics committees.[17]

Strategy at the RNA Level

Classic gene therapy approaches for genetic disorders is based on the complementation of a functional deficiency via the transfer of the relevant wild-type nucleic acid sequence to cells and organs. A different methodological principle is to correct the endogenous genetic information itself to direct the biosynthesis of a functional protein product. The exon skipping strategy is based on the capacity of small antisense sequences to mask signals recognized by the spliceosome machinery, thus leading to the excision of the target exon or exons carrying the mutation or mutations. If the target exon sequence is dispensable and the process maintains the open reading frame, it produces a shortened protein, which is partly or completely functional, and which restores the phenotype.

This approach has been successfully applied to Duchenne muscular dystrophy (DMD) in animal models (for a review see the article by Aartsma-Rus and van Ommen[18]), and a phase 2 clinical trial for DMD is actually ongoing in patients in the Netherlands.[19,20]

Computational analysis of *COL7A1*-genomic sequence revealed that this gene is particularly suited for the exon skipping strategy. Indeed, targeted skipping of any of the 84 exons encoding the central collagenous region preserves the reading frame of the mRNA. Moreover, these exons encode multiples of the Gly-X-Y collagenous repeat, so that the shortening of the protein sequence resulting from exon skipping would preserve the periodicity of these collagenous repeats. Recently, the group of Hiroshi Shimizu has convincingly shown the dispensability of exon 70 of *COL7A1*, by transducing RDEB keratinocytes and fibroblasts using a retroviral vector encoding a *COL7A1* cDNA in which exon 70 was deleted.[21] This group has also induced in vivo targeted skipping of exon 70 using antisense oligoribonucleotides in RDEB skin equivalents grafted onto nude mice, albeit with low efficacy. Although the efficacy of this approach for RDEB remains to be shown, it offers the opportunity of a noninvasive systemic in vivo treatment using easy-to-manufacture compounds (oligoribonucleotides). Drawbacks are that it can be used only on a subset of patients carrying mutations within exons that are dispensable for type VII collagen function, and it would require lifelong periodic administration.

OBSTACLES TO THESE GENE THERAPY APPROACHES

For most of these approaches, clear proof-of-principle evidence has been provided, although the feasibility of other approaches remains to be established. Still, obstacles can prevent the development of clinical application or benefit.

Safety concerns of gene therapy have arisen from the serious adverse events observed in the X-SCID trial.[22,23] The risk of insertional mutagenesis is now being evaluated, and the SIN technology should lower the risk to an acceptable level. Recent articles have clearly shown that the major determinants of genotoxicity in the Retroviridae-derived viral vectors are the transcriptionally active LTRs (ie, non-SIN). Thus, SIN vectors, devoid of the strong enhancer sequence contained in the wild-type LTR, show greater safety and therapeutic potential.[24–26]

Therefore, none of the approaches discussed earlier are readily transferable into clinical applications because of the need for prokaryotic selectable markers, the use of classic retroviral vectors (non-SIN), or the use of the MND promoter in a SIN vector. This modified MoMuLV LTR-based promoter, which contains the strong enhancer responsible for the genotoxic effect, strongly reduces the advantage of the SIN technology.[25]

In addition, a major issue to gene, cell, or protein therapy for RDEB is the immune response against the cells producing type VII collagen or to the protein itself. In patients with RDEB, the risk of adverse immune response after treatment remains difficult to predict because the nature of the protein, the target cells, the level of expression, and the administration procedure play an important role in this phenomenon.

The skin is a model of graft rejection and has important immune-associated functions. This organ is directly involved in innate and adaptive immunity, through the recognition and destruction of foreign pathogens and the priming of professional antigen-presenting cells (Langherans cells and dendritic cells).

Studies on gene or protein therapy for genetic diseases such as hemophilia A and B, where a gene is either defective or missing, have shown that the therapeutic effect may be hampered by the host immune system[27,28]. This immune response against the newly introduced gene product could induce a treatment failure through the destruction of transduced cells or neutralization of the therapeutic protein.[29,30] Type VII collagen is known to be immunogenic because epidermolysis ullosa acquisita (EBA) is an autoimmune disease characterized by circulating autoantibodies directed against type VII collagen that deposit at the dermal-epidermal junction and cause skin blistering.[31,32] In addition, Remington and colleagues[33] have detected type VII collagen antibodies after injection of recombinant type VII collagen in Col7a1-knockout mice. Although these antibodies did not bind to the dermal-epidermal junction and thus do not seem to be pathogenic, this study confirms that patients with RDEB who have been treated are at risk of developing an immune response against type VII collagen. Moreover, for many autoimmune diseases, the presence of circulating autoantibodies can be found many years before disease onset.[34]

Therefore, the authors have developed enzyme-linked immunosorbent and immunospot (ELISA and ELISPOT) assays using the full-length–type VII collagen molecule to assess the risk for patients with RDEB to present with either humoral or cytotoxic immune responses against type VII collagen or the cells that secrete it. These very sensitive and specific tests have been validated using sera and T cells of patients with EBA, and have been designed to select and monitor patients with RDEB for gene/cell/protein therapy protocols.[35]

Thus, the prevention of an immune rejection using immunosuppression, or more likely the induction of immune tolerance, might be necessary to achieve successful gene therapy. For this purpose, injection or oral administration of the exogenous protein has been shown to induce tolerance in hemophilia.[36,37] Alternatively, recent studies have shown that targeting regulatory T cells can induce immune tolerance.[38,39]

SUMMARY

Skin gene therapy is a dynamic field of investigation, and already tremendous progress toward efficient gene transfer has been accomplished. The success of gene therapy for JEB will lead to therapeutic trials for RDEB in the near future, using SIN retroviral or lentiviral vectors. However, questions regarding the risk of immune responses against the newly synthesized type VII collagen molecules in patients completely lacking these proteins remain to be answered.

Overall, the authors think that these approaches are not mutually exclusive, and that patients could benefit from their combined use, as well as from cell therapy and protein approaches (see the articles by Yan and Murrell, and Kiuru and colleagues elsewhere in this issue for further exploration of this topic.) as part of a therapeutic arsenal for the treatment of RDEB. Recently, the authors have developed SIN retroviral vectors expressing COL7A1 under human promoters which are suitable for clinical application.[40]

REFERENCES

1. Mavilio F, Pellegrini G, Ferrari S, et al. Correction of junctional epidermolysis bullosa by transplantation of genetically modified epidermal stem cells. Nat Med 2006;12:1397–402.

2. Barrandon Y, Green H. Three clonal types of keratinocyte with different capacities for multiplication. Proc Natl Acad Sci U S A 1987;84:2302–6.

3. Rheinwald JG, Green H. Serial cultivation of strains of human epidermal keratinocytes: the formation of keratinizing colonies from single cells. Cell 1975;6:331–43.

4. Ronfard V, Rives JM, Neveux Y, et al. Long-term regeneration of human epidermis on third degree burns transplanted with autologous cultured epithelium grown on a fibrin matrix. Transplantation 2000;70:1588–98.

5. Llames SG, Del Rio M, Larcher F, et al. Human plasma as a dermal scaffold for the generation of a completely autologous bioengineered skin. Transplantation 2004;77:350–5.

6. Navsaria HA, Myers SR, Leigh IM, et al. Culturing skin in vitro for wound therapy. Trends Biotechnol 1995;13:91–100.

7. Mecklenbeck S, Compton SH, Mejia JE, et al. A microinjected COL7A1-PAC vector restores synthesis of intact procollagen VII in a dystrophic epidermolysis bullosa keratinocyte cell line. Hum Gene Ther 2002;13:1655–62.

8. Ortiz-Urda S, Thyagarajan B, Keene DR, et al. Stable nonviral genetic correction of inherited human skin disease. Nat Med 2002;8:1166–70.

9. Chen M, Kasahara N, Keene DR, et al. Restoration of type VII collagen expression and function in dystrophic epidermolysis bullosa. Nat Genet 2002;32:670–5.

10. Woodley DT, Krueger GG, Jorgensen CM, et al. Normal and gene-corrected dystrophic epidermolysis bullosa fibroblasts alone can produce type VII collagen at the basement membrane zone. J Invest Dermatol 2003;121:1021–8.

11. Goto M, Sawamura D, Ito K, et al. Fibroblasts show more potential as target cells than keratinocytes in COL7A1 gene therapy of dystrophic epidermolysis bullosa. J Invest Dermatol 2006;126:766–72.

12. Gache Y, Baldeschi C, Del Rio M, et al. Construction of skin equivalents for gene therapy of recessive dystrophic epidermolysis bullosa. Hum Gene Ther 2004;15:921–33.

13. Ortiz-Urda S, Lin Q, Green CL, et al. Injection of genetically engineered fibroblasts corrects regenerated human epidermolysis bullosa skin tissue. J Clin Invest 2003;111:251–5.

14. Woodley DT, Keene DR, Atha T, et al. Injection of recombinant human type VII collagen restores collagen function in dystrophic epidermolysis bullosa. Nat Med 2004;10:693–5.

15. Titeux M, Zanta-Boussif A, Rochat A, et al. Ex vivo gene therapy for recessive dystrophic epidermolysis bullosa using safe retroviral vectors expressing type VII collagen under the control of its promoter. J Invest Dermatol 2005;125:110.

16. Woodley DT, Keene DR, Atha T, et al. Intradermal injection of lentiviral vectors corrects regenerated human dystrophic epidermolysis bullosa skin tissue in vivo. Mol Ther 2004;10:318–26.

17. Spink J, Geddes D. Gene therapy progress and prospects: bringing gene therapy into medical practice: the evolution of international ethics and the regulatory environment. Gene Ther 2004;11:1611–6.

18. Aartsma-Rus A, van Ommen GJ. Antisense-mediated exon skipping: a versatile tool with therapeutic and research applications. RNA 2007;13:1609–24.

19. Aartsma-Rus A, Fokkema I, Verschuuren J, et al. Theoretic applicability of antisense-mediated exon skipping for Duchenne muscular dystrophy mutations. Hum Mutat 2009;30:293–9.

20. van Deutekom JC, Janson AA, Ginjaar IB, et al. Local dystrophin restoration with antisense oligonucleotide PRO051. N Engl J Med 2007;357:2677–86.

21. Goto M, Sawamura D, Nishie W, et al. Targeted skipping of a single exon harboring a premature termination codon mutation: implications and potential for gene correction therapy for selective dystrophic epidermolysis bullosa patients. J Invest Dermatol 2006;126:2614–20.

22. Hacein-Bey-Abina S, von Kalle C, Schmidt M, et al. A serious adverse event after successful gene therapy for X-linked severe combined immunodeficiency. N Engl J Med 2003;348:255–6.

23. Hacein-Bey-Abina S, Von Kalle C, Schmidt M, et al. LMO2-associated clonal t cell proliferation in two patients after gene therapy for SCID-X1. Science 2003;302:415–9.

24. Cornils K, Lange C, Schambach A, et al. Stem cell marking with promotor-deprived self-inactivating retroviral vectors does not lead to induced clonal imbalance. Mol Ther 2009;17:131–43.

25. Maruggi G, Porcellini S, Facchini G, et al. Transcriptional enhancers induce insertional gene deregulation independently from the vector type and design. Mol Ther 2009;17:851–6.

26. Montini E, Cesana D, Schmidt M, et al. The genotoxic potential of retroviral vectors is strongly modulated by vector design and integration site selection in a mouse model of HSC gene therapy. J Clin Invest 2009;119:964–75.

27. Dasgupta S, Navarrete AM, Delignat S, et al. Immune response against therapeutic factor VIII in hemophilia A patients—a survey of probable risk factors. Immunol Lett 2007;110:23–8.

28. Wang L, Cao O, Swalm B, et al. Major role of local immune responses in antibody formation to factor IX in AAV gene transfer. Gene Ther 2005;12:1453–64.

29. Ghazizadeh S, Kalish RS, Taichman LB. Immune-mediated loss of transgene expression in skin: implications for cutaneous gene therapy. Mol Ther 2003;7:296–303.

30. Tripathy SK, Black HB, Goldwasser E, et al. Immune responses to transgene-encoded proteins limit the stability of gene expression after injection of replication-defective adenovirus vectors. Nat Med 1996;2:545–50.

31. Woodley DT, Remington J, Chen M. Autoimmunity to type VII collagen: epidermolysis bullosa acquisita. Clin Rev Allergy Immunol 2007;33:78–84.

32. Woodley DT, Briggaman RA, Gammon WR. Acquired epidermolysis bullosa. A bullous disease associated with autoimmunity to type VII (anchoring fibril) collagen [review]. Dermatol Clin 1990;8(4):717–26.

33. Remington J, Wang X, Hou Y, et al. Injection of recombinant human type VII collagen corrects the

disease phenotype in a murine model of dystrophic epidermolysis bullosa. Mol Ther 2009;17:26–33.

34. Scofield RH. Autoantibodies as predictors of disease. Lancet 2004;363:1544–6.

35. Pendaries V, Gasc G, Titeux M, et al. Immune reactivity to type VII collagen: implications for gene therapy of recessive dystrophic epidermolysis bullosa. Gene Therapy 2010, in press.

36. Faria AM, Weiner HL. Oral tolerance: therapeutic implications for autoimmune diseases. Clin Dev Immunol 2006;13:143–57.

37. Rocino A, Santagostino E, Mancuso ME, et al. Immune tolerance induction with recombinant factor

VIII in hemophilia A patients with high responding inhibitors. Haematologica 2006;91:558–61.

38. Eghtesad S, Morel PA, Clemens PR. The companions: regulatory T cells and gene therapy. Immunology 2009;127:1–7.

39. Joffre O, Santolaria T, Calise D, et al. Prevention of acute and chronic allograft rejection with CD4+CD25+Foxp3+ regulatory T lymphocytes. Nat Med 2008;14:88–92.

40. Titeux M, Pendaries V, Zanta-Boussif MA, et al. SIN retroviral vectors expressing COL7A1 under human promoters for ex vivo gene therapy of recessive dystrophic epidermolysis bullosa. Mol Ther 2010, in press.

Fibroblast-Based Cell Therapy Strategy for Recessive Dystrophic Epidermolysis Bullosa

W.F. Yan, MBBS, MSc[a,b],
Dédée F. Murrell, MA, BMBCh, FAAD, MD[a,b,*]

KEYWORDS
- Fibroblasts • Dystrophic epidermolysis bullosa
- Cell therapy

Dystrophic epidermolysis bullosa (DEB) is a severe skin fragility disorder associated with trauma-induced blistering, progressive soft tissue scarring, and increased risk of skin cancer. DEB is caused by mutations in the COL7A1 gene which result in reduced, truncated, or absent type VII collagen, and anchoring fibrils at the dermal-epidermal junction (DEJ). Although various topical wound-healing agents have been examined, including autologous cultured keratinocytes and skin bioequivalents, none has shown unequivocal benefits in the treatment of dystrophic forms of EB. Alternative approaches are needed.

CLINICAL MANIFESTATIONS

The spectrum of disease is very wide, ranging from minor dystrophy in the nails to the more severe forms in which there is a significant fragility of the skin with recurrent wounds, infection, scarring, deformity, failure to thrive, and premature death from squamous cell carcinoma.[1] The most severe varieties of the disease characteristically begin at birth with both cutaneous and mucosal involvement. Severe generalized blistering produces erosions that heal slowly, with atrophic scarring and milia formation. Nails become dystrophic and are lost early in life. Repeated cycles of blistering followed by scarring lead to digital fusion and mittenlike epidermal encasements of the fingers and toes, and flexural contractures of the knees, elbows, and wrist joints. Other features include esophageal stenosis,[2] dilated cardiomyopathy,[3] fractures,[4] and dental deformities.[5] Recurrent denudation of the skin, with chronic inflammation, causes anemia and growth retardation in severe recessive dystrophic epidermolysis bullosa (RDEB).

CLASSIFICATION OF RECESSIVE DYSTROPHIC EPIDERMOLYSIS BULLOSA

RDEB is classified into 2 subtypes, namely generalized severe (RDEB-GS) and generalized, other; the former lacks anchoring fibrils, whereas the latter exhibits reduced or rudimentary-appearing anchoring fibrils.[6] RDEB-GS is easily one of the most devastating, chronic diseases known to humanity. Characterized by mechanical fragility and repeated blister formation within potentially all epithelial-surfaced or lined structures, patients with generalized subtypes of RDEB who survive recurrent bacterial sepsis during early infancy are at high risk of later developing one or more severe complications, including profound growth retardation, multifactorial anemia, esophageal strictures, corneal scarring or blindness, poststreptococcal glomerulonephritis and renal failure, and progressive mutilation and loss (pseudosyndactyly) of the fingers and toes.[7]

[a] Department of Dermatology, St George Hospital, Gray Street, Kogarah, Sydney, NSW 2217, Australia
[b] University of New South Wales, Sydney, NSW 2050, Australia
* Corresponding author. Department of Dermatology, St George Hospital, Gray Street, Kogarah, Sydney, NSW 2217, Australia.
E-mail address: d.murrell@unsw.edu.au

Dermatol Clin 28 (2010) 367–370
doi:10.1016/j.det.2010.01.015

ETIOLOGY AND PATHOGENESIS

Two possible mechanisms for blister formation have been proposed: (1) destruction of dermal connective tissue by excessive amount of a protease,[8] and (2) a defective structural protein in the dermis that is responsible for the normal integrity of the skin at the epidermal-dermal junction.[9–11] Electron microscopy shows destruction of collagen fibrils in association with blister formation, as well as phagocytosis of collagen by macrophages in the skin adjacent to clinical blisters.[12]

The pathogenesis of DEB and structure of collagen VII are reviewed by Bruckner-Tuderman[13] and Uitto.[14] The purpose of "cell therapy" for RDEB is to increase the amount of collagen VII in the basement membrane zone (BMZ) to heal wounds and prevent further wound formation. Many DEB patients have multiple wounds with a large area of involvement, and all of these areas ideally should be treated, along with internal blistering such as may appear in the esophagus.

Compared with gene therapy, cell therapy has many advantages. The most important feature is that fibroblast cell therapy is safe and easy to work with. Several experiments have been performed with allogeneic fibroblasts, autologous fibroblasts, or parent donor fibroblasts in mouse models and in one study in RDEB patients in recent years. Only minor side effects such as temporary erythema, pruritus, mild hypertrophic scarring at the injection sites, and local skin inflammation have been found in some cases. All of these side effects resolved spontaneously.[15] Fibroblasts are more robust and easier to propagate than keratinocytes,[16] are less susceptible to growth arrest and differentiation, and can be frozen, packaged, and stored. Fibroblasts can be used by intradermal injection into skin and no special subsequent wound care is required. Furthermore, unlike stem cell transplantation, in which human leukocyte antigen (HLA) typing is important because the degree of HLA compatibility between donor and recipient will influence the outcome of the transplant, the donor of fibroblasts can be unrelated to the patient. Graft-versus-host disease did not occur when allogeneic fibroblasts were injected in the pilot study of 5 patients.[15] These advantages of fibroblast-based cell therapy give hope to RDEB patients and their families for improving therapy in the near future.

TARGET CELLS CHANGED FROM KERATINOCYTES TO FIBROBLASTS

Keratinocytes and dermal fibroblasts both express collagen VII, but keratinocytes are the primary source of collagen VII in the developing skin.[17,18] Many investigators have used keratinocytes as the target cells of RDEB gene therapy. Of note, intradermal injection of normal human fibroblasts or gene-corrected RDEB fibroblasts alone were found capable of synthesizing and secreting stable deposition of type VII collagen in mouse DEJ, thus contributing to the formation of anchoring fibrils.[19,20]

FIBROBLAST-BASED CELL THERAPY IN MOUSE STUDIES

Intradermal Injection of RDEB Fibroblasts Overexpressing Type VII Collagen

In 2003, RDEB fibroblasts overexpressing collagen VII (RDEB+ fibroblasts), RDEB fibroblasts, and normal fibroblasts were injected into mouse intact skin and the expression of collagen VII in mouse skin was determined. Compared with normal fibroblasts, which only produce a low level of collagen VII centered around murine dermal hair follicles, and RDEB fibroblasts, which yielded undetectable protein, the results showed that RDEB+ fibroblasts can produce correctly localized collagen VII at the epidermal-dermal junction, which can be stable for 16 weeks.[21]

Intradermal Injection of Normal Allogeneic Human Fibroblasts

Based on the supposition that the administration of actual fibroblasts would result in more sustained type VII collagen deposition, gene-corrected RDEB fibroblasts and normal human fibroblasts alone were administered to immunodeficient mouse skin or transplanted human skin equivalent. The expression of new human collagen VII by gene-corrected fibroblasts were detected stably for at least 4 months, and formation of anchoring fibrils was present in the mouse DEJ after injection. Nevertheless, unlike what had been found by Ortiz-Urda, this study also found that normal human fibroblasts are capable of producing, secreting, and depositing collagen VII at the DEJ as effectively as gene-corrected fibroblasts, which seems to be dependent on the number of cells injected, that is, 5×10^6 cells versus 1×10^6 cells.[19,21]

Bruckner-Tuderman's group succeeded in creating a mouse model for RDEB that expressed collagen VII at about 10% normal level, and their phenotype closely resembled characteristics of RDEB.[22] Intradermal injection of wild-type (WT) fibroblasts resulted in restoration of the DEJ, and increased deposition of collagen VII and resistance to induced stress compared with untreated areas. Recently, a long-term study of fibroblast-based cell therapy has been performed on a mouse model for RDEB. Collagen VII expression at the DEJ was increased by 3.5- to 4.7-fold for at least 100 days after intradermal injection of WT fibroblasts, and injected fibroblasts were the major source of newly deposited collagen VII, although injected fibroblasts gradually become apoptotic within 28 days. Skin integrity and resistance to mechanical forces also improved for at least 100 days. This preclinical test paves the way for human clinical trials.[23]

Intravenous Injection of Normal Human Fibroblasts

Severe RDEB patients usually have widespread lesions and multiple wounds spanning large areas as well as internal esophageal erosions; hence, a systemic delivery mode for cell therapy would be ideal. One problem with therapy involving intradermal injection of fibroblasts is that many intradermal injections need to be performed into numerous wound sites for each patient. An alternative strategy might be to inject allogeneic fibroblasts into the patient's circulation that home to the skin wounds and deposit the transgene product. A recent study showed that intravenously injected normal human fibroblasts home to the sites of wounded human RDEB skin engrafted onto immunosuppressed mice, and continually synthesize and secrete collagen VII to the BMZ of the human skin, forming anchoring fibril structures.[24,25] Thus, the mouse had a heterogeneous population of anchoring fibrils made up of both mouse collagen VII α chains and human collagen VII α chains. Of note, the investigators found that collagen VII delivered to the wound sites significantly enhanced wound healing. This study provides the first demonstration of the potential use of intravenously injected normal fibroblasts to restore collagen VII in DEB patients who have multiple open wounds.

FIBROBLAST-BASED CELL THERAPY FOR RDEB PATIENTS

Among the current cell therapies for RDEB using skin fibroblasts are the use of allogeneic fibroblasts (cultured from the patients' parents or unrelated individuals) or autologous fibroblasts (cultured from the patients themselves). Specifically, investigators evaluated the clinical benefits that may accrue from a single intradermal injection of these cells in subjects with RDEB. To assess potential clinical benefits in humans, Wong and colleagues[15] gave single intradermal injections of allogeneic fibroblasts to nonwounded skin on the backs of 5 subjects with collagen VII positive

RDEB. These investigators noted a 1.5- to 2-fold increase of type VII collagen at the DEJ at 2 weeks and at 3 months following injection, and a 1.5-fold increase of anchoring fibrils. Molecular analysis suggested that the major effect of allogeneic fibroblasts is to increase the recipients' own COL7A1 mRNA levels, with greater deposition of mutant type VII collagen at the DEJ and formation of additional rudimentary anchoring fibrils. No significant immune reactions were observed in skin biopsies, and none of these patients developed autoantibodies to collagen VII.

In a clinical trial of allogeneic cultured dermal substitute for the treatment of skin wounds in patients with RDEB, Hasegawa and colleagues[26,27] employed an allogeneic cultured dermal substitute (CDS) prepared by plating normal human fibroblasts on a double-layer spongy matrix of hyaluronic acid (HA) and Atelo-collagen (Col) to treat RDEB patients. During a 6-week treatment, abundant granulation was found on the wound surface within a week and epithelialization began from the margins of the ulcer after 4 weeks. This study indicated that cryopreserved human fibroblasts in the CDS are able to release vascular endothelial growth factor and fibronectin, which in turn induce prompt granulation in the wound beds. These data demonstrated the feasibility of fibroblast-based therapeutic approaches in a preclinical setting, and lay a basis for further dissection of quantitative and qualitative details associated with development of a clinically applicable therapy regimen.

McGrath's group have been conducting an open-label study of cultured foreskin fibroblasts obtained from Intercytex to RDEB wounds with encouraging results (EB 2009, Vienna, oral communication). The authors' group has conducted a double-blind randomized placebo-controlled trial of allogeneic fibroblasts versus their transport media in paired symmetric wounds in RDEB, demonstrating efficacy and safety of the technique.[28]

SUMMARY AND FUTURE OVERVIEW

RDEB is caused by recessive mutations in the human type VII collagen gene. The current lack of specific treatment for RDEB is the impetus to develop fibroblast-based cell therapy strategies that have many advantages including technical ease of use, wide application, and minor side effects. Over the past 10 years, tremendous progress has been made in fibroblast-based cell therapy for RDEB. Fibroblast-based cell therapy can dramatically restore stable collagen VII at the DEJ and normalize the substructure changes of DEB for at least a few months. Even though the mechanism and the duration of newly produced collagen VII at the DEJ are still unknown, cell therapy provides a new effective approach to therapy for RDEB.

REFERENCES

1. Mallipeddi R. Epidermolysis bullosa and cancer. Clin Exp Dermatol 2002;27(8):616–23.
2. Okada T, Sasaki F, Shimizu H, et al. Effective esophageal balloon dilation for esophageal stenosis in recessive dystrophic epidermolysis bullosa. Eur J Pediatr Surg 2006;16(2):115–9.
3. Fine JD, Hall M, Weiner M, et al. The risk of cardiomyopathy in inherited epidermolysis bullosa. Br J Dermatol 2008;159(3):677–82.
4. Fewtrell MS, Allgrove J, Gordon I, et al. Bone mineralization in children with epidermolysis bullosa. Br J Dermatol 2006;154(5):959–62.
5. De Benedittis M, Petruzzi M, Favia G, et al. Orodental manifestations in Hallopeau-Siemens-type recessive dystrophic epidermolysis bullosa. Clin Exp Dermatol 2004;29(2):128–32.
6. Fine JD, Eady RA, Bauer EA, et al. The classification of inherited epidermolysis bullosa (EB): report of the Third International Consensus Meeting on Diagnosis and Classification of EB. J Am Acad Dermatol 2008; 58(6):931–50.
7. Fine JD, Johnson LB, Weiner M, et al. Chemoprevention of squamous cell carcinoma in recessive dystrophic epidermolysis bullosa: results of a phase 1 trial of systemic isotretinoin. J Am Acad Dermatol 2004;50(4):563–71.
8. Takamori K, Ikeda S, Naito K, et al. Proteases are responsible for blister formation in recessive dystrophic epidermolysis bullosa and epidermolysis bullosa simplex. Br J Dermatol 1985;112(5):533–8.
9. Uitto J, Pulkkinen L, McLean WH. Epidermolysis bullosa: a spectrum of clinical phenotypes explained by molecular heterogeneity. Mol Med Today 1997;3(10):457–65.
10. Korge BP, Krieg T. The molecular basis for inherited bullous diseases. J Mol Med 1996;74(2):59–70.
11. Chan LS, Fine JD, Hammerberg C, et al. Defective in vivo expression and apparently normal in vitro expression of a newly identified 105-kDa lower lamina lucida protein in dystrophic epidermolysis bullosa. Br J Dermatol 1995;132(5):725–9.
12. Tidman MJ, Eady RAJ. Evaluation of anchoring fibrils and other components of the dermal-epidermal junction in dystrophic epidermolysis by a quantitative ultrastructural technique. J Invest Dermatol 1985;84:374–7.
13. Bruckner-Tuderman L. Dystrophic epidermolysis bullosa: pathogenesis and clinical features. Dermatol Clin 2010;28(1):107–14.
14. Chung HJ, Uitto J. Type VII collagen: the anchoring fibril protein at fault in dystrophic epidermolysis bullosa. Dermatol Clin 2010;28(1):93–105.
15. Wong T, Gammon L, Liu L, et al. Potential of fibroblast cell therapy for recessive dystrophic epidermolysis bullosa. J Invest Dermatol 2008;128(9):2179–89.
16. Chen M, Woodley DT. Fibroblasts as target cells for DEB gene therapy. J Invest Dermatol 2006;126(4):708–10.
17. Ryynänen M, Ryynänen J, Sollberg S, et al. Genetic linkage of type VII collagen (COL7A1) to dominant dystrophic epidermolysis bullosa in families with abnormal anchoring fibrils. J Clin Invest 1992; 89(3):974–80.
18. Ghazizadeh S, Taichman LB. Virus-mediated gene transfer for cutaneous gene therapy. Hum Gene Ther 2000;11(16):2247–51.
19. Woodley DT, Krueger GG, Jorgensen CM, et al. Normal and gene-corrected dystrophic epidermolysis bullosa fibroblasts alone can produce type VII collagen at the basement membrane zone. J Invest Dermatol 2003;121(5):1021–8.
20. Goto M, Sawamura D, Nishie W, et al. Targeted skipping of a single exon harboring a premature termination codon mutation: implications and potential for gene correction therapy for selective dystrophic epidermolysis bullosa patients. J Invest Dermatol 2006;126(12):2614–20.
21. Ortiz-Urda Susana, Lin Qun, Green Cheryl L, et al. Injection of genetically engineered fibroblasts corrects regenerated human epidermolysis bullosa skin tissue. J Clin Invest 2003;111(2):251–5.
22. Fritsch A, Loeckermann S, Kern JS, et al. A hypomorphic mouse model of dystrophic epidermolysis bullosa reveals mechanisms of disease and response to fibroblast therapy. J Clin Invest 2008;118(5):1669–79.
23. Kern JS, Loeckermann S, Fritsch A, et al. Mechanisms of fibroblast cell therapy for dystrophic epidermolysis bullosa: high stability of collagen VII favors long-term skin integrity. Mol Ther 2009, Jun 30 [online].
24. Woodley DT, Remington J, Huang Y, et al. Intravenously injected human fibroblasts home to skin wounds, deliver type VII collagen, and promote wound healing. Mol Ther 2007;15(3):628–35.
25. Uitto J. Epidermolysis bullosa: prospects for cell-based therapies. J Invest Dermatol 2008;128(9):2140–2.
26. Hasegawa T, Suga Y, Mizoguchi M, et al. Clinical trial of allogeneic cultured dermal substitute for the treatment of intractable skin ulcers in 3 patients with recessive dystrophic epidermolysis bullosa. J Am Acad Dermatol 2004;50(5):803–4.
27. Yamada N, Uchinuma E, Kuroyanagi Y. Clinical trial of allogeneic cultured dermal substitutes for intractable skin ulcers of the lower leg. J Artif Organs 2008;11(2):100–3.
28. Yan WF, Venugopal SS, Frew JW. Igawa S, Ishida-Yamamoto A, Murrell DF: Investigation of cell therapy for generalized severe recessive dystrophic epidermolysis bullosa by intradermal allogeneic fibroblasts randomized against placebo injections. J Invest Dermatol 2009;129:S28.

Bone Marrow Stem Cell Therapy for Recessive Dystrophic Epidermolysis Bullosa

Maija Kiuru, MD, PhD[a], Munenari Itoh, MD, PhD[a],
Mitchell S. Cairo, MD[b,c,d], Angela M. Christiano, PhD[a,e,*]

KEYWORDS

- Recessive dystrophic epidermolysis bullosa
- Bone marrow transplantation • Bone marrow stem cells
- Stem cell microenvironment • Clinical trial

The dystrophic forms of epidermolysis bullosa are a group of inherited blistering disorders caused by mutations in the type VII collagen gene (COL7A1).[1] Recessive dystrophic epidermolysis bullosa (RDEB) is characterized by severely reduced or complete lack of type VII collagen protein production, frequently resulting from premature termination codon mutations.[1] Type VII collagen, produced by both keratinocytes and fibroblasts, is the predominant component of anchoring fibrils, which connect the cutaneous basement membrane to the dermis, thereby maintaining the integrity of the epidermal-dermal connection.[2] Severe defects of anchoring fibrils in RDEB result in impaired dermal-epidermal cohesion as well as defective adhesion of mucosal surfaces in the gastrointestinal tract. Clinically, the patients show tense blisters and erosions that heal with extensive and mutilating scarring.[3] Scarring eventually leads to joint contractures and pseudosyndactyly. Repeated lifelong blistering and aberrant tissue repair results in aggressive and metastatic squamous cell carcinoma, one of the causes of early death in these patients.[3]

At present, there is no definitive treatment for RDEB. Clinical management is mainly supportive, aiming at protection of skin from friction, prevention of infections and loss of body fluids, analgesia, and optimal nutritional status.[4] Tremendous progress in understanding the molecular basis of RDEB has provided the basis for development of novel genetic and cellular therapies targeted at restoring the defective anchoring fibrils. The techniques include local or systemic delivery of collagen type VII gene using viral and nonviral vehicles, collagen type VII protein, genetically modified autologous cells, and allogeneic cells from unaffected donors.[5,6]

This review focuses on the development of bone marrow stem cell therapies for RDEB. The rationale for bone marrow stem cell therapies is based on the capacity of bone marrow–derived cells to differentiate into skin cells given the right microenvironment.[7–19] The hypothesis is that chronic skin

[a] Department of Dermatology, Columbia University, 630 West 168th Street VC15-204, New York, NY 10032, USA
[b] Department of Pediatrics, Morgan Stanley Children's Hospital of New York-Presbyterian Hospital, Columbia University, 3959 Broadway, CHN 10-03, New York, NY 10032, USA
[c] Department of Pathology, Morgan Stanley Children's Hospital of New York-Presbyterian Hospital, Columbia University, 3959 Broadway, CHN 10-03, New York, NY 10032, USA
[d] Department of Medicine, Morgan Stanley Children's Hospital of New York-Presbyterian Hospital, Columbia University, 3959 Broadway, CHN 10-03, New York, NY 10032, USA
[e] Department of Genetics & Development, Columbia University, 630 West 168th Street VC15-204, New York, NY 10032, USA
* Corresponding author. Department of Dermatology, Columbia University, 630 West 168th Street VC15-204, New York, NY 10032.
E-mail address: amc65@columbia.edu

Dermatol Clin 28 (2010) 371–382
doi:10.1016/j.det.2010.02.004

injury in RDEB generates a microenvironment that promotes homing of bone marrow–derived stem cells, which can then differentiate into skin cells, produce type VII collagen, and restore the anchoring fibrils defective in RDEB. Bone marrow cell therapy provides several advantages compared with other genetic and cellular therapies. Transplantation of wild-type allogeneic stem cells obviates the need for exogenous viral gene delivery and the risks associated with it, including insertional mutagenesis[20] and the eventual loss of gene expression. Furthermore, because bone marrow cell therapy can be delivered systemically via bone marrow transplantation, the therapy enables targeting of extensively affected skin as well as internal organs in RDEB. Here we review the data on the capacity of bone marrow–derived cells to become skin cells, the substantial progress both in preclinical and ongoing clinical studies, and the future directions in developing bone marrow stem cell therapies as a potential cure for RDEB.

BONE MARROW STEM CELL REPROGRAMMING INTO SKIN CELLS

Pluripotent embryonic stem cells are capable of differentiating into all cell types of the body.[21,22] By contrast, adult stem cells are capable of differentiating into some or all major cell types of the tissue or organ in which they reside. Bone marrow is the major source of adult hematopoietic stem cells (HSCs), which are capable of reconstituting the entire circulating population of hematopoietic cells.[23] The bone marrow also contains mesenchymal stem cells (MSCs), which contribute to the regeneration of mesenchymal tissues, including bone, cartilage, muscle, and adipose tissues.[24] In addition, bone marrow stem cells appear to have the capacity to differentiate into other cell types such as endoderm (eg, liver) and ectoderm (eg, epidermis).[7,25–28] This property has been attributed to bone marrow stem cell reprogramming or heterogeneity of stem cell types within bone marrow, although debate existed initially on the contribution of cell fusion and technical limitations to these observations.[29–32] Of importance is that the property of bone marrow cells differentiating into other cell types is thought to be relatively rare, guided by signals from a given microenvironment and promoted by selective advantage, as in the case of tissue injury.

Bone Marrow–Derived Stem Cells Exhibit Homing to the Skin

Bone marrow–derived stem cells have the capacity to migrate to the skin and become skin cells (Table 1).[7–15,17,18,33] The studies are largely retrospective data on transplantation of genetically marked or sex-mismatched donor bone marrow into wild-type recipients. Engraftment and differentiation of donor-derived cells has been shown by detection of donor-derived DNA, mRNA, or protein. Substantial variability in study design exists, most importantly in methods used for isolation of donor cells and characterization of engrafted donor cells. In some studies the transplant has been enriched for HSCs or MSCs, whereas others have used total bone marrow. Furthermore, the studies have focused on detection of either bone marrow–derived keratinocytes or fibroblasts, or both (see Table 1).

In their pioneering work, Krause and colleagues[7] demonstrated engraftment of bone marrow–derived stem cells to multiple organs, including the skin, after sex-mismatched transplants of a single bone marrow–derived stem cell harvested after serial transplantation. To isolate the HSC population, the donor cells were enriched through multiple sophisticated steps including lineage depletion, elutriation (a process involving gas or liquid that separates particles based on their size), bone marrow homing, and separation of G0/G1 cells. The frequency of donor-derived XY-positive cells with characteristics of keratinocytes, determined by expression of keratins and lack of expression of lymphocyte and macrophage markers, was 1% to 3%. In a later study, the investigators further demonstrated that the event was not due to cell fusion.[34] Instead, the finding was argued to result from either reprogramming or the presence of an uncharacterized epithelial or multipotent bone marrow stem cell population.

The concept of engraftment of bone marrow–derived cells to the skin was further proven in a small retrospective clinical study using skin from bone marrow transplant recipients.[9] The study included 11 patients who had received high-dose chemotherapy either alone or in combination with radiotherapy, followed by transplantation of allogeneic peripheral blood stem cells (PBSCs) in 10 patients or autologous PBSCs in 1 patient. Long-term engraftment and hematopoietic chimerism after transplantation was demonstrated by microsatellite marker analysis. Skin, liver, and gastrointestinal tract biopsies were studied for the presence of Y-chromosome–containing cells in the tissues of female recipients. Donor-derived keratin-positive cells were found in the epidermis of the skin as far as 3 years after PBSC transplantation, demonstrating that bone marrow cells can be reprogrammed into skin cells in human.[9]

Keratin-positive bone marrow–derived donor cells are often found scattered in the skin, including the epidermis, hair follicles, and sebaceous glands, as keratin-positive cells or adjacent cells.[7–15,17,18] Of note, each of these locations harbor a specified skin stem cell niche for the different epithelial lineages, specifically epidermis, hair follicle, and sebaceous gland.[35] Whereas some studies do not report donor-derived cells in the vicinity of the hair follicles,[19] others show preferential localization of the cells to the hair follicle bulge, one of the specialized skin stem cell niches.[36,37] Tamai[37] transplanted newborn mouse skin with developing hair follicles onto the back of a mouse with prior green fluorescent protein (GFP)-positive bone marrow transplantation. A significant number of GFP-positive bone marrow–derived cells engrafted into the hair follicle bulge region and the epidermis, supporting the hypothesis that ectopic cells home to one of the skin stem cell niches.

Role of the Microenvironment in Promoting Homing, Engraftment, and Differentiation of Bone Marrow–Derived Stem Cells into Skin Cells

The microenvironment has a critical role in regulating the differentiation potential of stem cells. Stem cell microenvironments, or niches, are specific anatomic locations that regulate the function of stem cells during tissue generation, maintenance, and repair.[38,39] A variety of factors contribute to the niche composition, including anatomic structures, cellular interactions, extracellular matrix proteins, products of cellular metabolism, and secreted factors.[40–42] The niche provides the physical interaction, and the inhibitory and stimulatory signals required to maintain stem cell numbers, and to modulate their response to changes in physiologic conditions, such as in wound repair. A commonly used example of modification of the microenvironment is conditioning for bone marrow transplantation, which creates "space" for the donor stem cells by freeing the stem cell niches.[23]

In *Drosophila*, an empty stem cell niche was shown to reactivate the proliferation of ectopic cells.[43] The investigators postulated that after loss of their normal stem cells, the stem cell niches will likely maintain the potential to stimulate the proliferation of foreign stem cells or other cell types for a defined period. Related findings were reported by Booth and colleagues,[44] who demonstrated that neural stem cells and their progeny enter mammary epithelium–specific niches and adopt the function of mammary cells. Intriguingly, Lako and colleagues[45] reported that hair follicle dermal cells have the capacity to repopulate the mouse hematopoietic system in a lethally irradiated animal, demonstrating an unexpected differentiation potential of these cells guided by the signals of an empty, irradiated hematopoietic stem cell niche. Together, these studies support the concept that tissue-specific signals originating from the stroma and the differentiated somatic cells of a given niche can redirect ectopic stem cells to produce cellular progeny committed to cell fates of the tissue in which the niche resides. The authors hypothesize that the skin microenvironment in RDEB, characterized by severe recurrent blistering and erosions, may function in a related fashion by providing a depleted skin stem cell niche for ectopic stem cells, thereby improving their engraftment and proliferation.

In addition to the role of bone marrow–derived inflammatory cells in the initial phases of wound repair, other bone marrow–derived cells are known to participate in the homeostasis and regeneration of skin during wound healing.[10–12,15,18] With few exceptions,[14] most studies show that wounded skin stimulates engraftment of bone marrow–derived cells to the skin and induces them to incorporate and differentiate into nonhematopoietic skin structures.[10–12,15,18] In comparison with skin at homeostasis, wounding increases the percentage of bone marrow–derived cells with keratinocyte characteristics by more than twofold.[12]

One of the studies showing the differentiation potential of bone marrow–derived cells into the components of the skin and the role of the microenvironment during wound repair was performed by Kataoka and colleagues,[11] who mixed fresh, unfractionated bone marrow from a GFP-transgenic mouse with embryonic epidermal and dermal cells and transplanted this mixture onto skin defects of nude mice. GFP-positive cells costained with keratinocyte, sebaceous gland, and endothelial cell markers and respective cell types were detected in the suprabasal layers of the epidermis, hair follicles, sebaceous glands, and in the dermis associated with blood vessels. Bone marrow cells alone were unable to reconstitute the skin defect, emphasizing the importance of the interactions in the microenvironment necessary for bone marrow cell engraftment. Different populations of bone marrow cells were not tested separately, but these investigators proposed that the unfractionated marrow may contain a common progenitor population producing endodermal, mesodermal, and ectodermal progeny.

In humans, topical application of bone marrow cells to chronic wounds similarly led to closure of the wounds.[10] Autologous bone marrow cells were applied directly to chronic wounds in 3 patients. These patients had not previously responded to standard or advanced therapies,

Table 1
Studies showing bone marrow–derived cell homing to the skin

References	Model	Isolation of Cells	Wound	Results
Krause et al[7]	Mice; BMT; Sex-mismatched; Transplantation of a single cell after serial transplantation	Lineage depletion, elutriation, bone marrow homing, separation of small G0/G1 cells	No	Bone marrow–derived cells in variable epithelial tissues including the skin; 1%–3% cytokeratin+ Y+ cells localizing to the bulge and epidermis
Korbling et al[9]	Human; PB HSC transplantation to treat malignancy (leukemia/lymphoma etc); Retrospective	CD34+ cells	No	Transplant-derived cells in various organs; Cytokeratin+ XY+ CD45− epithelial cells in the skin in stratum spinosum, granulosum and close to dermal-epidermal junction
Hematti et al[8]	Human; PB HSC transplantation to treat hematologic malignancy; Sex-mismatched	CD34+ cells	No	No donor –derived DNA in keratinocyte cultures analyzed by PCR for Y chromosome markers
Badiavas & Falanga[10]	Mice; BMT; Donor GFP transgenic mice	Unfractionated	Full-thickness wound with/without G-CSF pre-treatment	No wound: Scattered GFP+ cells in dermis Wound ± G-CSF: GFP+ inflammatory cells on day 2, GFP+ keratin+ cells in the hair follicle, sebaceous glands, epidermis on day 21
Badiavas et al[33]	Human; Transplantation of autologous bone marrow cells to chronic wounds	Unfractionated	Chronic wound	Wound closure and dermal rebuilding by inspection and histology
Kataoka et al[11]	Mice; Transplantation of a mixture of GFP+ bone marrow cells and embryonic dermal and epidermal cells into a full-thickness skin defect	Unfractionated	Wound	Bone marrow cells only: Wound not epithelialized Bone marrow cells with embryonic dermal and epidermal cells: Wound epithelialized, GFP+ cells in hair follicles (K6+), sebaceous glands (Oil red O+), epidermis (K1+), dermis
Borue et al[12]	Mice; BMT; Sex-mismatched	Unfractionated	Wound	Increase from <1% to 8% in cytokeratin+ XY+ epithelial cell number; No evidence of fusion

Reference	Model	Cell type	Wound	Findings
Fathke et al[13]	Mice; BMT; Donor GFP transgenic mice	Unfractionated	No/wound	Bone marrow–derived cells contribute to the skin and express both collagen types I and III
Rovo & Gratwohl[17]	Human; PB Allogenic HSC transplantation	Not specified	No	PCR of microsatellite markers revealed no evidence of donor DNA in plucked hairs
Fan et al[14]	Mice; BMT; Donor LacZ or GFP transgenic mice	Unfractionated	No/wound	No wound: Bone marrow–derived keratinocytes could not be detected in the epidermis; Wound: epidermis contained rare bone marrow–derived keratinocytes
Inokuma et al[15]	Mice; BMT; Donor GFP transgenic mice	Unfractionated	Full-thickness wound ± CCL27 intradermal injection	GFP^+ keratin14$^+$ CD11c$^-$ CD45$^-$ cells in basal epidermis and around hair follicle bulge; Intradermal injection of CCL27 chemokine enhanced bone marrow–derived keratinocyte migration and accelerated wound healing; Neutralizing antibody inhibited migration
Sasaki et al[18]	Mice; MSC transplantation; Donor GFP transgenic mice	Cultured adherent cells from bone marrow; CD29$^+$, CD44$^+$, CD90$^+$, CD34$^+$, CD31$^+$; adipogenic/osteogenic/chondrogenic potential	Full-thickness wound ± CCL21 intradermal injection	GFP^+ pancytokeratin$^+$ cell 0.14%, GFP^+ CD31$^+$ cells 4.7%, GFP^+ SMA$^+$ cells 0.2%, GFP^+ CD11b$^+$ cells 1.5%; Intradermal injection of chemokine CCL21 increased GFP^+ cell migration and accelerated wound repair

Abbreviations: BMT, bone marrow transplantation; CCL21, chemokine, C-C motif, ligand 21; CCL27, chemokine, C-C motif, ligand 27; G-CSF, granulocyte-colony stimulating factor; GFP, green fluorescent protein; HSC, hematopoietic stem cell; PB, peripheral blood; PCR, polymerase chain reaction.

including bioengineered skin application and grafting with autologous skin. Complete closure and evidence of dermal rebuilding was observed in all 3 patients. Findings suggestive of engraftment of applied cells were observed in biopsy specimens of treated wounds. Clinical and histologic evidence of reduced scarring was also observed. These studies suggest that bone marrow–derived cells can lead to dermal rebuilding and closure of nonhealing chronic wounds.

Woodley and colleagues[46] further demonstrated the role of the wounded microenvironment in promoting homing of transplanted cells and the use of fibroblasts as a vehicle to deliver type VII collagen to the wounded skin. The investigators used murine skin defects or grafted human skin as a model system, and showed that systemically delivered fibroblasts, derived from an RDEB patient and engineered to overexpress type VII collagen, have the capacity to home to skin wounds, deliver type VII collagen to the wound, and promote wound healing.

To search for factors contributing to homing of bone marrow–derived cells to the skin, Inokuma and colleagues[15] hypothesized that recruitment of bone marrow–derived cells to the skin is regulated by chemokine-chemokine receptor interactions. CCL27 (chemokine, C-C motif, ligand 27) is a small cytokine belonging to the CC chemokine family, and its receptor is CCR10 (chemokine, C-C motif, receptor 10). CCL27 is predominantly expressed by epidermal keratinocytes, and is associated with infiltration of circulating cells in immunologic disease.[47] Capitalizing on this property, Inokuma and colleagues[15] showed that it can also increase recruitment of bone marrow–derived cells to the epidermis after introduction into the wound bed and accelerate wound healing. Sasaki and colleagues[18] similarly injected CCL21 (chemokine, C-C motif, ligand 21) intradermally to mice transplanted with GFP-positive MSCs. CCL21 increased migration of MSCs to the skin and accelerated wound healing. These findings suggest that specific chemokines such as CCL27 and CCL21 may facilitate chemoattraction of circulating stem cells into the skin for therapeutic purposes.

CORRECTION OF THE RDEB PHENOTYPE IN MICE BY BONE MARROW TRANSPLANTATION

Stemming from the data on reprogramming of marrow cells into skin cells, several groups have conducted bone marrow transplantation to treat RDEB in an animal model of RDEB (Table 2).[16,19,48] Chino and colleagues[16] investigated whether bone marrow–derived fibroblasts can ameliorate RDEB phenotype in a mouse model using embryonic bone marrow cell transplantation. These investigators performed embryonic bone marrow cell transplantation into RDEB mice with T-cell–depleted GFP-transgenic bone marrow cells via the vitelline vein,

Table 2
Studies using bone marrow cell transplantation for RDEB treatment in mice

References	Model	Cells Used	Results
Tolar et al[19]	BMT to Col7a1−/− mice	MSC, MAPC, EpiSC, TAC, unfractionated BM, BM CD150+CD48−, BM CD150−	BM CD150+CD48− cells homed to skin, produced type VII collagen and anchoring fibrils, ameliorated skin fragility, and reduced lethality; no effect with other cell types
Chino et al[16]	Embryonic BMT to Col7a1−/− mice	CD90–depleted bone marrow cells	BMT ameliorated severity of phenotype in neonatal mice; type VII collagen deposited primarily in follicular basement membrane zone in vicinity of BMDFs
Woodley et al[48]	BMT and intradermal injection to Col7a1−/− mice	MSC	Improved dermal-epidermal adherence, decreased skin fragility, reduced new blister formation, markedly prolonged survival (40% up to 4 months); type VII collagen expression not detected

Abbreviations: BM, bone marrow; BMDF, bone marrow–derived stem cell; BMT, bone marrow transplantation; EpiSC, epidermal stem cell; MAPC, multipotent adult progenitor cell; MSC, mesenchymal stem cell; TAC, transient amplifying cell.

which is connected to the fetal circulation. The study showed that type VII collagen was detected in the basement membrane zone in the vicinity of the GFP-positive bone marrow–derived fibroblasts positive for fibroblast markers fibronectin, vimentin, type I collagen, and type VII collagen. Embryonic bone marrow cell transplantation also significantly ameliorated the lethal pathology in the neonate mice, with average survival of 15 to 20 days in the treated group and 2 days in the nontreated group.

Tolar and colleagues[19] assessed the beneficial effects of bone marrow transplantation for RDEB by infusing HSC and non-HSC populations into unconditioned RDEB (Col7a1−/−) mice. Strikingly, 3 of 13 (23%) HSC recipients survived for several months. Surviving animals had evidence of skin engraftment of donor cells and production of type VII collagen in the skin, with healing of skin blisters. Anchoring fibrils, composed of type VII collagen, were detected at the basement membrane zone, providing evidence of functional restoration. These data demonstrated that bone marrow–derived cell engraftment in the appropriate skin microenvironment results in sufficient numbers of engrafted cells to provide correction of the type VII collagen deficiency in mice.

Based on the knowledge that bone marrow–derived MSCs may serve as a source of skin progenitor cells and contribute to healing of skin wounds, Woodley and colleagues[48] isolated MSCs from wild type mice and injected them intravenously and intradermally into RDEB mice that had blisters on their paws, skin, and mucosa, recapitulating the human phenotype. The therapy improved dermal-epidermal adherence, decreased skin fragility, reduced new blister formation, and markedly prolonged survival (40% displayed an increased survival of up to 4 months). Intriguingly, collagen VII expression was not detected, and therefore the investigators concluded that MSC-based cell therapy may improve the RDEB phenotype via another mechanism.

In addition to the RDEB mouse models, stem cell transplantation was successfully performed in a collagen XVII knockout mouse, a model for human junctional epidermolysis bullosa (JEB).[49] The investigators transplanted bone marrow cells from GFP-transgenic mice into collagen XVII knockout mice. Immunohistochemistry and reverse transcription-polymerase chain reaction demonstrated collagen XVII expression underneath donor-derived keratinocytes. The mice showed fewer erosions and increased survival rate (73.2% vs 20.6% at 150 days post transplantation).

Together, these data demonstrate that adoptive transfer of type VII collagen–producing and type XVII collagen–producing bone marrow–derived cell populations ameliorate the basement membrane zone defect in RDEB and JEB murine models, respectively, and established the basis for clinical trials in different forms.

CLINICAL TRIALS USING BONE MARROW–DERIVED CELLS FOR RDEB

At present, at least 4 clinical trials are ongoing around the world to investigate the therapeutic potential of bone marrow transplantation for RDEB (Table 3). The preliminary data from these studies is discussed here.

Palisson and colleagues (Palisson F, Rodriguez F, González S, et al, personal communication, 2009) used intradermal injection of MSCs to treat RDEB in humans. MSCs were isolated from the bone marrow of healthy donors and cultured in vitro before injection into one side of the edge of selected RDEB wounds; the control was to not inject the other side of the wound. Recipients included 3 RDEB patients of age 13 to 25 years. The results showed that MSC administration promoted healing of ulcerated skin. Total reepithelialization was observed in 1 patient and new blistering was not observed in the other 2 patients. At the molecular level, MSC administration resulted in restoration of type VII collagen at the basement membrane zone.

To investigate the role of bone marrow MSCs for treatment of RDEB, El Darouti and colleagues (El Darouti M, personal communication, 2009) enrolled 14 RDEB patients in a clinical trial. Bone marrow donor cells were harvested and cultured in vitro to isolate adherent cells for the transplant. To investigate potential additional benefits of cyclosporine treatment, 7 of 14 patients received cyclosporine infusion in addition to the stem cell transplant. Comparisons were made between the severity of the disease before and after treatment as well as between treatment with stem cells only and stem cells combined with cyclosporine treatment. Preliminary results demonstrated that blister eruption was significantly decreased in both treatment groups and rate of blister healing was significantly increased. No differences were detected between stem cell transplantation only and cyclosporine combination therapy.

Wagner and colleagues[50] enrolled RDEB patients on a trial of bone marrow or cord blood transplantation consisting of myeloablative conditioning with busulfan (12.8–16 mg/kg), fludarabine (75 mg/m^2), and cyclophosphamide (200 mg/kg), followed by the infusion of bone marrow or cord blood. Three

Table 3
Clinical trials using bone marrow or cord blood–derived cells for treatment of RDEB

References	Model	Cells	BM Conditioning	Results
Wagner et al[50]	BM or CB transplantation	BM or CB	Myeloablation	Three of 4 patients received transplant; one patient died of cardiomyopathy before cell infusion; 3 of 4 patients showed increased type VII collagen production, increased anchoring fibrils; 2 of 4 patients alive at 434 days and 33 days after transplant
Christiano et al[51]	BM or CB transplantation	BM or CB	Reduced-intensity conditioning	Ongoing
El Darouti (personal communication)	BMT ± cyclosporine	MSCs enriched from bone marrow by in vitro culture	Not described	Blister eruption significantly decreased in both treatment groups; rate of blister healing significantly increased; no differences between stem cell transplantation only and cyclosporine combination therapy
Palisson et al (personal communication)	Intradermal injection of MSCs	MSCs	None	Improved healing of ulcerated skin; restoration of type VII collagen at the basement membrane zone

Abbreviations: BM, bone marrow; BMT, bone marrow transplantation; CB, cord blood; MSC, mesenchymal stem cell.

of 4 patients have completed the treatment plan. One of the 4 patients with significant renal impairment secondary to perinatal cardiac arrest received a reduced dose of fludarabine but died of cardiomyopathy before bone marrow infusion. The patients who completed the trial demonstrated marked clinical improvement, with a gradual decrease in blister formation. Preliminary data from immunohistochemistry and electron microscopy currently available for 2 patients showed increase in collagen VII expression and anchoring fibril number and maturity. Two of 3 patients are alive, 434 and 33 days after transplant, and 1 of 3 died 183 days after transplant. These data provide preliminary evidence that allogeneic bone marrow/cord blood transplant can be successfully used for curative benefit in RDEB, but may carry a high risk of mortality. These preliminary data, presence of collagen VII and anchoring fibrils, along with clinical improvement suggest that systemic bone marrow or cord blood transplantation or local administration of MSCs can ameliorate RDEB.

In addition to the aforementioned studies, we have begun a clinical trial investigating the curative potential of bone marrow/cord blood transplantation.[51] Along with demonstrating a potential curative therapy for RDEB, the study will examine a strategy of reduced-intensity conditioning (RIC) prior to bone marrow/cord blood transplantation, which may provide reduced risks and ethical concerns compared with myeloablative conditioning.[52,53] Myeloablative conditioning prior to bone marrow transplantation is associated with significant morbidity and mortality,[52] and RDEB patients have increased risks due to suboptimal nutritional status and poor barrier function of the skin. RIC regimens are used at extremes of age as well as for disorders in which myeloablative conditioning is associated with high rates of nonrelapse mortality. RIC is typically associated with lower rates of severe toxicity and nonrelapse mortality. Infections, graft-versus-host disease, and relapse of primary disease remain the most common obstacles to a successful outcome. Bradley and colleagues[54] studied the ability of RIC to induce long-term chimerism in children with nonmalignant diseases. RIC consisted of fludarabine (150–180 mg/m^2) with either busulfan (≤8 mg/kg) and rabbit antithymocyte globulin or cyclophosphamide and rabbit antithymocyte immunoglobulin ± etoposide. In a subset of patients, results were suggestive of rapid engraftment with potentially decreased severe graft-versus-host-disease and transplant-related mortality. Our study involves RIC with busulfan, fludarabine, and alemtuzumab on RDEB patients,[51] and will provide useful information on the use of RIC for genetic skin diseases such as RDEB.

FUTURE DIRECTIONS
Enrichment for Optimal Donor Cell Populations

A substantial degree of variability exists in the current preclinical literature regarding bone marrow cell isolation for transplantation purposes. Some groups have chosen to use total bone marrow cells, whereas others have purified subpopulations with different methods varying from simple culture to multiple steps to enrich the stem cell population, either hematopoietic or mesenchymal.[7–19] Tolar and colleagues[19] tested several different stem cell populations for curative effect in the RDEB mouse model, including MSCs, multipotent adult progenitor cells, epidermal stem cells, transient amplifying cells, nonenriched bone marrow, CD150$^+$ CD48$^-$ HSCs, and CD150$^-$ control fraction. Notwithstanding a difference in the number of cells in each group, only CD150$^+$ CD48$^-$ hematopoietic stem cells were able to ameliorate RDEB, suggesting that HSCs have a high potential for treatment of RDEB. In 2 of the clinical trials with available preliminary data, HSCs from either bone marrow or cord blood were used,[50,51] while in 2 others MSCs were used. The future results from these studies will provide essential information on choosing the optimal donor cell type for treatment of RDEB.

Enhancing Bone Marrow Stem Cell Homing to the Skin

What are the signals that recruit bone marrow–derived cells to home to the skin? Physiologic conditions such as chronic wound healing clearly recruit bone marrow–derived cells to the skin. Some of the factors mediating recruitment of bone marrow–derived cells to the wound and accelerating wound healing have been identified. These factors include chemokines, such as CCL27 and CCL21.[15,18] Other cytokines known to promote wound healing, including granulocyte macrophage-colony stimulating factor (GM-CSF),[55] may play a role in homing capacity. In clinical hematology, a variety of molecules are successfully used to mobilize peripheral blood stem cells for stem cell transplantation, including granulocyte colony-stimulating factor (G-CSF or fligrastim), the chemokine (C-X-C motif) ligand 2 (CXCL2 or GRO-β), and chemokine (C-X-C motif) receptor 4 (CXCR4) antagonist (AMD3100).[56] Identification of similar factors for recruitment of bone marrow–derived cells to the skin and their preclinical testing in additional epidermolysis bullosa

mouse models would be useful for the overall understanding of the mechanisms involved in ectopic cell recruitment to the skin and for development of corresponding clinical applications.

Furthermore, as evidenced in the *Drosophila*[43] and mouse models,[44,45] the presence of an empty niche itself may promote ectopic cell proliferation and redirect their differentiation. It is possible that the RDEB skin microenvironment with severe recurrent blistering and erosions generates a microenvironment depleted of stem cells, thereby promoting the engraftment and proliferation of ectopic stem cells. Further studies are needed to examine the skin stem cells and their microenvironment in RDEB skin before and after transplantation.

Tumorigenesis

Epithelial cancers, that is, gastric cancer, can originate from bone marrow–derived cells.[57] To investigate whether the same is true for skin cancers, Cogle and colleagues[58] identified 4 women who developed skin cancers after gender-mismatched hematopoietic cell transplants. None of the skin cancer cells analyzed for expression of keratins and presence of Y chromosome demonstrated donor-derived cells incorporated within the cancer. Ando and colleagues[59] observed only a low percentage of bone marrow–derived cells (0.03%) in UVB-induced skin cancer in a murine model. However, in human kidney transplant recipients, donor-derived cells were detected in 5 of 15 squamous cell carcinomas and in 3 of 5 basal cell carcinomas, with 1 tumor composed largely of donor-derived cells.[60] Whether these differences are due to the distinction between hematologic and solid organ transplants remains to be investigated. Furthermore, the effect of bone marrow transplantation on cancer development in RDEB patients, who typically develop squamous cell cancer without bone marrow transplantation, needs to be followed long term as an outcome measure after transplantation.

SUMMARY

Despite 15 years of progress since the identification of the first mutations in the type VII collagen gene in RDEB, there remains no curative treatment for RDEB. Several lines of evidence about reprogramming of stem cells have prompted us and others to consider novel approaches for the treatment of RDEB. Bone marrow stem cell therapies for RDEB are based on the hypothesis that bone marrow–derived cells are guided into becoming skin cells, given the right microenvironment. Cellular reprogramming of allogeneic cells would offer significant advantages over conventional gene replacement strategies, which are currently dependent on the introduction of the exogenous gene as well as the ability to generate long-term expression and engraftment via stem cells. Using donor cells from bone marrow of immunologically compatible healthy individuals would overcome both of these obstacles, because the gene of interest would already be present, and the exogenous tissue would be incorporated into new skin tissue. However, as allogeneic transplants require conditioning and are therefore not without risks, simultaneous development of transplants derived from safely gene-corrected autologous cells is necessary.

The preclinical data and the preliminary clinical data in both mouse and human models of epidermolysis bullosa have demonstrated the feasibility of bone marrow transplantation, showing longer-term survival and reversion of the phenotype with normalization of the skin basement membrane and the formation of anchoring fibrils. In addition to the ongoing clinical trials, further work is needed to identify the optimal bone marrow cell population for stem cell therapy, to identify factors that improve bone marrow cell homing to the skin, to investigate the quality and quantity of stem cells in RDEB skin, to investigate the potential effects of transplantation on tumorigenesis, and to develop safe and efficient methods for gene correction of autologous cells.

The authors believe the strategy of stem cell transplantation and reprogramming holds great promise in achieving the goal of a cure for RDEB.

ACKNOWLEDGMENTS

The authors are grateful to several colleagues for sharing their unpublished work for this review, in particular, Dr F. Pallison and Dr M. El-Darouti. We appreciate the valuable and stimulating conversations with Drs C. Jahoda, J. Uitto, J. McGrath, K. Tamai, H. Shimizu, A. Hovnanian, D. Woodley and M. Chen, among others, who have been generous with the sharing of ideas about stem cells, reprogramming, and new therapies for EB.

REFERENCES

1. Varki R, Sadowski S, Uitto J, et al. Epidermolysis bullosa. II. Type VII collagen mutations and phenotype-genotype correlations in the dystrophic subtypes. J Med Genet 2007;44(3):181–92.
2. Burgeson RE. Type VII collagen, anchoring fibrils, and epidermolysis bullosa. J Invest Dermatol 1993; 101(3):252–5.
3. Fine J, Bauer EA, McGuire J, et al. Epidermolysis bullosa: clinical, epidemiologic, and laboratory advances and the findings of the national epidermolysis bullosa registry. Baltimore (MD): The Johns Hopkins University Press; 1999.
4. Bello YM, Falabella AF, Schachner LA. Management of epidermolysis bullosa in infants and children. Clin Dermatol 2003;21(4):278–82.
5. Uitto J. Epidermolysis bullosa: prospects for cell-based therapies. J Invest Dermatol 2008;128(9): 2140–2.
6. Tamai K, Kaneda Y, Uitto J. Molecular therapies for heritable blistering diseases. Trends Mol Med 2009;15(7):285–92.
7. Krause DS, Theise ND, Collector MI, et al. Multi-organ, multi-lineage engraftment by a single bone marrow-derived stem cell. Cell 2001;105(3):369–77.
8. Hematti P, Sloand EM, Carvallo CA, et al. Absence of donor-derived keratinocyte stem cells in skin tissues cultured from patients after mobilized peripheral blood hematopoietic stem cell transplantation. Exp Hematol 2002;30(8):943–9.
9. Korbling M, Katz RL, Khanna A, et al. Hepatocytes and epithelial cells of donor origin in recipients of peripheral-blood stem cells. N Engl J Med 2002; 346(10):738–46.
10. Badiavas EV, Falanga V. Treatment of chronic wounds with bone marrow-derived cells. Arch Dermatol 2003;139(4):510–6.
11. Kataoka K, Medina RJ, Kageyama T, et al. Participation of adult mouse bone marrow cells in reconstitution of skin. Am J Pathol 2003;163(4):1227–31.
12. Borue X, Lee S, Grove J, et al. Bone marrow-derived cells contribute to epithelial engraftment during wound healing. Am J Pathol 2004;165(5):1767–72.
13. Fathke C, Wilson L, Hutter J, et al. Contribution of bone marrow-derived cells to skin: collagen deposition and wound repair. Stem Cells 2004;22(5):812–22.
14. Fan Q, Yee CL, Ohyama M, et al. Bone marrow-derived keratinocytes are not detected in normal skin and only rarely detected in wounded skin in two different murine models. Exp Hematol 2006; 34(5):672–9.
15. Inokuma D, Abe R, Fujita Y, et al. CTACK/CCL27 accelerates skin regeneration via accumulation of bone marrow-derived keratinocytes. Stem Cells 2006;24(12):2810–6.
16. Chino T, Tamai K, Yamazaki T, et al. Bone marrow cell transfer into fetal circulation can ameliorate genetic skin diseases by providing fibroblasts to the skin and inducing immune tolerance. Am J Pathol 2008; 173(3):803–14.
17. Rovo A, Gratwohl A. Plasticity after allogeneic hematopoietic stem cell transplantation. Biol Chem 2008; 389(7):825–36.
18. Sasaki M, Abe R, Fujita Y, et al. Mesenchymal stem cells are recruited into wounded skin and contribute

to wound repair by transdifferentiation into multiple skin cell type. J Immunol 2008;180(4):2581–7.

19. Tolar J, Ishida-Yamamoto A, Riddle M, et al. Amelioration of epidermolysis bullosa by transfer of wild-type bone marrow cells. Blood 2009; 113(5):1167–74.

20. Hacein-Bey-Abina S, Von Kalle C, Schmidt M, et al. LMO2-associated clonal T cell proliferation in two patients after gene therapy for SCID-X1. Science 2003;302(5644):415–9.

21. Evans MJ, Kaufman MH. Establishment in culture of pluripotential cells from mouse embryos. Nature 1981;292(5819):154–6.

22. Thomson JA, Itskovitz-Eldor J, Shapiro SS, et al. Embryonic stem cell lines derived from human blastocysts. Science 1998;282(5391):1145–7.

23. Domen J, Wagers AJ, Weissman IL. Bone marrow (hematopoietic) stem cells. Stem cells: scientific progress and future research directions; 2006. Available at: http://www.stemcells.nih.gov/info/2006report/2006 Chapter2.htm. Accessed February 4, 2010.

24. Prockop DJ. Marrow stromal cells as stem cells for nonhematopoietic tissues. Science 1997;276(5309): 71–4.

25. Eglitis MA, Mezey E. Hematopoietic cells differentiate into both microglia and macroglia in the brains of adult mice. Proc Natl Acad Sci U S A 1997;94(8): 4080–5.

26. Petersen BE, Bowen WC, Patrene KD, et al. Bone marrow as a potential source of hepatic oval cells. Science 1999;284(5417):1168–70.

27. Brazelton TR, Rossi FM, Keshet GI, et al. From marrow to brain: expression of neuronal phenotypes in adult mice. Science 2000;290(5497):1775–9.

28. Orlic D, Kajstura J, Chimenti S, et al. Mobilized bone marrow cells repair the infarcted heart, improving function and survival. Proc Natl Acad Sci U S A 2001;98(18):10344–9.

29. Abkowitz JL. Can human hematopoietic stem cells become skin, gut, or liver cells? N Engl J Med 2002;346(10):770–2.

30. Orkin SH, Zon LI. Hematopoiesis and stem cells: plasticity versus developmental heterogeneity. Nat Immunol 2002;3(4):323–8.

31. Herzog EL, Chai L, Krause DS. Plasticity of marrow-derived stem cells. Blood 2003;102(10):3483–93.

32. Wagers AJ, Weissman IL. Plasticity of adult stem cells. Cell 2004;116(5):639–48.

33. Badiavas EV, Abedi M, Butmarc J, et al. Participation of bone marrow derived cells in cutaneous wound healing. J Cell Physiol 2003;196(2):245–50.

34. Harris RG, Herzog EL, Bruscia EM, et al. Lack of a fusion requirement for development of bone marrow-derived epithelia. Science 2004;305(5680): 90–3.

35. Fuchs E, Horsley V. More than one way to skin. Genes Dev 2008;22(8):976–85.

36. Brittan M, Braun KM, Reynolds LE, et al. Bone marrow cells engraft within the epidermis and proliferate in vivo with no evidence of cell fusion. J Pathol 2005;205(1):1–13.

37. Tamai K. Bone marrow replenishes de novo keratinocytes in the regenerating hair follicles via circulating blood. J Invest Dermatol 2008;128:S93.

38. Schofield R. The relationship between the spleen colony-forming cell and the haemopoietic stem cell. Blood Cells 1978;4(1–2):7–25.

39. Scadden DT. The stem-cell niche as an entity of action. Nature 2006;441(7097):1075–9.

40. Adams GB, Scadden DT. The hematopoietic stem cell in its place. Nat Immunol 2006;7(4):333–7.

41. Moore KA, Lemischka IR. Stem cells and their niches. Science 2006;311(5769):1880–5.

42. Wilson A, Trumpp A. Bone-marrow haematopoietic-stem-cell niches. Nat Rev Immunol 2006; 6(2):93–106.

43. Kai T, Spradling A. An empty Drosophila stem cell niche reactivates the proliferation of ectopic cells. Proc Natl Acad Sci U S A 2003;100(8): 4633–8.

44. Booth BW, Mack DL, Androutsellis-Theotokis A, et al. The mammary microenvironment alters the differentiation repertoire of neural stem cells. Proc Natl Acad Sci U S A 2008;105(39):14891–6.

45. Lako M, Armstrong L, Cairns PM, et al. Hair follicle dermal cells repopulate the mouse haematopoietic system. J Cell Sci 2002;115(Pt 20):3967–74.

46. Woodley DT, Remington J, Huang Y, et al. Intravenously injected human fibroblasts home to skin wounds, deliver type VII collagen, and promote wound healing. Mol Ther 2007;15(3):628–35.

47. Nibbs RJ, Graham GJ. CCL27/PESKY: a novel paradigm for chemokine function. Expert Opin Biol Ther 2003;3(1):15–22.

48. Woodley DT, Wang X, Zhou H, et al. Bone marrow stem cells improve survivability of RDEB mice but do not correct the fundamental type VII collagen defect. J Invest Dermatol 2008;128:S126.

49. Fujita Y, Abe R, Inokuma D, et al. Bone marrow transplantation restores deficient epidermal basement membrane protein and improves the clinical phenotype in epidermolysis bullosa model mice. J Invest Dermatol 2008;128:S114.

50. Wagner JE, Ishida-Yamamoto A, McGrath JA, et al. Adult stem cells for treatment of recessive dystrophic epidermolysis bullosa (RDEB). J Invest Dermatol 2009(S1);129:S55.

51. Christiano AM, McGrath JA, Hillman E, et al. Reduced intensity conditioning and allogenic stem cell transplantation in recessive dystrophic epidermolysis bullosa. J Invest Dermatol 2009(S1);129: S56.

52. Giralt S. Reduced-intensity conditioning regimens for hematologic malignancies: what have we learned

over the last 10 years? Hematology Am Soc Hematol Educ Program 2005;384–9.

53. Satwani P, Morris E, Bradley MB, et al. Reduced intensity and non-myeloablative allogeneic stem cell transplantation in children and adolescents with malignant and non-malignant diseases. Pediatr Blood Cancer 2008;50(1):1–8.

54. Bradley MB, Satwani P, Baldinger L, et al. Reduced intensity allogeneic umbilical cord blood transplantation in children and adolescent recipients with malignant and non-malignant diseases. Bone Marrow Transplant 2007;40(7):621–31.

55. Mann A, Breuhahn K, Schirmacher P, et al. Keratinocyte-derived granulocyte-macrophage colony stimulating factor accelerates wound healing: stimulation of keratinocyte proliferation, granulation tissue formation, and vascularization. J Invest Dermatol 2001;117(6):1382–90.

56. Pelus LM. Peripheral blood stem cell mobilization: new regimens, new cells, where do we stand. Curr Opin Hematol 2008;15(4):285–92.

57. Houghton J, Stoicov C, Nomura S, et al. Gastric cancer originating from bone marrow-derived cells. Science 2004;306(5701):1568–71.

58. Cogle CR, Theise ND, Fu D, et al. Bone marrow contributes to epithelial cancers in mice and humans as developmental mimicry. Stem Cells 2007; 25(8):1881–7.

59. Ando S, Abe R, Sasaki M, et al. Bone marrow-derived cells are not the origin of the cancer stem cells in ultraviolet-induced skin cancer. Am J Pathol 2009;174(2):595–601.

60. Aractingi S, Kanitakis J, Euvrard S, et al. Skin carcinoma arising from donor cells in a kidney transplant recipient. Cancer Res 2005;65(5): 1755–60.

Interdisciplinary Management of Epidermolysis Bullosa in the Public Setting: The Netherlands as a Model of Care

José C. Duipmans, MScN, RN,
Marcel F. Jonkman, MD, PhD*

KEYWORDS

- Epidermolysis bullosa • Carrousel model
- Interdisciplinary approach • Dermatologist

Epidermolysis bullosa (EB) is an umbrella term for a group of rare genetic blistering skin disorders characterized by blister formation, from birth on, in response to minimal trauma or friction. Fragility can also involve the internal mucosa and the eyes in some forms of EB.[1] The symptoms experienced by patients with EB vary, but blistering and pain are common symptoms to all types of the disease. This chronic skin blistering affects the physical, personal, emotional, and socioeconomic aspects of patients' life; it is no wonder that EB has a severe impact on the quality of life and impairs the health status in most patients.[2] EB is one of the most devastating chronic diseases known to mankind.[3] Because of the myriad of medical and nonmedical complications that patients with EB endure, all patients and their families should be evaluated in a specialized center familiar with the many complications of EB. Obviously, medical services for people with EB demand a multidisciplinary approach.

AIMS OF THE DUTCH INTERDISCIPLINARY EB TEAM

In many countries medical services have a large multidisciplinary EB team, headed by a dermatologist. The Dutch EB service in the Center for Blistering Diseases in the University Medical Center, Groningen was established in 1990 and services both children and adults. The EB service, including all EB team activities and the nurse coordinator's salary, is funded by the university medical center from its standard academic care budget because it is recognized as a top reference service. Not all expert centers experience a comparably funded, convenient situation.

In addition, Dystrophic Epidermolysis Bullosa Research Association (DEBRA) Netherlands funds an outreach service with an EB social worker. Home outreach nurses are lacking in this program; the hospital-based nurse specialist will visit a patient at home on occasion. Thus, the EB service in this small country is hospital based.

The aim of the interdisciplinary EB team is to provide excellent, comprehensive care and treatment for patients with EB, to help in the process of managing the condition and enhancing comfort and patient autonomy. One of the activities of the EB team is to make early and precise diagnosis and thus be able to inform the patients in the first weeks about prognosis and treatment. An important part of the Dutch EB center is its diagnostic and research laboratory that provides routine diagnostics, including immunofluorescence

Center for Blistering Diseases, Department of Dermatology, University Medical Center Groningen, University of Groningen, Groningen, The Netherlands
* Corresponding author.
E-mail address: m.f.jonkman@derm.umcg.nl

Dermatol Clin 28 (2010) 383–386
doi:10.1016/j.det.2010.02.005

antigen mapping, electron microscopy, and mutation analysis. In addition, the EB team aims to provide state-of-the-art medical advice and treatment, both during hospital admissions and EB-clinic visits, and in the community. Finally, one of the goals is to conduct scientific research.

VISION OF THE INTERDISCIPLINARY TEAM

The vision of the team is to work patient-centered, that is, to acknowledge the situation of the patient and to tailor the treatment (age appropriate) to both the severity of the condition and the symptoms and problems experienced. When undertaking treatments the EB professional negotiates with the patient over what is acceptable to him or her and what the professional feels able to undertake within the bounds of professional accountability, always remembering that the patient is also an expert in his or her own condition. All professionals involved in the treatment of EB can participate in the International EB forum (http://www.internationalebforum.org), to consult, to educate, or to inform medical professionals worldwide about the best possible care for patients with EB. There are good links with other EB centers in Europe and other continents. This international communication and cooperation is very helpful in successful delivery of care.

RAPID DIAGNOSIS

Newborns suspected of having EB are immediately referred to the children's hospital of the University Medical Center Groningen and admitted to the neonatal ward or intensive care unit. Diagnosis is obtained by writing down the family history, physical examination, taking skin biopsies, collecting blood samples of the newborn and parents for DNA testing, and physical examination, taking medical photographs. Two punch biopsies (2 and 4 mm) are taken from a fresh blister (<24 hours); secondly, another 2 biopsies are taken from the intact skin of the inner aspect of the upper arm. The 2-mm biopsies are fixed in 2% glutaraldehyde and analyzed by electron microscopy; the 4-mm biopsies are snap frozen in liquid nitrogen to conduct rapid IF antigen mapping. Within 24 to 48 hours, diagnosis is obtained and informed to the parents. During the hospital admission, parents are provided with accommodation and learn, step by step, to perform dressing changes and to care for their child. In the meantime the specialist nurse organizes all the care at home, which is provided by a community nurse, with or without the parents. On average, after 1 week of support, instruction, training, and information about diagnosis, prognosis, and care, the parents and their child are discharged.

REFERRALS

All patients with EB should, at least once, be referred to the EB center for the making of an exact diagnosis and the setting up of a care plan. Dutch patients and those from within the European Union can consult the EB team at the expense of their health insurance. Notwithstanding incidences, consultations are scheduled twice a year for the more severely affected patients, and once per year for those with milder EB. New children are invited more often, 3 or 4 times per year. The need and frequency of the different consultations are determined depending on the severity and type of EB and the associated problems. In the case of limited follow-up being needed, for example only a wound assessment and growth checkup, the patient can visit the weekly "small" EB-clinic run by the dermatologist and pediatrician.

THE DUTCH CARROUSEL MODEL

For more than 10 years the interdisciplinary EB team offers, in addition to the standard weekly outpatient EB clinics, so-called all-in-one-day clinics 6 times a year.[4] The Dutch interdisciplinary team includes long-term appointed, dedicated professionals, representing 19 disciplines (Box 1). At present, the authors have 10 years of experience with a carrousel model. A maximum of 6 patients, prioritized according to their clinical problems, are scheduled per clinic, and an examination room on the ambulatory clinics is assigned to each family. The medical professionals, sometimes put together in a subteam, all start at 12:30 PM and visit the patients serially, by rotating every 30 minutes, as in a carrousel. During these clinics, the patient and family can consult different specialists in sequence within 4 hours. In these all-in-one-day clinics, the following medical items are evaluated: pain and itch, wound healing and infections (parents and patients bring photographs to examine some wounds; bad wounds will be examined during the EB clinic), nutritional aspects, growth and development, presence of squamous cell carcinoma (as there is no bath, only wounds thought to be suspicious by the community nurses or family are examined and if necessary, biopsies can be done during the EB clinic), level of function in fine motor and life skills (including need for adaptive equipment and techniques), mobility,

Box 1
Specialists involved in the Dutch EB team
Specialist nurse
Dermatologist
Pediatrician
Internist
Dietician
Ear/nose/throat surgeon
Orthopedic surgeon
Pediatric gastroenterologist
Speech therapist
Plastic surgeon
Dentist
Anesthesiologist
Pain relief doctor
Occupational therapist
Pathologist
Ophthalmologist
Social worker (1 hospital based and 1 DEBRA funded)/psychologist
Psychologist
Clinical geneticist

Box 2
Parameters of routine blood test
Complete blood count
Urea
Electrolytes
Liver function tests
Erythrocyte sedimentation rate
C-reactive protein
Iron
Iron-binding capacity
Ferritin
Calcium
Phosphate
Zinc
Selenium
Vitamins A, B6, C 25(OH)-vitamin D3
Folate

hand function, gastrointestinal and genitourinary complications, anemia, fatigue, cardiac problems, bone metabolism, eye problems, oral problems, and hematologic issues. Also, the psychological and social aspects are always a part of the evaluations. As part of the regular 6- to 12-monthly follow-ups, the following investigations can be performed: weight and height measurements, medical photographs (eg, of the hands, to evaluate problems such as fusion of the fingers), measurements of the web spaces, routine blood tests (**Box 2**), measurements focused on mobility of the mandible, lips and tongue including mouth width parameters, orthopantogram, barium swallow to examine the esophagus, skin biopsies, swab cultures (antibiotic sensitivity), radiographs, bone scintigrams, and other tests. Each specialist decides which specific investigations are needed. Apart from measurements of weight and height, no investigations are performed ahead of the multidisciplinary EB clinic.

Directly following the EB clinic, all professionals communicate their findings, and the advice and treatments are collected during a 1.5-hour patient conference, chaired by the dermatologist. An integrated care plan is established, written down by the specialist nurse in the multidisciplinary patient record and in a collective medical letter, which is presented to the patient or family and to all professionals involved. Each member of the EB team has the responsibility of liaising with his or her appropriate counterpart to optimize communication and patient care. Telephone support, e-mail contacts with local and regional hospitals and practitioners, occasional home visits, and information, all provided by the EB nurse, are supportive in implementing the integral integrated plan. Furthermore, the interdisciplinary approach is used when EB patients need to have surgery or other procedures done under anesthesia. If possible, two or more interventions (eg, dental treatment, hand surgery, oncology screening) are scheduled in one theater session; this means that only one anesthetic session is needed (also called "all-in-one surgery"[4]). The EB nurse is present during the procedures, and the professionals adhere to the EB protocol for theater management.

COORDINATION AND CONTINUITY IN CARE

To achieve the aforementioned goals, the dermatologist acts as a medical coordinator of the team, and is responsible for creating consensus in proposals for treatments and for the quality of the team. Besides, the nurse coordinator plays a key role in the treatment; he or she is permanently in close contact with the patients, caregivers, and all professionals involved, and lists and prioritizes the problems, coordinates and communicates the needed care, and refers to relevant carers, combining the unique expertise of all professionals. It is clear that without a (nurse) coordinator, the interdisciplinary approach will fail.

The Netherlands is a small country with a population of about 16.5 million inhabitants; an estimated 700 people are affected with EB. In the last 20 years, 335 sufferers of EB have been diagnosed. Although the EB center is located in the northern part of the country, for almost all families it is still feasible to visit the EB clinics and travel back home in one day. Furthermore, whereas most well-informed interdisciplinary EB teams are located in children's hospitals, the Dutch EB team also delivers care to young patients who survive into adulthood. This means that the adult EB patients do not need to change hospital or doctors, except for the pediatrician. The relatively small numbers of patients and the location of a center within easy reach for patients of all ages contribute to a well-organized delivery of interdisciplinary care.

In summary, until the day comes when a cure can be found for this devastating condition, all that can be offered is support in management of the condition through good interdisciplinary teamwork.[5] The Dutch interdisciplinary EB team performs at a high level that is appreciated by the patients and parents. The possibility of rapid, precise diagnosis, the efficient carrousel-like clinics, and the continuity in care are characteristic elements of the Dutch method of delivering EB care. Judging by the rewards of the patients, this approach is very successful and it stimulates efforts to continue and to optimize the EB care. Nevertheless, the most important part of the EB patient's care is given by the parents, primarily the mother, in cooperation with local caregivers and practitioners.

REFERENCES

1. Uitto J, Eady R, Fine JD, et al. The DEBRA International Visionary/Consensus Meeting on Epidermolysis Bullosa: summary and recommendations [review]. J Invest Dermatol 2000;114(4):734–7.
2. Tabolli S, Sampogna F, Di Pietro C, et al. Quality of life in patients with epidermolysis bullosa. Br J Dermatol 2009;161(4):869–77.
3. Fine JD, Johnson LB, Weiner M, et al. Genitourinary complication of inherited epidermolysis bullosa: experience of the national epidermolysis bullosa registry and review of the literature. J Urol 2004; 172(5 Pt 1):2040–4.
4. Pohla-Gubo G, Riedl R, Hintner H. DEBRA-Austria and the EB-hause Austria. In: Fine JD, Hintner H, editors. Life with epidermolysis bullosa (EB): etiology, diagnosis, multidisciplinary care and therapy. Vienna (Austria): Springer; 2009. p. 241–5.
5. Abercombie E, Mather C, Hon J, et al. Care of the adult patient with recessive dystrophic EB. (Tissue Viability Supplement). BJN 2008;17(6):10–7.

Epidermolysis Bullosa Care in the United States

H. Alan Arbuckle, MD[a,b,*]

KEYWORDS

- Epidermolysis bullosa • EB centers
- Interdisciplinary • Immunomapping

There is a wide range of health care delivery systems within the United States for patients with epidermolysis bullosa (EB). They range from nonexistent, primarily because of remote geographic locations, to 4 comprehensive interdisciplinary EB centers. Table 1 lists the 5 large interdisciplinary centers, clinic directors, and the services available either as part of the care team or via consultation. In addition to these 5 centers, the University of Miami has an EB program, directed by Lisa Connelly, MD, which can provide care and resources to individuals with EB.

According to the US National EB Registry, the prevalence of EB is 4.6 cases per million of the population and 10.75 per million live births.[1] The number of cases cared for by the 5 interdisciplinary teams (Table 2) is certainly much lower than the present total number of individuals with EB in the United States. The reason for this discrepancy is that the vast majority of individuals with EB are cared for by either their primary care provider or pediatric dermatologist. In the United States, there are many outstanding pediatric dermatologists and dermatologists who care for EB patients.

There is a concerted effort by the 4 centers not only to provide direct patient care but also to be advocates for patients and provide other health care delivery system access to resources and expertise. All 4 centers work closely with local and national advocacy organizations. All Medical Directors, including Dr Connelly, are members of the Scientific Advisory Board of the Dystrophic Epidermolysis Bullosa Research Association of America (www.DeBRA.org). In addition, they are also members of the Epidermolysis Bullosa Interest Group (EBIG), which is a list-serve–based organization composed of EB health care providers from around the world. The mission of EBIG is to provide collaboration and expert opinion to all EB heath care providers to improve the lives of persons with EB.

In the United States, the standard workup for an individual suspected of having EB is immunomapping and electron microscopy on an induced blister. Some centers will also do routine histology if other diseases are being considered. Although not all centers have the capability of performing all tests, all the centers have access to testing. Two centers, the Lucile Packard Children's Hospital at Stanford and the Children's Hospital in Colorado, have the capability of providing other centers with both immunomapping and electron microscopy.

Although most governmental and private insurers will pay for the initial workup, very few pay for genetic testing. There are a few centers that are able to do genetic testing if a research protocol is available, but most samples are sent to GeneDx (www.GeneDx.com). Given that most insurers do not pay for genetic testing in the United

[a] Epidermolysis Bullosa Clinic, The Children's Hospital, 13123 East 16th Avenue, B570, Aurora, CO 80045, USA
[b] Department of Dermatology, Dermatology Services, Denver VA Medical Center, 1055 Clermont Street, Denver, CO 80220, USA
* Department of Dermatology, Dermatology Services, Denver VA Medical Center, 1055 Clermont Street, Denver, CO 80220.
E-mail address: Alan.Arbuckle@ucdenver.edu

Dermatol Clin 28 (2010) 387–389
doi:10.1016/j.det.2010.02.012
0733-8635/10/$ – see front matter. Published by Elsevier Inc.

Table 1
EB centers in the United States and the subspecialties available either as part of the care team or through consultation

Name of Institutions	Lucile Packard Children's Hospital at Stanford	The Children's Hospital, Aurora, CO	Cincinnati Children's Hospital	Columbia University, New York
Director, Interdisciplinary Center	Anna Bruckner, MD	H. Alan Arbuckle, MD	Anne Lucky, MD	Kim Morel, MD
Subspecialties at Centers				
Dermatology	Y	Y	Y	Y
EB Nurse Specialist	Y	Y	Y	Y
Gastroenterology/Nutrition	Y	Y	Y	Y
Pediatric Surgery	a	a	Y	Y
Pain Management	Y	Y	Y	Y
Occupational Therapy	Y	Y	Y	Y
Physical Therapy	Y	Y	Y	Y
Genetics	Y	Y	a	Y
Infectious Disease	a	a	a	Y
Social Work	Y	Y	Y	Y
Psychology/Psychiatry	Y	a	Y	a
Child Life	a	Y	Y	Y
Dental	b	Y	Y	Y
Hematology	Y	a	a	Y
Cardiology	a	a	a	a
Oncology	a	a	a	a
Ophthalmology	Y	a	a	a
Nephrology	a	a	a	a
Orthopedics	a	a	a	a
Interventional Radiology	a	a	a	a
Endocrinology	a	a	a	a

Abbreviation: Y, yes, subspecialty is part of the interdisciplinary care team.

a Subspecialty is not part of the routine EB clinic but is available to the center via consultation.

b The center does not have a dental clinic, but pediatric dental services are available at the University of California San Francisco and/or in the local community.

Table 2
The 4 centers and their EB population based on subtype

Subtypes	Lucile Packard Children's Hospital at Stanford	The Children's Hospital, Aurora, CO	Cincinnati Children's Hospital	Columbia University, New York	Total
Simplex	8	20	33	18	79
Junctional	2	1	28	4	35
DDEB	7	4	26	7	44
RDEB	33	15	58	15	121

Abbreviations: DDEB, dominant dystrophic epidermolysis bullosa; RDEB, recessive dystrophic epidermolysis bullosa.

States, most patients never have gene mapping as part of their workup.

REFERENCE

1. Fine JD, Johnson LB, Suchindran C, et al. The epidemiology of inherited epidermolysis bullosa. In: Fine JD, Bauer EA, McGuire J, et al, editors. Epidermolysis bullosa clinical, epidemiologic and laboratory advances and the findings of the National Epidermolysis Bullosa Registry. Baltimore: Johns Hopkins University Press; 1999. p. 101–13.

Epidermolysis Bullosa Care in Canada

Elena Pope, MD, MSc

KEYWORDS

- Epidermolysis bullosa • Canada
- Universal health care • Specialists

Based on the described prevalence and size of the population, approximately 300 to 500 patients with epidermolysis bullosa (EB) reside in Canada. There are specific challenges faced by patients and families as well as the practitioners looking after patients with EB. Canada follows the Universal Canada Health Act, which guarantees universal medical access to care patients and families. As a result, patients do not have to pay to see a practitioner or for in-hospital care; however, they have to pay for prescribed (unless they have private insurance) and over-the-counter medications, dressings, and other medical supplies, which reach a significant amount for patients with high, chronic needs. To date, there is a lack of government (federal or provincial) funding that prevents the development and sustenance of specialized EB centers. It is also difficult to centralize EB care at a national level (as in the United Kingdom, Chile, and other countries) because the EB population is spread over a large territory. In addition, because of the funding formula of the pediatric hospitals, care over age 18 years is discouraged. As children with EB live longer, their care ideally should be transferred to an adult EB specialized center. Currently, there is no formal adult specialized EB care in Canada; most adults continuing to be followed in the pediatric centers beyond their 18th birthday. This scenario has limitations in that specific adult issues, such as sexuality, employment, independence, and skin cancer, are not part of the traditional pediatric expertise.

The EB care is currently provided primarily in the major pediatric centers, such as those in Toronto, Vancouver, and Montreal. Recognizing the challenges associated with caring for patients with EB, SickKids hospital in Toronto established the first multidisciplinary specialized EB clinic in Canada in January 2004. This specialized EB clinic takes a coordinated, collaborative approach involving many subspecialties, all focused on improving the quality of care delivered and health outcomes for patients with EB and their families. Housed within the dermatology program, the EB clinic is supported by a team of physicians and nurses from dermatology, wound care, plastic surgery, gastroenterology, hematology, ophthalmology, cardiology, dentistry, pediatrics, and chronic pain as well as social work, occupational therapy, and physiotherapy. The team manages the outpatient care of 50 to 60 pediatric patients (0–25 years of age) with EB and provides inpatient consultations for admitted patients, prenatal counseling for affected families, and advice and consultations to other providers across Canada. The EB clinic offers improved access and delivery of care, coordinating appointments on the same day, leading to increased patient and family satisfaction and improved clinical outcomes. A list of EB specialists is in **Table 1**.

Dystrophic Epidermolysis Bullosa Research Association (DEBRA) Canada is the national support group for patients with EB.

SickKids hospital has access to a local EM and immunohistochemistry laboratory for pathology diagnosis. Molecular diagnosis is done through Genedx for a fee, currently covered under the Ontario Health Insurance Plan.

The Hospital for Sick Children, 555 University Avenue, Toronto, ON M5G 1X8, Canada
E-mail address: elena.pope@sickkids.ca

Dermatol Clin 28 (2010) 391–392
doi:10.1016/j.det.2010.02.013

Table 1
Canadian EB Specialists

Toronto	Dr Elena Pope, MSc, FRCPC, Medical Director, Epidermolysis bullosa clinic, The Hospital for Sick Children
Vancouver	Dr Julie Prendiville, BC Children's Hospital
Montreal	Dr Catherine McCuaig, St Justine Hospital

Epidermolysis Bullosa Care in Mexico

Carmen Liy-Wong, MD[a], Rodrigo Cepeda-Valdes, MD[b],
Julio Cesar Salas-Alanis, MD[b],*

KEYWORDS

• EB • Epidermolysis • Bullosa • Mexico

Epidermolysis bullosa (EB) in Mexico continues to be a rare genodermatosis that is still unknown to most of the health care professionals in the country; many patients are treated without the specialist's health care that they need and in some cases, we still see how they receive wrong treatment and even wrong diagnosis. Regarding this situation, the severity of some cases, the chronic evolution of the disease, and the financial and social burden that it brings, Dystrophic Epidermolysis Bullosa Research Association (DebRA) of MEXICO was founded as a charity in February 1998[1]; however, the spirit of organization was born in 1994 when a small group of volunteers and dermatologists started to see patients with the main purpose to provide medical care, genetic counseling, and advice to patients with EB and their families; to promote collaboration and exchange information among people with EB; to research and find new therapeutic approaches; and finally, to diffuse knowledge and raise awareness of the issues of EB in general public and health care professionals. This spirit is alive in the current organization, whereby day by day there are more patients and people interested in helping the "butterfly kids" or "NIÑOS PIEL MARIPOSA" in Spanish.

DebRA MEXICO has established its main office in Monterrey city and has dedicated health care services for people with EB around Mexico, mainly in cities and villages around Monterrey, in conjunction (directly and indirectly) with national health services (Instituto Mexicano del Seguro Social). Unfortunately, national health services do not cover all the cost of the disease and private insurances do not include coverage for the disease. DebRA MEXICO health care team is formed by dermatologist; pediatric dermatologist; pediatrician; pediatric gastroenterologist; a team of plastic surgeon, geneticist, and psychologist; nutritionals team; and a physical therapist, all of them working as volunteers donating their time to provide patients with EB the highest standards of care, regardless of the patients' place of living, religion, or even economy.

DebRA MEXICO improved the quality of life of individuals and families affected by EB by providing them dressing materials, drugs, nutritional supplements, transportation and accommodations for foreign patients, and even hand surgeries for pseudosyndactyly, thanks to the fund-raising activities from sporting to social events, taking place mainly in Monterrey city. In the same manner, nutrition and medical students interact with patients and their families in each meeting to educate and involve the new health care workers with the disease.

In the last years, DebRA MEXICO has been gaining experience in managing patients with EB, thanks to the significant contributions made by the support and help from the professional colleagues of DebRA UK, DebRA USA, and DebRA International, specially in symptom relief and optimal management of the condition as well as in clinical research.

DebRA MEXICO works closely with 4 hospital centers of excellence: Centro Dermatológico "Dr Ladislado de la Pascua" and Instituto Nacional

---

[a] Department of Dermatology, Hospital Universitario "Dr Jose E. Gonzalez" UANL, Monterrey, Nuevo León 64460, México
[b] DebRA MEXICO AC, Otomie 206, Colonia Azteca Guadalupe, Nuevo León 67150, México
* Corresponding author.
E-mail address: drjuliosalas@gmail.com

Dermatol Clin 28 (2010) 393–394
doi:10.1016/j.det.2010.02.014
0733-8635/10/$ – see front matter © 2010 Elsevier Inc. All rights reserved.

de Pediatria, both located in Mexico city, Instituto Dermatológico de Jalisco in Guadalajara city, and Hospital Universitario UANL in Monterrey.

The prevalence of EB in Mexico is still unknown; the main problem is the lack of an immunolaboratory for immunomapping for the diagnosis of EB in Mexico. To address this, DebRA MEXICO, in conjunction with those centers, has been trying to do a National Registry of Patients with EB (Registro Nacional de las Epidermolisis Bullosas [RENAC-eb]).

The Instituto Nacional de Pediatria, the unique center with electronic microscopic diagnosis for EB in Mexico, in the last 5 years has had 29 patients: 9 (32%) with EB simplex, 5 (17%) with junctional EB, and 15 (51%) with dystrophic EB. The Centro Dermatológico " Dr Ladislao de la Pascua" in the last 20 years has 107 patients: 51 with (47%) EB simplex, 1 (0.93%) with junctional EB, 33 (30.8%) with dystrophic EB, and 23 (21%) with no specific classification. In this Centro, as in the beginnings of DebRA MEXICO (which controls the Northwest and receives patients from all over the country), the diagnosis is based on clinical and histologic findings when available.

DebRA MEXICO, since 1995, has on its clinical registry the following information: 6 (4%) cases of EB simplex, 2 (1.3%) junctional EB, 41 (27%) dominant dystrophic EB, 74 (50%) recessive dystrophic EB, and 23 (15%) without diagnosis. Unfortunately, in the Instituto Dermatológico de Jalisco "Dr José Barba Rubio", there are no data available.

DebRA MEXICO has been supported by DebRA UK, DebRA International, DebRA America, and recently by DebRA Austria that have been keen to help with immunomapping and molecular studies.

To achieve one of the goals of the organization, DebRA MEXICO has made different research projects in collaboration with DebRA UK, finding a new mutation for COL7A1 in 21 Mexican families. In 1998, the 2470insG/2470insG mutations in type VII collagen gene (COL7A1) were found using molecular analysis. Since then, some papers have published with international collaboration.[2–8] Furthermore, between 2007 and 2008, the charity performed 30 hand reconstructive surgeries in patients with pseudosyndactyly.

The organization expects to provide dental help and surgeries for patients with EB, promote public understanding of the illness, supply continuous multidisciplinary education, and train the new health care workers to extend throughout the country and spread out DebRA's spirit to encourage and help the formation of new national EB groups in Latin American countries, such as Costa Rica, Chile, and México have initiated a cooperation to set up the charity DebRA Latinoamerica since 2005, with the firm idea to help patients with EB from all America Latina.

We do believe in our dream and we are sure that with our little help, we can move mountains and make fly "los niños mariposa."

ACKNOWLEDGMENTS

Special thanks to Dra Angelica Beirana, Dr Mario Amaya, Dra Carola Duran, Dr Andy South, (Dundee University, Scotland, UK), Dra Gabriela Pohla-Gubo (Paracelsus Private Medical University, Salzburg, Austria), Dra Angela Christiano, (Columbia University, NY, USA), Dr John McGrath (St John's Institute of Dermatology, London, UK) and Dr Helmut Hintner (Paracelsus Private Medical University, Salzburg, Austria) for their help and support.

REFERENCES

1. Julio C, Salas-Alanis CE, Carta AL, editors, In: Nace Fundación DEBRA México AC, 42. Mexico D.F.: Revista Mexicana de Dermatología; 1998. p. 172–3.
2. Salas-Alanis JC, Mellerio JE, Amaya-Guerra M, et al. Frameshift mutations in the type VII collagen gene (COL7A1) in five Mexican cousins with recessive dystrophic epidermolysis bullosa. Br J Dermatol 1998;138(5):852–8.
3. Salas-Alanis JC, McGrath JA. 2470insG, represents the commonest mutation in Mexican patients with epidermolysis bullosa. A study of 21 families. Gac Med Mex 2006;142(1):29–34.
4. Mellerio JE, Salas-Alanis JC, Talamantes ML, et al. A recurrent glycine substitution mutation, G2043R, in the type VII collagen gene (COL7A1) in dominant dystrophic epidermolysis bullosa. Br J Dermatol 1998;139(4):730–7.
5. Cserhalmi-Friedman PB, McGrath JA, Mellerio JE, et al. Restoration of open reading frame resulting from skipping of an exon with an internal deletion in the COL7A1 gene. Lab Invest 1998;78(12):1483–92.
6. Wessagowit V, Ashton GH, Mohammedi R, et al. Three cases of de novo dominant dystrophic epidermolysis bullosa associated with the mutation G2043R in COL7A1. Clin Exp Dermatol 2001;26(1): 97–9.
7. Pourreyron C, Cox G, Mao X, et al. Patients with recessive dystrophic epidermolysis bullosa develop squamous-cell carcinoma regardless of type VII collagen expression. J Invest Dermatol 2007; 127(10):2438–44.
8. Salas-Alanis JC. El proyecto DEBRA; state of the arts. Med Cut Iber Lat Am 2007;35(4):165–6. 8.

Epidermolysis Bullosa Care in the United Kingdom

Jemima E. Mellerio, MD, FRCP[a,b],*

KEYWORDS

• Epidermolysis bullosa • National Diagnostic EB Laboratory
• National Commissioning Group

Since 2002, epidermolysis bullosa (EB) services in England (see list below) have been nationally funded by the National Commissioning Group (NCG), which also funds the National Diagnostic EB Laboratory. This provides a comprehensive multidisciplinary service including relevant medical and nursing specialists, therapists, investigations, and treatments. This service also covers Welsh and Scottish patients although there is also a clinical center in Edinburgh, and keratin gene testing for EB simplex is undertaken in Dundee. The NCG-funded centers and laboratory have close links with each other and DebRA (Dystrophic Epidermolysis Bullosa Research Association), meeting regularly to discuss protocols, audit, and service developments. A national EB database has also been set up as part of the NCG service and a Scottish EB register has also been established for a number of years. DebRA UK funds some of the adult and pediatric EB clinical nurse specialists in the United Kingdom and a team of social care managers.

There are thought to be approximately 5000 people with EB in the United Kingdom, of whom around 350 have a severe form. Currently, approximately 900 of these patients regularly attend a specialist center for EB.

The National Health Service (NHS) funds all aspects of clinical care for patients with EB, including dressings, drugs, and hospital treatments.

The National Diagnostic EB Laboratory in London undertakes skin biopsy (immunofluorescence and electron microscopy) and molecular testing (except keratin 5 or 14 in EB simplex cases) for United Kingdom patients (and overseas patients, although a fee is charged). They also carry out prenatal testing for severe forms of EB from chorionic villus sampling or fetal skin biopsy. Preimplantation genetic diagnosis is also licensed for Herlitz junctional EB (with *LAMA3* or *LAMB3* mutations) and recessive dystrophic EB. EB simplex *KRT5* and *KRT14* gene testing is performed at Ninewell's Hospital, Dundee.

Contacts

Birmingham Children's Hospital NHS Foundation Trust (Prof Celia Moss), Pediatric EB Service, Steelhouse Lane, Birmingham, W Midlands B4 6NH, UK. Tel: +44 (0) 121 333 8224, e-mail: eb.team@bch.nhs.uk.

Birmingham Heartlands and Sollihull NHS Trust (Dr Adrian Heagerty), Adult EB

Funding: The author acknowledges financial support from the Department of Health via the National Institute for Health Research (NIHR) comprehensive Biomedical Research Centre award to Guy's and St Thomas' NHS Foundation Trust, in partnership with King's College London and King's College Hospital NHS Foundation Trust.

[a] St John's Institute of Dermatology, Guy's and St Thomas' NHS Foundation Trust, St Thomas' Hospital, Westminster Bridge Road, London SE1 7EH, UK
[b] Department of Dermatology, Great Ormond Street Hospital for Children NHS Trust, Great Ormond Street, London WC1N 3JH, UK
* Department of Dermatology, Great Ormond Street Hospital for Children NHS Trust, Great Ormond Street, London WC1N 3JH, UK.
E-mail address: jemima.mellerio@kcl.ac.uk

Dermatol Clin 28 (2010) 395–396
doi:10.1016/j.det.2010.02.015

Service, Bordesley Green East, Birmingham, W Midlands B9 5SS, UK. Tel: +44 (0) 121 424 4563, e-mail: Adrian.heagerty@heartofengland.nhs.uk.

Great Ormond Street Hospital for Children NHS Trust (Dr Anna Martinez, Dr Jemima Mellerio), Pediatric EB Service, Great Ormond Street, London WC1N 3JH, UK. Tel: +44 (0) 20 7829 7808, e-mail: martia@gosh.nhs.uk, mellej@gosh.nhs.uk.

Guy's and St Thomas' NHS Foundation Trust (Prof John McGrath, Dr Jemima Mellerio, Dr Ann Marie Powell), Adult EB Service, St Thomas' Hospital, Westminster Bridge Road, London SE1 7EH, UK. Tel: +44 (0) 20 7188 6399, e-mail: jemima.mellerio@gstt.nhs.uk.

EB Service (Dr Mike Tidman, Dr Olivia Schofield, Dr Helen Horn), Department of Dermatology, Old Royal Infirmary of Edinburgh, Lauriston Building, Lauriston Place, Edinburgh EH3 9HA, UK. Tel: +44 (0) 131 536 2414, e-mail: helen.horn@luht.scot.nhs.uk.

Robin Eady National Diagnostic EB Laboratory (Trish Dopping-Hepenstal Head of Laboratory), St John's Institute of Dermatology, Basement, South Wing Stair C, St Thomas' Hospital, Westminster Bridge Road, London SE1 7EH, UK. Tel: +44 (0) 20 7188 7229, e-mail: EBLab@gstt.nhs.uk.

East of Scotland Regional Genetics Service (Dr David Baty, Dr Ana Terron-Kwiatkowski), Level 6, Ninewells Hospital and Medical School, Dundee DD1 9SY, UK, Tel: +44 (0) 1382 496261, e-mail: dbaty@nhs.net, aterron-kwiatkowski@nhs.net.

DebRA UK, DebRA House, 13 Wellington Business Park, Duke's Ride, Crowthorne, Berkshire RG45 6LS, UK, Tel: +44 (0) 1344 771961, e-mail: debra@debra.org.uk.

Care of Epidermolysis Bullosa in Ireland

Rosemarie Watson, MD, FRCPI[a,b,c,]*

KEYWORDS

• DEBRA • EB • Health care • Diagnosis

Advances in the medical care of epidermolysis bullosa (EB) have led to the development of National Service Centers for EB in many countries worldwide. The exemplary model of care to children and adults with EB in the United Kingdom, combined with the knowledge that people with EB were travelling to the United Kingdom for treatment, encouraged us to develop the Irish national service. Dystrophic Epidermolysis Bullosa Research Association (DEBRA) of Ireland, founded in 1988, played a pivotal role in the development of our service.

Ireland (North and South) is an island of almost 6 million people, and it is conservatively estimated that approximately 200 families in Ireland are affected by EB. The EB service caseload is outlined in **Table 1**. Patients living in Northern Ireland (governed by the UK National Health Service) and those living in the south of the country have access to this service. In addition, those patients with skin fragility disorders other than EB have access because of the specialist care required.

The service for children with EB is based at Our Lady's Children's Hospital, Crumlin, Dublin, where we have held dedicated clinics since 1996. The adult service is based at St James' Hospital, Dublin and has been in existence since 2002. The current funding of the core multidisciplinary team for adults and children is outlined in **Table 2**. The aims of the multidisciplinary team are to provide high-quality medical care meeting international standards of excellence for our patients, to minimize disabilities, and to offer support necessary to maintain patients' daily lives as normal as possible.

OUTLINE OF SERVICE

Both the adult and children's hospitals provide quarterly multidisciplinary outpatient clinics and a coordinated and preplanned admission service. A dedicated EB-patient treatment room is available at both locations for drop-in visits. Monthly team meetings are held at both sites. There is an active outreach service that includes home visits by the core team with general review and intensive education for parents, carers, public health nurses, community services, and general practitioners. The outreach service also includes rapid response for all maternity units. Visits to schools and colleges ensure an appropriate adaptive environment. The adult service has allowed many of our patients to achieve an independent lifestyle with the appropriate supports. Several patients with severe EB have achieved university education and subsequent employment (**Fig. 1**).

MOLECULAR DIAGNOSIS

More than 90% of our patients/families have molecular diagnoses pending or complete. The diagnostic laboratory used for EB simplex molecular diagnostics is the Scottish Molecular Genetics Consortium, Human Genetics Department of Pathology, Ninewells Hospital, Dundee, Scotland. For immunofluorescence, electron microscopy, and molecular diagnosis of junctional and dystrophic EB, the laboratory we refer to is The National Diagnostic EB Laboratory, St John's Institute of Dermatology, St Thomas' Hospital, Westminster Bridge Road, London SE1 7EH, United Kingdom.

[a] National EB Service, St James' Hospital, James' Street, Dublin 8, Ireland
[b] Our Lady's Children's Hospital Crumlin, Dublin 12, Ireland
[c] Trinity College, Dublin, Ireland
* Our Lady's Children's Hospital Crumlin, Dublin 12, Ireland.
E-mail address: RWatson@STJAMES.IE

Dermatol Clin 28 (2010) 397–399
doi:10.1016/j.det.2010.02.017

Table 1
Irish EB service caseload (adult & pediatric)

Diagnosis	Number of Patients
EB simplex	
Localized	40
Dowling-Meara	3
Junctional EB	
Herlitz	2[a]
Non-Herlitz	
Dystrophic EB	
Recessive	24
Severe generalized	12[b]
Non–Hallopeau-Siemens	12
Dominant	13
Unclassified	1
Total	83

[a] Deaths N = 2.
[b] Deaths N = 7.

Professor Alan Irvine, in conjunction with the department of genetics, directs genetic counseling for our patients.

SERVICE LINKS

Further information on our service is available at http://www.stjames.ie/departments/department sato3/e/epidermolysisbullosa.

The service has close links with colleagues in the United Kingdom; in particular, staff at Great Ormond Street Hospital (with funding support from DEBRA UK) played a pivotal role in the development of the service and continue to attend our clinics on an intermittent basis. The service also has close links with DEBRA Ireland (http://www.debraireland.org), which has supplied funding for equipment and continue to fund a portion of our nurse specialist's appointment in the children's hospital. They have also provided funds for travels to international EB meetings. Links to the international EB forum and EB care network have afforded us invaluable advice on EB care.

FUNDING OF THE SERVICE

In 1996, initial funding from DEBRA Ireland provided a 0.5 whole-time equivalent EB nurse specialist in the children's hospital. This position was increased to a full-time position in 2004, with the second half being funded by the health service. We have applied for dedicated funding for a multidisciplinary service for children with EB. The service is currently provided by the necessary health care professionals on an ad hoc basis; unfortunately, budgetary cuts in health care have resulted in restricted access of these services to EB.

In contrast, funding for the adult multidisciplinary service was obtained from the health service in 2002. Both our patients and we have seen the benefits of dedicated funding for the multidisciplinary adult service and continue to seek dedicated funding for children with EB. Provision of core staff is outlined in **Table 2**.

PATIENT COSTS

All patients on this island have free access to medical care and a number have additional private insurance. We are fortunate that all of our patients with recessive dystrophic EB, (with the help of the multidisciplinary team, in terms of application to the relevant health boards) have free access to silicone, dressings, prescription and nonprescription drugs and topical agents (ie, manuka honey). In

Table 2
Current provision of core staff

Specialty	Adult Service WTE	Pediatric Service WTE
EB nurse specialist	1.0	1.0[a]
Medical social worker	0.5	NDF
Occupational therapy	0.25[a]	NDF
Physiotherapy	0.2	NDF
Psychology	0.25	NDF
Clinical nutrition	0.5	NDF
Secretary	0.5	NDF

Abbreviations: WTE, whole-time equivalent; NDF, no dedicated funding.
[a] Partially funded by DEBRA Ireland.

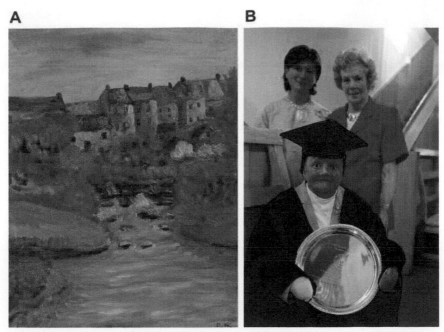

Fig. 1. (*A*) Painting of Ennistymon Falls, Co. Clare by Patti Lynch (RIP). Patti had severe generalized recessive dystrophic EB. (*B*) Merit award given by faculty of medicine, Trinity College, Dublin 2005 to Patti (seen with her mother and sister) for her role as educator in the development of the Irish National EB service.

addition, a significant portion of our other patients are eligible for a medical card, which is means tested and allows for free drugs and a limited number of dressings. In addition, the local health centers provide needles, sharps container, tubifast (Mölnlycke Health Care, Sweden), and some dressings. Our patients in Northern Ireland have free access to all supplies, including dressings, medications, and topical products via the UK National Health System. Hospital doctor visits are also free for our patients, but there is a charge in primary care for those who do not have a medical card. DEBRA Ireland has also supported patients who do not have complete cover.

ADVANTAGES OF THE IRISH SERVICE

The joint appointment of Professor Alan Irvine and myself to both the adult and children's hospitals allows for continuity of care for our patients. This is particularly useful during the transition period from child to adult services, which is normally a very stressful time for patients and their families. The development of the outreach services with greater communication and involvement of community care for our patients has resulted in care closer to home. Our proximity to the United Kingdom and Scotland has afforded us the access to excellent diagnostic centers and referral in addition to joint consultations on patients with complex problems. The financial burden for our patients because of government support is significantly less than in other countries.

FUTURE DIRECTIONS

We will continue to request funding for the children's EB service. Curative care, which is becoming a distinct reality for EB, will place increased pressure on the service, and thus it is imperative that our patients are ready and well enough when this becomes available. In this regard, the service is currently developing an Irish EB registry.

ACKNOWLEDGMENTS

I would like to acknowledge the unwavering commitment of the core team and our other hospital colleagues to the EB service. I would also like to acknowledge our patients who have taught us much and DEBRA Ireland for its continued support.

Epidermolysis Bullosa in France: Management in the National Reference Center for Genodermatosis

Christine Bodemer, MD, PhD[a,b,c,]*, MAGEC-Necker Team[1]

KEYWORDS

- National reference center • MAGEC • Genodermatosis
- Rare diseases • Epidermolysis bullosa
- Genodermatosis database • CEMARA

Since more than 20 years, the coordination of an epidermolysis bullosa (EB)–specific multidisciplinary management has been organized by our department of dermatology, in Necker Enfants Malades Hospital (Paris). There were 2 reasons for that: (1) We have a specific unit for children with severe dermatologic diseases (from birth to 18 years of age), and (2) the Necker Enfants Malades Hospital is a very famous and important pediatric hospital, with more than 400 beds for children and 200 beds for adults. This hospital is highly specialized in the treatment of genetic diseases and permits a multidisciplinary management of the pediatric patients with a qualified technical platform. Genetic counseling, prenatal diagnosis, and preimplantation genetic diagnosis are also possible. Therefore, a multidisciplinary medical and paramedical staff for EB has been meeting every month for 20 years.

In 2004, the French Ministry of Health decided to distinguish reference centers for rare diseases and to support them financially. Reference centers (RCs) have been distinguished because of their (1) ability to establish the right diagnosis of the types and subtypes of a rare disease, (2) ability to manage the patients correctly because of their experience and their highly adapted technical platform, and (3) research programs and publications.[1–11] They are supposed to develop a national network for the rare diseases and elaborate precise guidelines, which should be followed by their partners called competence centers (CCs). RCs have also to develop new national and international programs of research, new therapeutics, and an epidemiologic registry. CCs follow the recommendations of the RCs, work closely with them to collect epidemiologic data, and take part in their research programs.

In 2004, our center was recognized as an RC for genodermatosis. The name of this RC is MAGEC, for the French name Maladies Genetiques à Expression Cutanée. MAGEC comprises of 3 dermatologic departments in Paris (departments of Necker Enfants Malades, St Louis hospital, and Avicenne hospitals). In 2005 and 2006, two other RCs have been identified for genodermatosis (Bordeaux-Toulouse with Alain Hovnanian for EB; Nice with Jean-Philippe Lacour and Gim

a Department of Dermatology, Necker Enfants Malades Hospital, 149 Rue de Sèvres, APHP Paris 75015, France
b University René Descartes, Paris V, France
c Institut National de la Santé et de la Recherche Médicale U781, Paris, France
1 www.magec.eu
* Corresponding author. Department of Dermatology, Necker Enfants Malades Hospital, 149 Rue de Sèvres, APHP Paris 75015, France.
E-mail address: christine.bodemer@nck.aphp.fr

Dermatol Clin 28 (2010) 401–403
doi:10.1016/j.det.2010.02.007
0733-8635/10/$ – see front matter © 2010 Elsevier Inc. All rights reserved.

Meneguzzi for molecular diagnosis concerning junctional EB). Since September 2009, Alain Hovnanian and his research team joined Necker Hospital in Paris.

MAGEC-Necker aims to offer the best medical and social EB management, with a rapid clinical, histologic, and molecular diagnosis. In the same vein, we have developed an active clinical research program in close correlation with a more fundamental one. Our aim is to improve, hoping to soon offer innovative therapies, such as genetic therapies. The clinical research consists of programs concerning pain management, nutrition, surgery/anesthesia, and skin management. The financial supports are insufficient but helpful for the development of EB-specific programs of therapeutic education and social integration (school and professional).

The organization of MAGEC-Necker consists of (1) a managing team formed by 5 specialized physicians (3 pediatric dermatologists, an anesthetist, and 1 for epidemiologic studies); 1 specialized nurse for EB nursing and therapeutic education; 1 social worker for the social integration; 1 secretary; 1 technician for the technical management of the skin biopsies; (2) a multidisciplinary task force of experts, including pediatric dermatologists, molecular and genetic specialists, a dietician and a nutritionist, a physical therapist, an occupational therapist, a plastic surgeon, a psychologist, and an anatomic pathologist, associated with the managing team (the managing team meets weekly, the task force monthly); (3) a specific space with adapted bathtubs for the organization of the homecoming, management of chronic conditions, and therapeutic education (Fig. 1).

Therapeutic education is organized for families but, before all, for all medical and paramedical professionals concerned with the care of patients with EB in France. Regular sessions for education are organized. There is an important lack of qualified professionals close to the patients' homes. For this reason, homecoming remains an important problem. The cost of the care partly explains these difficulties. There is a lack of respite centers when hospitalizations are no longer necessary.

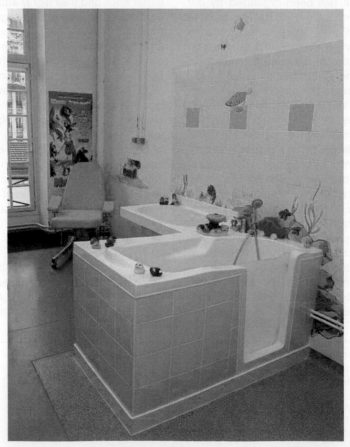

Fig. 1. Two bathtubs, one for newborns and young children and another for adolescents and adults.

All the information concerning MAGEC, its programs, and its guidelines are available in www.magec.eu, which will soon be translated into English.

Diagnosis of the type and subtype of EB is established by the combination of the study of clinical characteristics and the histologic, immunohistologic, and, if necessary, ultrastructural skin analysis in Necker's anatomic pathology laboratory (Dr S. Fraitag and S. Leclerc-Mercier). Molecular diagnoses of patients followed up by MAGEC are performed in Alain Hovnanian's laboratory (Paris, Necker) for epidermolytic and dystrophic EB and Gim Menneguzzi's laboratory for junctional EB (Nice).

French EB epidemiologic data are not yet completely available. An epidemiologic database for rare diseases, called CEMARA, was recently constructed. This database is essential for the activity recording, epidemiologic data, and monitoring of the RC and also contributes to specific projects of the centers, such as follow-up of cohorts and clinical research. CEMARA is now available for all French RCs and CCs. We expect that precise clinical and molecular epidemiologic data will be available in the nearest future. In MAGEC-Necker we have followed up around 200 patients with EB; 150 of them are still alive and regularly followed up. This group consists of mainly patients with the dystrophic form (about 90). Data of all patients have not yet been collected in CEMARA; this work is underway.

One next essential step in the study of EB in Europe is the clinical trial for genetic therapy of recessive dystrophic epidermolysis bullosa (Therapeuskin) coordinated by A. Hovnanian, which will be conducted in France in the Necker Enfants Malades Hospital (in the important new institute for genetic research and innovating therapies, IMAGINE).

REFERENCES

1. Titeux M, Pendaries V, Tonasso L, et al. A frequent functional SNP in the MMP1 promoter is associated with higher disease severity in recessive dystrophic epidermolysis bullosa. Hum Mutat 2008;29(2):267–76.
2. Changotade SI, Assoumou A, Guéniche F, et al. Epigallocatechin gallate's protective effect against MMP7 in recessive dystrophic epidermolysis bullosa patients. J Invest Dermatol 2007;127(4):821–8.
3. Titeux M, Mazereeuw-Hautier J, Hadj-Rabia S, et al. Three severe cases of EBS Dowling-Meara caused by missense and frameshift mutations in the keratin 14 gene. J Invest Dermatol 2006;126(4):773–6.
4. Bodemer C, Tchen SI, Ghomrasseni S, et al. Skin expression of metalloproteinases and tissue inhibitor of metalloproteinases in sibling patients with recessive dystrophic epidermolysis and intrafamilial phenotypic variation. J Invest Dermatol 2003;121(2):273–9.
5. Gache Y, Allegra M, Bodemer C, et al. Genetic bases of severe junctional epidermolysis bullosa presenting spontaneous amelioration with aging. Hum Mol Genet 2001;10(21):2453–61.
6. Spirito F, Chavanas S, Prost-Squarcioni C, et al. Reduced expression of the epithelial adhesion ligand laminin 5 in the skin causes intradermal tissue separation. J Biol Chem 2001;276(22):18828–35.
7. Sakuntabhai A, Hammami-Hauasli N, Bodemer C, et al. Deletions within COL7A1 exons distant from consensus splice sites alter splicing and produce shortened polypeptides in dominant dystrophic epidermolysis bullosa. Am J Hum Genet 1998;63(3):737–48.
8. Hovnanian A, Rochat A, Bodemer C, et al. Characterization of 18 new mutations in COL7A1 in recessive dystrophic epidermolysis bullosa provides evidence for distinct molecular mechanisms underlying defective anchoring fibril formation. Am J Hum Genet 1997;61(3):599–610.
9. Callot-Mellot C, Bodemer C, Caux F, et al. Epidermolysis bullosa acquisita in childhood [review]. Arch Dermatol 1997;133(9):1122–6.
10. Hovnanian A, Hilal L, Blanchet-Bardon C, et al. DNA-based prenatal diagnosis of generalized recessive dystrophic epidermolysis bullosa in six pregnancies at risk for recurrence. J Invest Dermatol 1995;104(4):456–61.
11. Messiaen C, Le Mignot L, Rath A, et al. CEMARA: a Web dynamic application within a N-tier architecture for rare diseases. Stud Health Technol Inform 2008;136:51–6.

Epidermolysis Bullosa Care in Germany

Leena Bruckner-Tuderman, MD

KEYWORDS
- Rare diseases • Disease networks
- Molecular diagnostics • Epidermolysis bullosa

Until 2003, no structures existed in Germany for special care of patients with rare diseases, such as epidermolysis bullosa (EB). At that point, the Federal Ministry of Education and Research announced a clinical research program—networks for rare diseases. Competitive applications could be submitted for diseases with a prevalence of less than 5:10,000. The Network Epidermolysis Bullosa (EB Network), coordinated from the Department of Dermatology, University Medical Center Freiburg, has operated since October 2003 with the goal of improving diagnostics and clinical management, elucidating disease mechanisms, and development of novel therapies for EB (www.netzwerk-eb.de). The network currently has 6 partners, physicians and basic scientists, and its activities build on a combination of clinical and scientific expertise of the partners and the synergies generated between them. In the past 6 years, efficient clinical-diagnostic centers, multidisciplinary patient care, and a Web-based communication/information structure have been established. An EB patient registry exists as a prerequisite for research, which uses human tissues and mouse models and has generated significant new knowledge on dermal-epidermal adhesion and genotype-phenotype correlations in EB.

Two network centers, in Freiburg and Cologne, offer clinical and diagnostic services; 1 is responsible for the information technology (IT) infrastructure and 5 have experimental research projects. Fifteen collaborating clinical centers in Germany and in neighboring cities in Austria, Switzerland, and the Netherlands are associated with the network (**Fig. 1**). The clinicians in these centers represent different medical specialties (eg, dermatology, pediatric dermatology, pediatrics, genetics,

neurology, and dentistry); they refer patients, send diagnostic samples, and exchange information with the network. As a result, a multidisciplinary group of specialists interested in EB provides services in most of Germany, Austria, and Switzerland (see **Fig. 1**). Also the patient organizations, Dystrophic Epidermolysis Bullosa Research Association (DEBRA) Germany and DEBRA Europe, actively support the efforts to increase awareness on EB and the network activities.

Network meetings provide the partners and the collaborating centers with opportunities to report on progress, review and exchange data, and coordinate their activities. The 1-day meetings also include discussions in small groups and time for informal exchange. The activities of the network are supervised by an international advisory board, which attends 1 network meeting per year for evaluation and advice.

The network engages in dissemination of EB-relevant information to patients, health professionals, interested public, and the media. For this, the Web site is continuously updated, and the partners give talks in medical and scientific meetings, provide interviews in the media, organize actions days and training courses, and teach students of medicine/molecular medicine about skin biology and EB.

These efforts have resulted in a steady increase of diagnostic requests for suspected EB. Since 2004, several molecular diagnostic tests have been performed, including more than 300 immunofluorescence mappings on skin biopsies to determine the major EB category and more than 450 mutation analyses of EB genes. Requests for prenatal diagnosis for EB are not frequent in Germany, only about 5 each year. Immunofluorescence mapping and mutation

Funding support: EB Network grant from the Federal Ministry of Education and Research 2003–2011.
Department of Dermatology, University Medical Center Freiburg, Hauptstrasse 7, 79104 Freiburg, Germany
E-mail address: bruckner-tuderman@uniklinik-freiburg.de

Dermatol Clin 28 (2010) 405–406
doi:10.1016/j.det.2010.02.020

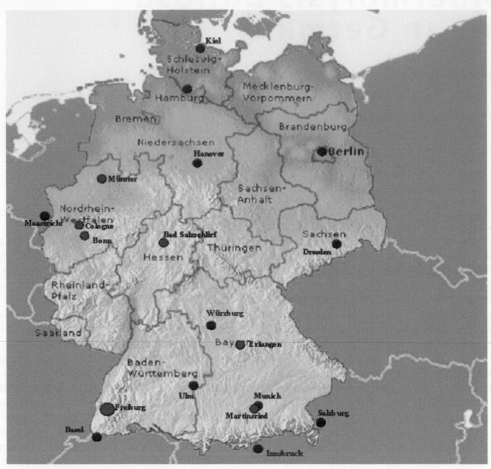

Fig. 1. The EB Network with its centers covers most of Germany and extends into some neighboring countries. Red: network partners; blue: collaborating clinical centers.

screening for EB genes are now offered by the University Medical Center Freiburg on a commercial basis. Thus, molecular EB diagnostics are readily available to all German patients, and the cost is covered by the health insurance.

The network with its centers has also achieved a significant improvement in standardized clinical care of EB in Germany. All clinicians associated with the network examine patients and have standard operating procedures on how to record personal and family history, document skin lesions photographically, obtain skin and blood specimens for diagnostics, and design an individual management plan based on a high standard of personal hygiene and daily skin care and protection from trauma and infection. In addition to primary care, coordinated multidisciplinary management is offered in Freiburg and in the collaborating center in Salzburg, with a broad range of medical specialties (dermatology, pediatrics, ophthalmology, surgery, human genetics, gastroenterology, neurology, oncology, dentistry,

psychology, and social work) for patients who visit for 1 to 2 days. This approach is often required to deal with many complications (eg, growth retardation, anemia, poor wound healing, joint contractures, infections, ocular, dental, social and psychological problems, or skin cancer).

Future goals of the EB Network include securing the clinical-diagnostic and IT structures established with grant support and focusing research on molecular disease mechanisms in EB and novel biologically valid therapies. Intensive collaborations with other networks for rare genetic diseases will generate durable structures in Germany and form a basis for future international consortia.

ACKNOWLEDGMENTS

The author gratefully acknowledges the assistance of Daniela Kirstein, the manager of the coordination center of the EB Network in preparation of this article.

Epidermolysis Bullosa Care in Italy

Daniele Castiglia, PhD, Giovanna Zambruno, MD*

KEYWORDS

- Rare diseases • Molecular diagnostics
- Disease registry • Diagnostic guidelines

In 2001, the Italian Ministry of Health issued a law for the creation of a national network of reference centers for the diagnosis and care of rare diseases, defined as diseases with a prevalence of less than 5:10,000. According to this law, reference centers for rare diseases are identified on a regional basis and are charged to (1) assure disease diagnosis, (2) release a specific certification to the patient, (3) ensure proper management and follow-up—also through collaboration with general practitioners, (4) keep patients' records and communicate all new disease cases to a regional registry for rare diseases, (5) organize training of health care personnel, (6) disseminate information and raise public awareness about rare diseases, and (7) keep contacts with patients' associations. The coordination of epidemiologic, clinical, and research activities on rare diseases, including the collection of epidemiologic data from regional registries and their organization in a national registry and the release of guidelines for disease diagnosis and care, is assigned to the National Institute of Health where a National Center for Rare Diseases (NCRD) has been created. According to this law, the National Health System covers costs related to (1) examinations required to establish the disease diagnosis, including molecular diagnosis and prenatal diagnosis; (2) laboratory examinations, specialists' consultations, and hospitalization; and (3) drugs. Other items that can be paid by the National Health System include medical devices and antiseptics, emollients, dietary supplements, dressings, etc.

As inherited epidermolysis bullosa (EB) is officially recognized as a rare disease in Italy, regional reference centers for EB have been created during the past years (the reference center list is available at the NCRD Web site: http://www.iss.it/cnmr/). These centers provide clinical services for patient primary care. In addition, coordinated multidisciplinary management is offered in some centers. In particular, the Pediatric Hospital Bambino Gesù in Rome has organized an outpatient clinic under the coordination of the Dermatology Unit where the patients are offered a wide range of medical specialties (dermatology, pediatrics, gastroenterologic and plastic surgery, anesthesiology, ophthalmology, dentistry, otorhinolaryngology, orthopedics, cardiology, nephrology, psychology, etc) according to the individual's needs. As for EB diagnosis, centers that perform both immunofluorescence antigen mapping and ultrastructural analysis include the Center for Inherited Skin diseases of the Institute of Dermatologic Sciences in Milan and the authors' laboratory (Laboratory of Molecular and Cell Biology, IDI-IRCCS) in Rome. Molecular testing for EB is assured by two centers: the Division of Biology and Genetics, Department of Biomedical Sciences and Biotechnology, University of Brescia, where the COL7A1 gene is screened and the authors' laboratory in Rome, where about 200 molecular diagnoses for various EB types have been performed in the last years. In particular, the genotyping of Italian patients with recessive dystrophic EB (RDEB) (89 cases), Herlitz junctional EB (HJEB) (20 cases), and Kindler syndrome (KS) (17 cases) has led to the

This work was supported by grants from the Istituto Superiore di Sanità (no. 526D/4 and E-Rare 1, acronym Kindlernet).

Laboratory of Molecular and Cell Biology, IDI-IRCCS, Via dei Monti di Creta 104, Rome 00167, Italy

* Corresponding author.

E-mail address: g.zambruno@idi.it

Dermatol Clin 28 (2010) 407–409

doi:10.1016/j.det.2010.02.016

Table 1
Recurrent mutations identified in Italian patients with recessive dystrophic EB (COL7A1), Herlitz junctional EB (LAMB3, LAMC2), and Kindler syndrome (FERMT1/KIND1)

Mutation	Number of Mutated Alleles	Percent of Mutated Alleles	Geographic Origin	Detection Method
COL7A1				
c.497insA	21	11.8	Widespread	Sequencing
c.4783-1G>A	6	3.4	Sicily	Sequencing
c.7344G>A	10	5.6	Widespread	HphI
c.425A>G	6	3.4	Widespread	StyI
p.G1664A	6	3.4	Apulia	PstI
c.8441-14del21	7	3.9	Sicily	Sequencing
c.8074delG	5	2.8	Apulia	Sequencing
LAMB3				
p.R635X	3	7.5	Widespread	BglII
p.R81X	3	7.5	Widespread	Sequencing
p.W143X	4	10.0	Campania	BstNI
c.31insC	4	10.0	Widespread	Sequencing
LAMC2				
p.R95X	4	10.0	Sicily	TaqI
p.Y355X	4	10.0	Calabria	Sequencing
p.R223X	3	7.5	Sicily	Sequencing
FERMT1/KIND1				
c.373delT	4	11.8	Central Italy	Sequencing
c.1161delA	6	17.6	Central Italy	Sequencing
g.70250_74168del	9	26.5	Calabria	PCR
c.958-1G>A	6	17.6	Central Italy	Sequencing

identification of a number of recurrent mutations in the causative genes (**Table 1**). The majority of these variants were detected in families from specific Italian regions and haplotype analysis of highly polymorphic intragenic single nucleotide polymorphisms or flanking polymorphic microsatellites in the patients carrying these mutations indicated a common ancestral origin for the corresponding mutant allele. At present, seven frequent mutations in COL7A1 cover the 34% of the RDEB alleles, eight mutations (four in LAMB3 and three in LAMC2) target the 62.5% of the mutant HJEB alleles, and four recurrent FERMT1 mutations comprise the 73.5% of Italian KS alleles (see **Table 1**). These findings have allowed the optimization of priority strategies for mutation detection in new Italian patients with EB.[1–4]

Although data on EB from the rare disease national registry are not yet available, the Center for Inherited Skin Diseases of the Institute of Dermatologic Sciences in Milan was started in 1991 and regularly updates an Italian registry for EB.[5] The registry at present comprises 897 EB cases, including 258 EB simplex, 82 JEB, 524 DEB, 17 KS, and 16 unclassified EB forms.

Regarding the development of guidelines for EB, a multidisciplinary task force of experts, comprising dermatologists, pediatricians, geneticists, molecular biologists, ethicists, and a representative of the EB patient organization (DebRA Italy), was convened in July 2007 under the coordination of the National Center for Rare Diseases with the aim to establish national guidelines for EB diagnosis. The task force has prepared, using a modified Delphi methodology, a consensus document that will be shortly made available at http://www.iss.it/cnmr/. Finally, the active role of DebRA Italy (http://www.debraitaliaonlus.org/) in increasing awareness of EB and supporting the reference center activities should be underlined.

REFERENCES

1. Gardella R, Castiglia D, Posteraro P, et al. Genotype-phenotype correlation in Italian patients with

dystrophic epidermolysis bullosa. J Invest Dermatol 2002;119(6):1456–62.

2. Posteraro P, Pascucci M, Colombi M, et al. Denaturing HPLC-based approach for detection of COL7A1 gene mutations causing dystrophic epidermolysis bullosa. Biochem Biophys Res Commun 2005;338(3):1391–401.

3. Has C, Wessagowit V, Pascucci M, et al. Molecular basis of Kindler syndrome in Italy: novel and recurrent Alu/Alu recombination, splice site, nonsense, and frameshift mutations in the KIND1 gene. J Invest Dermatol 2006;126(8):1776–83.

4. Castori M, Floriddia G, De Luca N, et al. Herlitz junctional epidermolysis bullosa: laminin-5 mutational profile and carrier frequency in the Italian population. Br J Dermatol. 2008;158(1): 38–44.

5. Tadini G, Gualandri L, Colombi M, et al. The Italian registry of hereditary epidermolysis bullosa. G Ital Dermatol Venereol 2005;140(4):359–72.

Epidermolysis Bullosa in the Netherlands

José C. Duipmans, MScN, RN*, Marcel F. Jonkman, MD, PhD

KEYWORDS

- Epidermous bullosa • Netherlands
- Registry • Expert Center

EPIDERMOLYSIS BULLOSA EXPERT CENTER

Center for Blistering Diseases, Department of Dermatology, University Medical Center Groningen, the Netherlands. Director: Prof. Dr M.F. Jonkman, P.O. Box 30.001, 9700 RB Groningen, the Netherlands; telephone: +31 50 3 612 520; e-mail address: m.f.jonkman@derm.umcg.nl (**Tables 1 and 2**).

DIAGNOSTICS

Diagnostic laboratory used for immunofluorescence microscopy and electron microscopy: Center for Blistering Diseases, Laboratory of Dermatology, University Medical Center Groningen, the Netherlands; Dr G.F.H. Diercks, P.O. Box 30.001, 9700 RB Groningen, the Netherlands; telephone: +31 50 3 612 520; e-mail address: g.f.h.diercks@path.umcg.nl.

Diagnostic laboratory used for genetic testing (EB simplex [EBS], junctional EB [JEB]): Department of Genetics, University Medical Center Groningen, P.O. Box 30.001, 9700 RB Groningen, the Netherlands, e-mail address: secr-dna@medgen.umcg.nl; Head of Section Genomics: Prof. Dr R.J. Sinke, e-mail address: r.j.sinke@medgen.umcg.nl.

Diagnostic laboratory used for genetic testing (dystrophic epidermolysis bullosa [DEB]): Department of Human Genetics, Radboud University Nijmegen Medical Center. DNA Diagnostics, P.O. Box 9101, 6500 HB Nijmegen, the Netherlands; Head of division DNA diagnostics: Dr H. Scheffer, PhD; telephone: +31 24 3 613 799; e-mail address: dna@umcn.nl; www.dna-diagnostieknijmegen.nl.

DEBRA

Linked with Dystrophic Epidermolysis Bullosa Research Association (DEBRA) the Netherlands, P.O. Box 3160, 3760 DD Soest, the Netherlands; telephone: +31 35 6 018 977; Web site: www.debra.nl; e-mail address: consulent@debra.nl.

FINANCIAL ASPECTS

All doctors' fees, hospital visits, and hospital admissions focused on EB care, including routinely performed mutation screenings, are covered by the insurance companies and social services. Drugs, dressings, and other therapeutic devices are (almost all) covered by the insurance company, except for materials, such as needles, gloves, disinfectants, and so forth. European citizens can visit an EB center and all costs of investigations are covered by the insurance company, if patients bring an E-112 form.

Center for Blistering Diseases, Department of Dermatology, University Medical Center Groningen, University of Groningen, Groningen, The Netherlands
* Corresponding author.
E-mail address: j.c.duipmans@derm.umcg.nl

Dermatol Clin 28 (2010) 411–413
doi:10.1016/j.det.2010.02.011
0733-8635/10/$ – see front matter © 2010 Elsevier Inc. All rights reserved.

Table 1
Registrations in Dutch EB Database

Major EB Type + nrs	Subtype + nrs	Mutation	Numbers
Suprabasal EBS (14)	Plakophilin (4)	PP1	4
	Lethal acantholytic (1)	DSP	1
		Unknown yet	9
Basal EBS (120)	EBS localized (60)	KRT5	20
		KRT14	16
		PLEC1	5
		Unknown yet	19
	EBS generalized (18)	KRT5	10
		Unknown yet	18
	EBS, Dowling Meara (24)	KRT5	3
		KRT14	11
		Unknown yet	10
	EBS, autosomal recessive (7)	KRT14	7
	EBS other (11)	KRT5	4
		PLEC1	2
		Unknown yet	5
JEB (66)	JEB, Herlitz (22)	LAMA3	2
		LAMB3	14
		Unknown yet	6
	JEB, non-Herlitz (39)	LAMA3	2
		LAMB3	5
		COL17A1	15
		ITGB4	1
		Unknown yet	16
	JEB-pyloric atresia (5)	ITGB4	1
		Unknown yet	4
DEB (99)	dominant DEB (64)	COL7A1	50
		Unknown yet	14
	Recessive DEB, severe generalized (18)	COL7A1	15
		Unknown yet	3
	Recessive DEB, other (17)	COL7A1	16
		Unknown yet	1
Kindler syndrome (2)	(2)	FERMT1	1
		Unknown yet	1
Unknown subtypes (15)	(15)		15
Total numbers (316)			316

Table 2
Summary of Dutch EB database

EB Types	Total Numbers	Deaths
Suprabasal EBS	14	2
Basal EBS	120	4
JEB	66	13
Dominant DEB	64	0
Recessive DEB	35	13
Kindler	2	0
Unknown subtypes	15	2
	316	34

Epidermolysis Bullosa Care in Austria and the Epidermolysis Bullosa House Austria

Gabriela Pohla-Gubo, PhD*, Helmut Hintner, MD

KEYWORDS
- Epidermolysis bullosa • Multidisciplinary care
- Epidermolysis Bullosa House Austria

In the European Union (EU) rare (orphan) diseases are defined by a prevalence of less than 5 per 10,000 persons. It is estimated that between 6% and 8% of the population (27–36 million people in the EU) have a distinct rare disease that is considerably reducing an individual's quality of life or socioeconomic potential. There are between 5000 and 8000 different rare diseases,[1] one of which is Epidermolysis bullosa (EB), an inborn and at this time incurable skin disease. EB affects approximately 500 patients in Austria out of a current population of 8.2 million. At present, the authors have registered 179 patients from Austria regularly seen in the Outpatient Unit of the EB House Austria. There may be a high number of unreported patients mainly diseased by dominant forms of EB.

For a long time the care of patients with EB was in the hands of pediatricians and dermatologists focusing mainly on the severe cutaneous problems. Because the gene defect may also involve conjunctivae, the mucosa of the gastrointestinal, urogenital or respiratory tract, and other internal organs, taking care of patients with EB means always following a multidisciplinary approach for a multisystem disease.

Disappointing experiences of EB families was among other the reasons for founding the support group DEBRA Austria in 1995 for those suffering from EB, their families, and caregivers. Debra was the name of a girl whose mother founded the first EB patient group in England more than 30 years ago. Meanwhile, there are more than 40 DEBRA groups worldwide. Today DEBRA Austria offers medical help, counseling, and information to those whose quality of life is significantly limited by this rare disease and its numerous complications.

At the Department of Dermatology, Paracelsus Medical University (PMU) Salzburg, the treatment of hereditary and acquired bullous dermatoses has a long history. Because there was and still is no official support for the development of a specific treatment for patients with rare diseases including EB, DEBRA Austria started a fundraising campaign. The term "butterfly children" is used for the youngest patients with EB because of their skin, which is as fragile as the wings of a butterfly and some of them also have a short life expectancy, like a butterfly. Because of this extremely successful campaign (**Fig. 1**), within the last few years patients affected by EB have been acknowledged and DEBRA Austria was able to open the EB House Austria in 2005. It is a unique clinical center situated on the campus of the General Hospital Salzburg that provides medical care, scientific research, and education for people affected by EB.

EPIDERMOLYSIS BULLOSA HOUSE AUSTRIA

The EB House Austria is as part of the Department of Dermatology of the PMU Salzburg, the world's first center of its kind (**Fig. 2**). Vast knowledge

Department of Dermatology, EB House Austria, Paracelsus Medical University Salzburg, Muellner Hauptstrasse 48, A-5020 Salzburg, Austria
* Corresponding author.
E-mail address: g.pohla-gubo@salk.at

Dermatol Clin 28 (2010) 415–420
doi:10.1016/j.det.2010.02.008

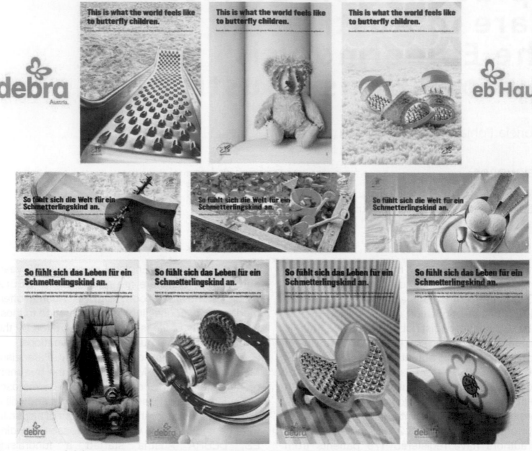

Fig. 1. Successful fundraising campaign from DEBRA Austria. *Courtesy of* DEBRA Austria, Vienna, Austria.

about EB was accumulated as the result of many years of cooperation between various medical disciplines and therapists of different departments of the PMU Salzburg. In addition, contact was sought and continued with a worldwide network of medical doctors and researchers working in the field of EB, who have elucidated clinical, epidemiologic, cellular, and molecular aspects of EB and have therefore initiated better treatments, even when those are still only symptomatic.

The EB House Austria consists of three major units (Fig. 3):

- The *EB Outpatient Unit* is where medical doctors and various therapists provide state-of-the-art medical advice and treatment.
- The *EB Research Laboratory* is where a research team works on various projects with the ultimate goal to find a cure by developing a successful molecular therapy.
- The *EB Academy* is where continuous multidisciplinary education and training for laypersons and experts is provided.

Even when there are several initiatives on a European level for rare diseases like EB, the running costs for the EB House Austria of about 500,000 euros per year are still covered completely by private donations given to DEBRA Austria.

CARE FOR EPIDERMOLYSIS BULLOSA IN AUSTRIA

The authors' experiences in the medical care of patients with EB in Austria have been included in the book *Life with Epidermolysis Bullosa (EB): Etiology, Diagnosis, Multidisciplinary Care and Therapy*.[2] In brief, physicians of various medical disciplines, who specialized in treating complications of EB, are familiar with the treatment modalities for each individual patient. Their expertise is absolutely crucial for optimal care. In addition to dermatologists and pediatricians, there are specialists for surgery, physical and occupational medicine and therapy, ophthalmology, ear-, nose- and throat-related illnesses, dental, and mouth and jaw treatment. Experts of pain management, nutritional care, and psychological guidance

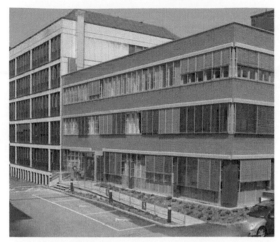

Fig. 2. The EB House Austria at the General Hospital Salzburg, Paracelsus Medical University.

are also involved. The multidisciplinary network is managed by two general practitioners (Anja Diem and Katharina Ude-Schoder) and two EB-specialized nurses (Manuela Langthaler and Alexandra Waldhör), all working at the Outpatient Unit of the EB House Austria.

Most of the patients from Austria, and many patients from neighboring countries (eg, Germany, Italy, Switzerland, and so forth) are seeking counseling and medical assistance in Salzburg. Following an appointment, the patients start at the Outpatient Unit where they are examined by one of the practitioners and then by experienced dermatologists. For patients visiting the EB House for the first time, a detailed medical and family history is obtained, and if necessary, a biopsy sample is taken for immunofluorescence (antigen) mapping (IFM) and sometimes transmission electron microscopy. See articles elsewhere in this issue to gain more information about specific types of EB. In many cases, the IFM allows a preliminary diagnosis, which is then confirmed by mutation analysis on blood samples of patients and of family members, mostly the parents. These results allow counseling for the patients and their families with regard to the outcome of their disease. Knowing the exact genetic alteration (ie, mutations) is also necessary for prenatal diagnosis in case the family wants to have another child.

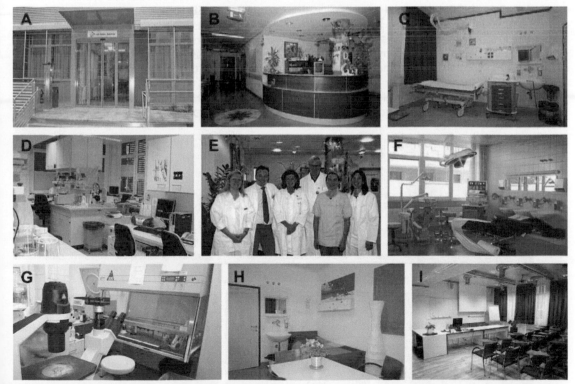

Fig. 3. Rooms at the EB House Austria. (*A*) Entrance. (*B*) Reception. (*C*) Outpatient room. (*D*) Research laboratory. (*E*) Members of the medical and scientific staff (left to right: Anja Diem, MD; Prof. Johann Bauer, MD; Gabriela Pohla-Gubo, PhD; Prof. Helmut Hintner, MD; Manuela Langthaler, Nurse; Katharina Ude-Schoder, MD). (*F*) Room for dental and surgical interventions. (*G*) Research laboratory. (*H*) Room for patients and consultations. (*I*) Seminar room, Academy.

In a care program, not only the skin but many other organs must be regularly and thoroughly monitored and examined for changes. The authors act upon the maxim to always pay attention to the entire human being and not only to their skin and they want to offer each of their patients the best possible individual care and advice. There are two types of patient care for individuals with EB seeking advice in the EB House in Salzburg:

- "All on one day" means that all necessary appointments on an outpatient base should be on one day to make their stay in Salzburg (ie, far from home) as short as possible.
- "All in one" implies that in case of an admittance to the hospital for a surgical intervention, as many operations as possible should be performed (eg, esophageal dilatation, hand surgery, or dental care under general anesthesia).

In addition to the multidisciplinary medical care, continuous patient training (together with the family) is offered at the EB House Austria.

Because EB is a rare disease, it is often difficult to find enough patients for clinical projects related to treatment. Nevertheless, the authors created a list of 27 major and minor clinical and therapeutic projects for patient-applied research. In this kind of research, including studies on the most severe symptoms of EB, interviews and written questionnaires serve as a tool to establish guidelines for better care of patients. The main topics include contractures and mutilations of fingers and toes; hand surgery and rehabilitation support; management of wounds, itching, and pain; photodynamic diagnostics and therapy for prevention of squamous cell carcinomas; nutritional aspects; psychological needs; and additional methods, such as laser therapy for wound healing, special clothing, or homeopathy (**Fig. 4**).

All our patient data are carefully monitored and the relevant results are, with the consent of the patients, put into the EB Registry, which the authors have operated since 1996. In September 2009, the authors have registered 276 patients from 15 different countries, 179 from Austria (**Fig. 5**A). The distribution of the different subtypes of EB in patients from Austria is shown in **Fig. 5**B.

MISSION

Major progress in EB therapy can only be achieved by correcting the genetic cause and the consequences of mutations on skin and mucous membranes. An Italian research team, led by Professor Michele de Luca at the University of Modena, has demonstrated for the first time that it is possible to correct the genetic defect and effectively cure the treated areas of skin of patients with EB. The EB House Austria is in contact with the worldwide network of EB therapists and researchers, and together, with numerous other scientists, we are also working to find a causative EB treatment. Careful monitoring of our patients will enable us to treat them as soon as a cure arises on the horizon. The successful work and support from DEBRA Austria allows not only to

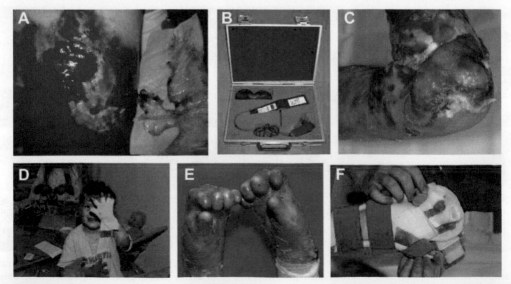

Fig. 4. Examples of patient-applied research. (*A*) Wound care. (*B*) Laser therapy set. (*C*) Prevention and therapy of cancer. (*D*) Prevention of contractures and mutilations of fingers. (*E*) Before hand surgery. (*F*) Postoperative rehabilitation support with splints.

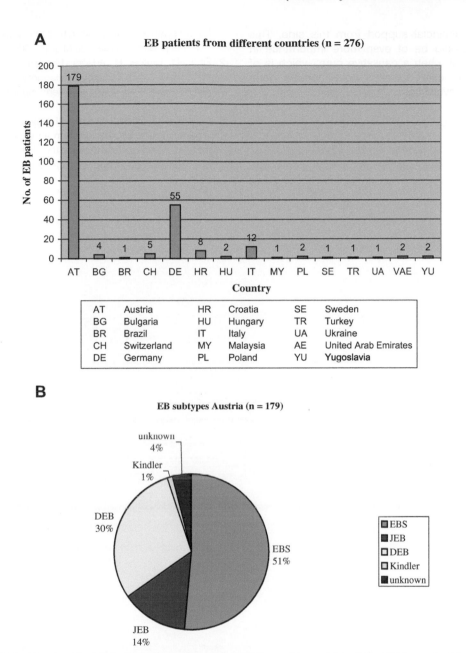

Fig. 5. EB Registry Austria. (*A*) Patients from different countries seeking advice at the EB House Austria (n = 276; data of September 2009). (*B*) EB subtypes from patients in Austria (n = 179; data of September 2009).

maintain the patient care at the EB House Austria but also to fund basic research in the field of EB, such as trans-splicing, that the authors are currently investigating.

SUMMARY

The EB House Austria is a special unit for the multi-disciplinary management of children and adults with EB. Major advances in EB care have been made possible by a multidisciplinary approach including most of the medical specialties offered at the General Hospital in Salzburg. The EB House Austria is independently funded by the support group DEBRA Austria. As the EB House Austria fulfills all criteria for a European Union reference center, as stated by the Rare Disease Task Force in 2005,[3] the authors hope that in the near future the EB House Austria will be accepted as such on a European Union level and that they can soon get financial support from this side. This support would be of even more importance in the moment when a causative cure, which is of course supposed to be a cost-intensive gene therapy, is available.

REFERENCES

1. The voice of 12,000 patients. Experiences and expectations of rare disease patients on diagnosis and care in Europe. A report based on the EurordisCare2 and EurordisCare3 surveys. March 2009. Available at: www.eurordis.org. Accessed March, 2009.

2. Fine JD, Hintner H, editors. Life with epidermolysis bullosa (EB). Etiology, diagnosis, multidisciplinary care and therapy. Wien: Springer-Verlag; 2008. p. 338.

3. Overview of current Centres of Reference on rare diseases in the EU. Report from an expert group of the Rare Diseases Task Force to the High Level Group on Health Services and Medical Care. September, 2005.

Epidermolysis Bullosa Care in Hungary

Márta Medvecz, MD, PhD[a,b],
Sarolta Kárpáti, MD, PhD, DSc[a,b,*]

KEYWORDS

- Epidermolysis bullosa • Genodermatoses
- Rare diseases • Molecular diagnostics

THE EPIDEMIOLOGIC CHARACTERISTICS OF EPIDERMOLYSIS BULLOSA IN HUNGARY

Hereditary epidermolysis bullosa (EB) is a rare skin disease that occurs worldwide and in all racial groups. European and North American surveys show that the incidence is 1 between 50,000 and 100,000 live births and its prevalence is approximately 25×10^{-6} to 50×10^{-6}, which reflects the cumulative frequency of EB; however, it can vary according to subtypes and subpopulations.[1]

There are currently 60 families affected by EB and about 150 patients with EB under care in Hungary, a Central Eastern European country of 10 million inhabitants. These figures correspond fairly well to international data.

Fifty-one percent of Hungarian patients with EB are diagnosed with EB simplex (EBS); junctional EB (JEB) accounts for only 3% of cases. The frequency of dominant dystrophic EB (DEB) is 33%, and recessive DEB occurs in 13% of EB patients.

ORGANIZATIONS REPRESENTING EB PATIENTS IN HUNGARY
National Epidermolysis Bullosa Center: DebRA Hungary

The National Epidermolysis Bullosa Center was founded in 1995, with the aim of creating a special environment for the treatment and care of EB patients. The Dermatological Clinic of Semmelweis University was among the founding organizations, and the Center still operates from there today. The EB Center, now called DebRA (Dystrophic Epidermolysis Bullosa Research Association) Hungary, later became part of DebRA Europe. Our official Web site is http://www.debra.hu.

The coworkers of DebRA Hungary have organized an interdisciplinary cooperation to provide high-quality care for patients with EB in the fields of internal medicine, surgery, otorhinolaryngology, dentistry, pediatrics, and dietetics. DebRA Hungary established the background for the clinical, histologic, and molecular genetic diagnostics of EB in Hungary, and also provides preventive DNA-based prenatal diagnostics.

The Center had the opportunity to employ a DebRA nurse from 2004 to 2008, which greatly contributed to the high-quality care of patients. The training of the DebRA nurse took place in London, with the support of DebRA Europe.

Epidermolysis Bullosa Foundation

DebRA Hungary is supported and financed by the Epidermolysis Bullosa Foundation, founded in 1997. The aims of the Foundation are to organize special health care that meets the needs of

Funding support: This work was supported by OTKA F049556, GENESKIN Coordination Action (LSHM-CT-2005-512117) and DebRA Hungary.

[a] Department of Dermato-Venereology and Dermatooncology, Semmelweis University, H-1085, Budapest, Mária u. 41, Hungary

[b] Molecular Medicine Research Group, Hungarian Academy of Sciences, H-1085, Budapest, Mária u. 41, Hungary

* Corresponding author. Department of Dermato-Venereology and Dermatooncology, Semmelweis University, H-1085, Budapest, Mária u. 41, Hungary.

E-mail address: karsar@bor.sote.hu

Dermatol Clin 28 (2010) 421–423
doi:10.1016/j.det.2010.02.022

patients with EB, perform research in genetics, provide professional and public education about EB, organize social activities, and provide social care for patients with EB.

OUR ACHIEVEMENTS

We established a unique center in Hungary for the care and the genetic analysis of patients with various EB subtypes. DebRA Hungary is not only investigating and taking care of patients with EB but also patients with other genodermatoses (Table 1). This has led to increased satisfaction and trust of patients, more accurate clinical trials, and new diagnostic opportunities.

As a result of our research, various new gene mutations were identified, the high-frequency recurrence of the COL7A1 gene 425A→G splice-site mutation was determined in the Central European region, and an easy method was established for the screening of keratin-14 gene amplification to exclude pseudogene sequences in EBS.[2-5]

Table 1
Genes are analyzed by DebRA Hungary

Genodermatoses	Online Mendelian Inheritance in Man (OMIM)	Target Gene	Protein
Epidermolysis bullosa simplex	MIM 131760 MIM 131800 MIM 131900	KRT5, KRT14	Keratin-5, keratin-14
Dowling-Degos disease	MIM 179850	KRT5	Keratin-5
Junctional epidermolysis bullosa	MIM 226700	LAMA3, LAMB3, LAMC2	Laminin-332 (laminin-5)
Dystrophic epidermolysis bullosa	MIM 131750 MIM 226600	COL7A1	Type VII collagen
Hailey-Hailey disease (benign familial pemphigus)	MIM 169600	ATP2C1	ATPase, Ca^{2+}-transporting, type 2C, member 1 (ATPase, Ca^{2+}-sequestering)
Darier disease (dyskeratosis follicularis)	MIM 124200	ATP2A2	Sarco-/endoplasmic reticulum Ca^{2+}-ATPase type 2 isoform (SERCA2)
Lamellar ichthyosis type 1	MIM 242300	TGM1	Keratinocyte transglutaminase
Ichthyosis congentia, Harlequin fetus type (lamellar ichthyosis type 2)	MIM 242500	ABCA12	ATP-binding cassette subfamily A, member 12
Comel-Netherton syndrome	MIM 256500	SPINK5, LEKTI	Serine protease inhibitor, Kazal type, 5
Conradi-Hünermann-Happle syndrome (chondrodysplasia punctata 2, X-linked dominant)	MIM 302960	EBP	Δ^8-Δ^7-sterol isomerase emopamil-binding protein (EBP)
Epidermolytic palmoplantar keratoderma (Vörner type)	MIM 144200	KRT9	Keratin-9
Monilethrix	MIM 15800	KRTHB1 (KRT81), KRTHB3 (KRT83), KRTHB6 (KRT86)	Hair cortex keratin genes

THE IMPORTANCE OF SELF-HELP ORGANIZATIONS FOR PATIENTS AND THEIR FAMILIES

EB is a rare disease, and therefore it has no priority from the point of view of public health. The burden of affected families is unproportionately high, and the management of comprehensive care seems more plausible through self-help organizations. The cooperation of professional and civilian resources is of utmost importance for DebRA Hungary. Thus, our organization endeavors to access modern diagnostics, therapy and education, increase patient motivation and activity, promote the representation of patient groups and the communication of special needs and aims.

REFERENCES

1. Volz A, Has C, Schumann H, et al. [Network epidermolysis bullosa: molecular pathomechanisms and novel therapeutic approaches]. J Dtsch Dermatol Ges 2007;5:274–9 [in German].

2. Csikós M, Szocs HI, Lászik A, et al. High frequency of the 425A–>G splice-site mutation and novel mutations of the COL7A1 gene in central Europe: significance for future mutation detection strategies in dystrophic epidermolysis bullosa. Br J Dermatol 2005;152(5):879–86.

3. Glász-Bóna A, Medvecz M, Sajó R, et al. Easy method for keratin 14 gene amplification to exclude pseudogene sequences: new keratin 5 and 14 mutations in epidermolysis bullosa simplex. J Invest Dermatol 2009;129(1):229–31.

4. Csikós M, Orosz Z, Bottlik G, et al. Dystrophic epidermolysis bullosa complicated by cutaneous squamous cell carcinoma and pulmonary and renal amyloidosis. Clin Exp Dermatol 2003;28(2):163–6.

5. Csikós M, Szalai Z, Becker K, et al. Novel keratin 14 gene mutations in patients from Hungary with epidermolysis bullosa simplex. Exp Dermatol 2004;13(3):185–91.

Epidermolysis Bullosa Care in Scandinavia

Anders Vahlquist, MD, PhD[a],*, Kaisa Tasanen, MD, PhD[b]

KEYWORDS

• EB • Gene • Mutation • Therapy

A SHORT HISTORY

One of the first papers published on epidermolysis bullosa (EB) in Scandinavia was that of Gillis Herlitz (1902–1982) who, when working as a pediatrician at Uppsala University Hospital in the early 1930s, described a lethal form of the disease now known as junctional EB (JEB) of the Herlitz type.

In the beginning of the 1960s, the Norwegian geneticist Tobias Gedde-Dahl (1938–2006) started his pioneering work on EB in Norway, whereby he personally visited and documented virtually all patients with EB, as well as described new forms of the disease, such as epidermolysis bullosa simplex (EBS)–Ogna.

Dermatologist Matti Kero,[1] in his thesis work, documented during the period between 1971 and 1980 the clinical and ultrastructural features of 121 patients affected by recessively inherited EB living in Finland. Research group of Professor Jouni Uitto, originally from Finland, was the first to discover the genetic linkage between the type VII collagen gene and dystrophic EB (DEB) in a large Finnish pedigree in 4 generations.[2–4]

EPIDEMIOLOGY

The recessive forms of EB are relatively common in Scandinavia, especially in the northern parts of Norway and Sweden where a founder effect for *LAMB3* gene mutation (R635X) causing JEB-Herlitz has been noted. **Table 1** shows very approximate figures for the number of Scandinavian families affected by EB reported during a period of 40 years. It can be seen that the prevalence of JEB and recessive DEB (RDEB) is highest in Norway and Sweden, whereas the other EB subtypes seem to be more evenly distributed among the Nordic countries. The figures for the mild forms of EBS and dominant DEB are probably grossly underreported in this type of compilation from the literature. In a more recent questionnaire sent to all Swedish dermatologists and pediatricians, 39 patients with EBS, 5 with JEB, and 28 with DEB were identified (Wittbolt and Vahlquist, unpublished data, 2005). Only 6 of the DEB cases were of the recessive type; however a few of these patients died prematurely. The highest death rate is no doubt among patients with JEB-Herlitz of whom practically all babies die within 1 to 2 years, thus heavily reducing the prevalence of this EB subtype. Historically, about 1 child per year with JEB-Herlitz was born in Sweden. However the incidence of this subtype and RDEB is increasing, particularly in Sweden receiving many immigrants from countries where cousin marriage is common. This also introduces new types of mutations.

THE ORGANIZATION OF EB HEALTH SERVICES

The care of EB in Scandinavia is organized around the patient via settings at the local hospital or health service. However, the diagnosis of EB and providing correct patient/family information usually require a specialized service, which in Sweden is provided at the Genodermatosis Center in Uppsala. This center mainly operates on an outpatient basis where patients come for 1 to 2 visits, either a couple of months after birth or in the case of older patients, whenever there is a need for improved diagnoses and information about EB. When a child with suspected EB is born in Sweden, there is usually

a Department of Medical Sciences, Uppsala University, University Hospital, SE-751 85 Uppsala, Sweden
b Department of Dermatology, Clinical Research Center, Oulu University Hospital, University of Oulu, Oulu, Finland
* Corresponding author.
E-mail address: Anders.Vahlquist@medsci.uu.se

Dermatol Clin 28 (2010) 425–427
doi:10.1016/j.det.2010.02.018
0733-8635/10/$ – see front matter © 2010 Elsevier Inc. All rights reserved.

Table 1
Estimated number of EB families in the Nordic countries (no data available from Iceland)

	Population Size (Millions)	(Total)	EBS	JEB	DDEB	RDEB
Sweden	9	(93)	13	53	9	18
Norway	5	(80)	30	27	13	10
Finland	5	(37)	24	3	8	2
Denmark	5	(19)	9	4	3	3
Total	24	(229)	76	87	33	33

From Kero M. Occurrence of epidermolysis bullosa in Finland. Acta Derm Venereol 1984;64:57–62; Gedde-Dahl T. Epidermolysis bullosa: a clinical, genetic and epidemiological study. Oslo (Norway): Scandinavian University Books; 1971. p. 180; and Gedde-Dahl T. Epidemiology of epidermolysis bullosa in Scandinavia [abstract]. Acta Derm Venerol 2002;82:238.

a telephone call or an e-mail contact within days after the delivery, whereby a preliminary diagnosis is discussed over digital pictures. Concurrently, a specially trained nurse is alerted to assist the hospital staff and the family by visiting the birthplace.

A skin biopsy is taken and send to the laboratory of Professor Leena Bruckner-Tuderman's department in Freiburg, Germany (http://www.netzwerk-eb. de/index_eng.html) for immunofluorescence (IF)-analysis of candidate proteins. In case of suspected JEB, a blood sample is send for screening of the *LAMB3* hotspot mutation, whereas in suspected EBS, a screening of keratin mutation is made usually in collaboration with a research laboratory. Only rarely do we take biopsies for electron microscopy analysis.

In Finland, the diagnostics and follow-up of patients with EB is focused in the dermatology clinics of 5 university hospitals where there is at least 1 dermatologist specialized in inherited skin diseases, especially Tampere University Hospital has long traditions in this field. After the birth, babies with severe EB are usually transferred to the pediatric intensive care units of the university hospitals, and dermatologists visit the newborns within 1 or 2 days after birth. Similar to Sweden, the diagnosis of EB in Finland is also based on IF-analysis of skin biopsies that is performed in Freiburg. The mutation analysis of patients with EB is made in collaboration with geneticists, and most of the samples are analyzed in Freiburg. Similar approaches are used in Denmark and in Norway where Rikshospitalet (in Oslo) is the leading center.

OTHER COLLABORATORS AND PATIENT EDUCATION

Pediatricians, physical therapists, geneticists, and dieticians are contacted whenever needed. For dental problems there are 2 specialized centers in Sweden (Jönköping and Gothenburg) to which patients are referred. Similar services are available in Norway at Rikshospitalet in Oslo together with the TAKO-center.

Psychological support and lengthy discussions (sometimes via interpreter) about the disease and its consequences are essential and should be provided as soon as feasible. Wound management is taught to parents, adult patients, and in some cases also to accompanying hospital staff. When desirable, contacts are made between the family and the appropriate patient organization (eg, DebRA-Sweden, DebRA-Norway, DebRA-Finland).

A special service for young patients that is very much appreciated by the families is provided by the Ågrenska and Frambue rehabilitation centers in Sweden and Norway, respectively. EB families are invited to stay for 1 week at these centers where they will meet specialists of all kinds teaching them about the disease and how to cope and deal with EB. The program also includes lectures and group discussions about the biology of skin and various inheritance patterns. General principles for wound care and future prospects for novel therapies are discussed.

In Finland, there are no rehabilitation centers for patients with EB or other rare skin diseases; instead, the Finnish Central Organization for Skin Patients (Iholiitto ry) is organizing regularly rehabilitation courses for adult and young patients with EB and their families.

EDUCATION OF HOSPITAL STAFF

Every 3 years the Nordic EB Association arranges a 2-day symposium to which doctors, nurses, dentists and social workers dealing with patients with EB are invited. These meetings are rotated among the 4 Nordic countries, and the faculty involves leading experts on EB from Scandinavia and abroad. This activity is also supported by the Nordic EB forum, which is a Web site where questions about EB can be asked and new information is distributed to professionals.

RESEARCH AND NEW IDEAS ABOUT THERAPY

Norway has a long tradition of EB research (see the section "A short history") and more recent activities.[5,6] In Finland, the current topics of the EB research include the molecular mechanisms of EB mutations and EB-associated squamous cell carcinomas.[7,8] In Denmark and Sweden, there is a special interest in keratin mutations causing EBS.[9,10] A new therapeutic concept was developed in Sweden to reduce hidrosis-induced precipitation of foot blisters in EBS. The idea to use plantar injections of botulinum toxin to prevent hyperhidrosis was originally described in patients with pachyonychia congenita,[11] but this therapy has also proved beneficial in cases of EBS with "summer blisters." A double-blind placebo controlled study of botulinum toxin in EBS is underway.

SUMMARY

Specialized EB care in Scandinavia is mainly provided by dermatologists, pediatricians, and dentists working together in a team. This type of health service is facilitated in Sweden by the establishment of a national center for genodermatoses in Uppsala 10 years ago and by working in a network with many international collaborators (the European GENESKIN project). The increasing number of EB families with foreign ethnic backgrounds and language problems is a challenge to the health service, especially in Sweden, and demands increased facilities. Also, the high expectations by parents of children with JEB and RDEB about new, revolutionizing therapies (stem cell therapy, bone marrow transplantation, gene therapy) are challenges that can only be met by international collaboration and more research in specialized centers for EB. A close collaboration with patient organizations and various charity organizations will be very helpful in this respect.

ACKNOWLEDGMENTS

The valuable discussions with Dr Anette Bygum Odense, Denmark and Dr Dorte Koss-Harness, Oslo, Norway are gratefully acknowledged.

REFERENCES

1. Kero M. Occurrence of epidermolysis bullosa in Finland. Acta Derm Venereol 1984;64:57–62.
2. Ryynänen M, Knowlton RG, Parente G, et al. Human type VII collagen: genetic linkage of the gene (COL7A1) on chromosome 3 to dominant dystrophic epidermolysis bullosa. Am J Hum Genet 1991;49: 797–803.
3. Lai-Cheong JE, Liu L, Sethuraman G, et al. Five new homozygous mutations in the KIND1 gene in Kindler syndrome. J Invest Dermatol 2007;127(9): 2268–70.
4. Fine JD, Eady RA, Bauer EA, et al. The classification of inherited epidermolysis bullosa (EB): report of the Third International Consensus Meeting on Diagnosis and Classification of EB. J Am Acad Dermatol 2008; 58(6):931–50.
5. Koss-Harnes D, Høyheim B, Jonkman MF, et al. Life-long course and molecular characterization of the original Dutch family with epidermolysis bullosa simplex with muscular dystrophy due to a homozygous novel plectin point mutation. Acta Derm Venereol 2004;84(2):124–31.
6. Koss-Harnes D, Høyheim B, Anton-Lamprecht I, et al. A site-specific plectin mutation causes dominant epidermolysis bullosa simplex Ogna: two identical de novo mutations. J Invest Dermatol 2002; 118(1):87–93.
7. Huilaja L, Hurskainen T, Autio Harmainon H, et al. Glycine substitution mutations cause intracellular accumulation of collagen XVII and its affect post-translational modifications. J Invest Dermatol 2009; 129:2302–6.
8. Kivisaari AM, Kallajoki M, Mirtti T, et al. Transformation-specific matric metalloproteinase (MMP)-7 nad MMP-13 are expressed by tumour cells in epidermolysis bullosa-associated squamous cell carcinomas. Br J Dermatol 2008;158:778–85.
9. Chamcheu JC, Pavez-Loriè E, Akgul B, et al. Characterization of immortalized human epidermolysis bullosa simplex (KRT5) cell lines: trimethylamine N-oxide protects the keratin cytoskeleton against disruptive stress conditions. J Dermatol Sci 2009; 53:198–206.
10. Sørensen CB, Andresen BS, Jensen UB, et al. Functional testing of keratin 14 mutant proteins associated with the three major subtypes of epidermolysis bullosa simplex. Exp Dermatol 2003;12(4): 472–9.
11. Swartling C, Vahlquist A. Treatment of pachyonychia congenita with plantar injections of botulinum toxin. Br J Dermatol 2006;154:763–5.

involves leading experts on EB from Scandinavia and abroad. This activity is also supported by the Nordic EB forum, which is a Web site where questions about EB can be asked and new information is distributed to professionals.

RESEARCH AND NEW IDEAS ABOUT THERAPY

Norway has a long tradition of EB research (see the section "A short history") and more recent activities. In Finland, the current topics of the EB research include the molecular mechanisms of EB mutations and EB-associated squamous cell carcinomas. In Denmark and Sweden, there is a special interest in keratin mutations causing EBS. A new therapeutic concept was developed in Sweden to reduce blisters-induced precipitation of cocal blisters in EBS. The idea to use plantar injections of botulinum toxin to prevent hyperhidrosis was originally described in patients with pachyonychia congenita, but this therapy has also proved beneficial in cases of EBS with "summer blisters". A double-blind placebo controlled study of botulinum toxin in EBS is underway.

SUMMARY

Specialized EB care in Scandinavia is mainly provided by dermatologists, pediatricians, and dentists working together in a team. This type of health service is facilitated in Sweden by the establishment of a national center for genodermatoses in Uppsala 10 years ago and by working in a network with many international collaborations like European GENESKIN project. The increasing number of EB families with foreign ethnic backgrounds and language problems is a challenge to the health service, especially in Sweden and Denmark. Also, the high expectations by parents of children with EB and RDEB about new revolutionizing therapies (stem cell therapy, bone marrow transplantation, gene therapy) are challenges that can only be met by international collaboration and more research in specialized centers for EB. A close collaboration with patient organizations and various charity organizations will be very helpful in this respect.

ACKNOWLEDGMENTS

The valuable discussions with Dr Anette Bygum, Odense, Denmark and Dr Doris Ross-Hames, Oslo, Norway are gratefully acknowledged.

REFERENCES

1. Nero TA. Occurrence of epidermolysis bullosa in Finland. Acta Dermatovenereol 1984;64:57-62

2. Ryynänen M, Knowlton RG, Parente G, et al. Human type VII collagen: genetic linkage of the gene (COL7A1) on chromosome 3 to dominant dystrophic epidermolysis bullosa. Am J Hum Genet 1991;49:797-803

3. Lai-Cheong JE, Liu L, Sethuraman G, et al. Five new homozygous mutations in the KIND1 gene in Kindler syndrome. J Invest Dermatol 2007;127(9):2268-70.

4. Fine JD, Eady RA, Bauer EA, et al. The classification of inherited epidermolysis bullosa (EB): Report of the Third International Consensus Meeting on Diagnosis and Classification of EB. J Am Acad Dermatol 2008;58(6):931-50.

5. Koss-Harnes D, Hoyheim B, Anton-Lamprecht I, et al. A novel and comprehensive characterization of the plectin Ogna family with a plectin gene basis: epidermolysis simplex with muscular dystrophy due to a primary gene mutation, plectin gene mutation. Acta Derm Venereol 2004;84(6):419-26.

6. Koss-Harnes D, Hoyheim B, Anton-Lamprecht I, et al. A site-specific plectin mutation causes dominant epidermolysis bullosa simplex Ogna: two identical de novo mutations. J Invest Dermatol 2002;118(1):87-93.

7. Pulkkinen L, Hennekam L, Abdul-Hasnayen H, et al. Glycine substitution mutations cause a intracellular accumulation of collagen XVII and its effect on transmembrane modifications. J Invest Dermatol 2002;123(2):626-8.

8. Rousselle AM, Keene DR, Ruggiero F, et al. Laminin-5 binds the NC-1 domain of type VII collagen. J Cell Biol 1997;138(3):719-28.

9. Christiano AM, Keffler M, Mulji T, et al. Homozygous for-specific marine dominant dystrophic epidermolysis bullosa. J Dermatol Sci 2002;28(2):85-95.

10. Chen M, Kasahara N, Keene DR, et al. Restoration of type VII collagen expression and function in dystrophic epidermolysis bullosa. Nat Genet 2002;32:670-5.

11. Sverdrup B, Vahlquist A. Treatment of recessive dystrophic epidermolysis bullosa: with dermal injections of botulinum toxin. Br J Dermatol 2007;156(1):172-4.

Epidermolysis Bullosa Care in Israel

Eli Sprecher, MD, PhD

KEYWORDS

- Epidermolysis bullosa • Keratin • Blisters
- Epidermis • Intermediate filaments • Mutation

EPIDEMIOLOGY OF EPIDERMOLYSIS BULLOSA IN ISRAEL

The Israeli population is composed of many ethnic communities, which have been living for centuries in a state of genetic isolation, one community relative to the other community. As a consequence, these communities, where consanguineous marriages are traditionally common, are characterized by genetic homogeneity, which in turn is associated with an excess prevalence of recessive disorders.[1] Thus, it is not entirely surprising that, although autosomal recessive epidermolysis bullosa simplex (EBS) is exceedingly rare worldwide, it accounts in Israel for approximately one-third of all EBS cases.[2] This in turn has significant implications for the genetic counseling of families at risk for EBS. Similarly, in contrast with the situation in Europe and in the United States, dominant forms of dystrophic epidermolysis bullosa (EB) are more rare in Israel than recessive forms of the disease.[2] Finally, the same demographic features may also underlie the fact that, although autosomal recessive junctional EB accounts in Western populations for less than 5% of the total number of EB cases, in Israel it comprises more than 25% of the cases.[2] Unfortunately, no official survey on EB in Israel has been performed, so the true prevalence of the disease in this region remains unknown.

MOLECULAR FEATURES OF EB IN ISRAEL

Several recurrent molecular features identified in Western populations are absent in Israeli patients with EB. For example, most cases of EBS result from mutations affecting *KRT14* R125 residue.

R125 mutations are rare in the Israeli populations.[2,3] Similarly, most cases of junctional EB are due to a few specific mutations in *LAMB3*. Not only are these mutations rare in the Israeli and Middle Eastern populations but also the proportion of cases resulting from mutations in LAMB3 as compared with LAMA3 and LAMC2 is different from in Western countries.[2,4] These peculiarities most certainly relate to the demographic features characteristic of Middle Eastern populations with a high coefficient of inbreeding ensuring the propagation of rare genetic variants within closed communities.

Similarly, most recessive forms of EB are due to homozygous mutations. This in turn can be exploited to screen affected families using homozygosity mapping, before formal mutation analysis,

---

Box 1

Laboratories offering molecular testing for EB in Israel and the Palestinian authority

Laboratory of Molecular Dermatology

Director: Dr Ofer Sarig

Department of Dermatology, Tel Aviv Sourasky Medical Center, 6, Weizmann Street, Tel Aviv 64239, Israel

Telephone: +972 3 697 3720; e-mail address: ofers@tasmc.health.gov.il

Hereditary Research Laboratory

Director: Dr Moien Kanaan

Life Science Department, Bethlehem University, POB 9 or Jerusalem POB 54866

Telephone: +972 2 274 4233; e-mail address: mkanaan@bethlehem.edu

---

Department of Dermatology, Tel Aviv Sourasky Medical Center, Tel Aviv, Israel
E-mail address: elisp@tasmc.health.gov.il

Dermatol Clin 28 (2010) 429–430
doi:10.1016/j.det.2010.02.019

resulting in significant cost and time saving Box 1.[5]

REFERENCES

1. Zlotogora J. Genetic disorders among Palestinian Arabs: 1. Effects of consanguinity. Am J Med Genet 1997;68(4):472–5.
2. Abu Sa'd J, Indelman M, Pfendner E, et al. Molecular epidemiology of hereditary epidermolysis bullosa in a Middle Eastern population. J Invest Dermatol 2006;126(4):777–81.
3. Ciubotaru D, Bergman R, Baty D, et al. Epidermolysis bullosa simplex in Israel: clinical and genetic features. Arch Dermatol 2003;139(4):498–505.
4. Nakano A, Lestringant GG, Paperna T, et al. Junctional epidermolysis bullosa in the Middle East: clinical and genetic studies in a series of consanguineous families. J Am Acad Dermatol 2002;46(4):510–6.
5. Mizrachi-Koren M, Shemer S, Morgan M, et al. Homozygosity mapping as a screening tool for the molecular diagnosis of hereditary skin diseases in consanguineous populations. J Am Acad Dermatol 2006;55(3):393–401.

Epidermolysis Bullosa in Japan

Satoru Shinkuma, MD*, Ken Natsuga, MD,
Wataru Nishie, MD, PhD, Hiroshi Shimizu, MD, PhD

KEYWORDS

• Epidermolysis bullosa • Japan • Epidemiology • DebRa

Epidermolysis bullosa (EB) is a group of hereditary disorders characterized by mechanical stress-induced blistering of the skin and mucous membranes.[1] EB is generally classified into the 3 main subtypes of EB simplex (EBS), junctional EB (JEB), and dystrophic EB (DEB), depending on the level of skin cleavage.[1] According to the National EB Registry (USA), the prevalence of EB in the Unites States in terms of cases per million population is estimated to be 8.22 (EBS, 4.60; JEB, 0.44; dominant DEB [DDEB], 0.99; recessive DEB [RDEB], 0.92).[1] The prevalence of EB in Japan in terms of cases per million is estimated to be 4.03 to 5.16 (EBS, 1.54; JEB, 0.34; DDEB, 1.02; RDEB, 1.60), based on data from the Japanese Study Group for Rare Intractable Skin Diseases in 1994.[2] However, the precise disease frequency of EB in Japan is still controversial.

Genetic studies of Japanese patients have revealed specific mutations and distinct tendencies in the genes responsible for the 3 EB subtypes. For example, the proportion of Japanese patients with EBS with *KRT5* mutations is 3 times higher than those with *KRT14*,[3] whereas outside of Japan, mutations in these 2 genes have been reported as equally prevalent. In the *LAMB3* gene, which is associated with JEB, the recurrent mutations R42X and R635X are more common among Caucasians than among ethnic Japanese.[4] The mutations 5818delC, 6573+1G>C, E2857X, and Q2827X have been regarded as recurrent *COL7A1* mutations associated with DEB in Japan.[5,6]

The medical expenses at the hospital for patients with JEB and DEB are covered under the public expenditure system, and 333 JEB and DEB patients in Japan are certified to receive medical care. However, the expense of the dressings and bandages, which is necessary for EB care, is not covered, and the patients have to purchase all that they need. Guidelines for the diagnosis and treatment of EB have been drafted by the Japanese Study Group for Rare Intractable Skin Diseases.[7] In March 2008, the Dystrophic Epidermolysis Bullosa Research Association (DebRA) of Japan was founded (http://www.ne.jp/asahi/eb-japan/com/english1.html), and more than 50 patients with EB and their families have been registered.

The environment surrounding patients with EB has been slowly improving, but support for such patients is still not sufficient (eg, the government finally begins moves to cover part of their dressing costs). EB patients, dermatologists, dermatologic researchers, and the government must interact more closely to improve the quality of life for these patients.

REFERENCES

1. Fine JD, Johnson LB, Suchindran C, et al. The epidemiology of inherited EB: findings within American, Canadian, and European study populations. In: Fine JD, Bauer EA, McGuire J, et al, editors. Epidermolysis bullosa: clinical, epidemiologic, and laboratory advances, and the findings of the National Epidermolysis Bullosa Registry. Baltimore (MD): Johns Hopkins University Press; 1999. p. 101–13.

2. Inaba Y, Kurosawa M, Hashimoto I, et al. Epidemiology of epidermolysis bullosa and generalized pustular psoriasis. Annual Report of the Intractable

Department of Dermatology, Hokkaido University Graduate School of Medicine, N15 W7, Sapporo 060-8638, Japan
* Corresponding author.
E-mail address: qxfjc346@ybb.ne.jp

Dermatol Clin 28 (2010) 431–432
doi:10.1016/j.det.2010.02.010
0733-8635/10/$ – see front matter © 2010 Elsevier Inc. All rights reserved.

Skin Diseases Study Group. Ministry of Welfare and Health of Japan, 1995;19–36 [in Japanese].

3. Yasukawa K, Sawamura D, Goto M, et al. Epidermolysis bullosa simplex in Japanese and Korean patients: genetic studies in 19 cases. Br J Dermatol 2006;155:313–7.

4. Shimizu H, Takizawa Y, McGrath JA, et al. Absence of R42X and R635X mutations in the LAMB3 gene in 12 Japanese patients with junctional epidermolysis bullosa. Arch Dermatol Res 1997;289:174–6.

5. Tamai K, Murai T, Mayama M, et al. Recurrent COL7A1 mutations in Japanese patients with dystrophic epidermolysis bullosa: positional effects of premature termination codon mutations on clinical severity. Japanese Collaborative Study Group on Epidermolysis Bullosa. J Invest Dermatol 1999; 112:991–3.

6. Sawamura D, Goto M, Yasukawa K, et al. Genetic studies of 20 Japanese families of dystrophic epidermolysis bullosa. J Hum Genet 2005;50:543–6.

7. Tamai K, Hashimoto I, Hanada K, et al. Japanese guidelines for diagnosis and treatment of junctional and dystrophic epidermolysis bullosa. Arch Dermatol Res 2003;295:S24–8.

Epidermolysis Bullosa in Australia and New Zealand

Dédée F. Murrell, MA, BMBCh, FAAD, MD

KEYWORDS
- Epidermolysis bullosa • Dystrophic epidermolysis bullosa
- Epidermolysis bullosa simplex

Australia has a population of about 24 million people, and New Zealand, separated from Australia by a 2-hour flight, and consists of the North Island and South Island, has about 5 million people. Australia is a larger land mass than the continental United States, and 90% of its population are concentrated in eight major cities, all of which, except the capital, Canberra, are on the coast. These are the capital cities of the former territories/colonies of the United Kingdom, which only federated into one nation in 1901. Hence, managing patients with an orphan disease presents particular difficulties of distance and tradition. The largest populations are Sydney, New South Wales (4 million); Melbourne, Victoria (3 million); Perth, Western Australia; Brisbane, Queensland; Adelaide, South Australia; Canberra, Australian Capital Territory; Hobart, Tasmania; and Darwin, Northern Territory (Fig. 1).

The first epidermolysis bullosa (EB) clinic to be established was in Sydney, by Mark Eisenberg, a general practitioner with a personal interest in EB. He had the support of the late Brien Walder,

head of dermatology at Sydney Children's Hospital (SCH), and Kieran Moran, a pediatrician was brought in as well. In 1996, I was invited by Walder to assist with this clinic as the dermatologist, since I had been taking care of the EB registry patients at Rockefeller University in New York from early 1994. At that stage there, was ad hoc electron microscopy (EM) in different units and no immunofluorescence mapping (IFM) in Australia. I set up a national diagnostic laboratory for IFM and EM for EB based at St George Hospital, Sydney, within the anatomic pathology department. From 1996, the laboratory has received specimens from around Australia and New Zealand and some surrounding Asian countries shipped in Michel's media.[1–4] EM is provided by C.W. Chow of Royal Children's Hospital, Melbourne. In addition, I began seeing adults with EB at St George Hospital and in my part-time private practice, assisted by my practice nurse, Lesley Rhodes.

Since this first EB clinic was established in Sydney, two other EB clinics started, one at Royal Children's Hospital, Melbourne, run by

Funding has been provided by the St George Hospital for salary support for clinical time at St George Hospital and Sydney Children's Hospital with epidermolysis bullosa (EB) patients. Premier Dermatology Clinical Trials, Kogarah, for salary support for EB nurse and research staff. University of New South Wales for medical students and scholarships for Masters of Science and PhD students.

Much of this work was supported by feeder grants from DebRA Australia, DebRA New Zealand and DebRA in New South Wales, South Australia, Victoria and Queensland. Premier Dermatology Clinical Trials have supported salaries and conference expenses for fellows and researchers Eleni Yiasemides, Linda Martin, Niken Trisnowati, Ningning Dang, Matt Kemp, Adam Rubin, Becca Cummins, Anna Liza Agero, Wenfei Yan, Supriya Venugopal, and Lizbeth Intong, and medical students John Frew, Julien Lahmar, Mary Alice Nading, Yong Kho, and EB nurse Lesley Rhodes. Support from SEALS, Anatomic Pathology, St George Hospital, Sydney, for the national EB diagnostic laboratory and the molecular diagnostic laboratory at Royal Brisbane Hospital, Brisbane, for storage and assistance with genetic testing and prenatal diagnosis.

Department of Dermatology, St George Hospital, University of New South Wales, Gray Street, Sydney, NSW 2217, Australia

E-mail address: d.murrell@unsw.edu.au

Dermatol Clin 28 (2010) 433–438
doi:10.1016/j.det.2010.02.009
0733-8635/10/$ – see front matter © 2010 Elsevier Inc. All rights reserved.

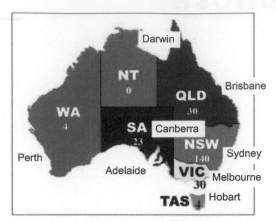

Fig. 1. Geographic distribution of the major cities and states/territories of Australia showing the numbers of EB patients in the Australasian EB registry from each area.

dermatologists George Varigos, John Su, and David Orchard, and in Adelaide at the Women's and Children's Hospital, originally by Julie Wesley and now by Lachlan Warren. The EB clinic at SCH was expanded with the addition of a medical geneticist, Anne Turner, in 2000, and an additional dermatologist, Orli Wargon, in 2003, after the death of Walder, and a part time EB nurse in 2007, Louise Stevens. In addition, physical, occupational, and pain therapists attend the clinic, which is held monthly as well as a social worker. Newborn infants with EB usually are transferred to SCH from other hospitals in the state of New South Wales.

When EB patients are 16 years of age, they transition to St George Hospital, Sydney, another teaching hospital of the University of New South Wales Medical School. Here the more severe patients with recessive dystrophic EB (RDEB) are reviewed every 3 months in the ambulatory care

unit, with a full skin check after a bath, possible biopsies, and infusions as needed, while they are reviewed by designated experts in hematology, renal, endocrinology, pain service, gastroenterology, as needed (**Fig. 2**).

In New Zealand, Nick Burchall established the service for EB, based in Auckland, now assisted by Deanna Purvis, and Dystrophic Epidermolysis Bullosa Research Association (DebRA) New Zealand raised funds for several regional EB nurses who assist with the management of EB patients around the country with him and regional dermatologists.

AUSTRALASIAN EB REGISTRY

In 2005, the author established a national EB registry based at St George Hospital. There are currently 242 patients enrolled, 140 of whom are in New South Wales (see **Fig. 1**). According to figures by the DebRA charities in New South Wales, Victoria, and SA and the newly formed DebRA Australia, there are likely to be about 400 patients with more severe forms of EB and probably 1000 or more if milder cases are included. DebRA New Zealand has about 40 members (A Kemble-Welch, personal communication, May 2009), and 11 are currently enrolled in the registry. To be enrolled, patients have to be examined by one of the EB clinic dermatologists and have confirmatory biopsies or genetic testing to confirm the subtype of EB. Currently the prevalence of EB is 10 per million population, but in reality it will be higher than this.[3]

PROVISION OF CARE

In Australia, the public hospital clinics are all free to patients with citizenship or permanent resident status. What is not covered is the cost of the

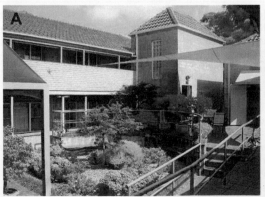
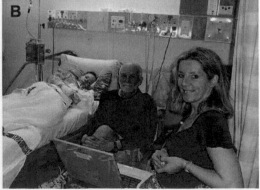

Fig. 2. Transition to adult care at St George Hospital with accommodation for patients at Bezzina House and review at the Ambulatory Care Center with infusions and patient education.

expensive dressings, which have been supplied ad hoc by some local hospitals/charities or DebRA. The registry has enabled the author and colleagues in conjunction with DebRA Australia to secure funding for the dressings for the next 4 years for EB patients, up to $16 million. Caregivers allowances are available for the more severe patients, but home nursing is difficult to obtain in Australia.

RESEARCH AND TEACHING ABOUT EB

The author's research has been performed at St George Hospital (**Fig. 3**) and has focused on geno-type to phenotype correlations in EB, skin cancers in EB, and novel therapies for EB. Regularly there are organized seminars and lectures at major national and international congresses and invited lectures about EB to improve awareness.[5–7]

Dystrophic EB

In RDEB, the author and colleagues have discovered nine novel COL7A1 mutations[8] and reviewed all collagen VII mutations causing dystrophic EB DEB.[9] In dominant dystrophic EB (DDEB), the most common mutation in Australia is G2043R, and the author and colleagues have published the first prenatal diagnosis case in DDEB[10] and the first Aboriginal family with DDEB and novel mutations underlying EB pruriginosa.[8] The author and colleagues attempted to use the baculovirus system to introduce the COL7A1 gene, which was able to incorporate the gene, but it did not transduce into human keratinocytes or fibroblasts.[11]

EB Simplex

A collaborative laboratory at Royal Brisbane Hospital has been confirming keratin 5 and 14 mutations identified in the author's research laboratory at St George Hospital as well as doing routine screening.[12] One of the author's patients has had an extremely severe form of Dowling-Meara EBS, and the author and colleagues explained how this had occurred due to the mismatch of the mutated amino acid and its position, Krt14 M119T, with another family with localized EBS, with Krt14 M119V.[13] The author and colleagues discovered a patient with EBS-DM caused by a unique deletion in Keratin 5[14] and also patients with codominant inheritance of Krt5 and Krt14 mutations.[15,16] Altogether, there are at least 10 novel keratin 5 or 14 mutations in the St George Hospital patient population with EBS.[17] The author and colleagues reviewed a keratin 14-negative case in the context of all K14-recessive EBS as the 14th reported case in the world.[18] Recently, the author and colleagues had their first case of EBS with late-onset muscular dystrophy caused by a novel plectin mutation[19] and another case from the Philippines referred with autosomal dominant EBS and ankyloblepharon.[20,21]

Junctional EB

Thanks to collaborators overseas, the author and colleagues have been able to have mutation studies done on the relevant genes, depending on IF mapping findings. Several new integrin B4 and laminin 332 mutations were published in conjunction with the Uitto group.[22,23] The author and colleagues set up a rapid screening test for the most common LAMB3 mutations seen in Australia, R42X and R635X, and other specific mutations with the help of laboratories overseas, at the laboratory in Brisbane to enable prenatal diagnosis of Herlitz JEB in Australia.[24–26] Other studies have led to papers on junctional EB (JEB) with pyloric atresia showing that integrin B4 mutations do not always cause this,[27] and the author's group was the first to find that heterozygote carriers of COL17A1 mutations

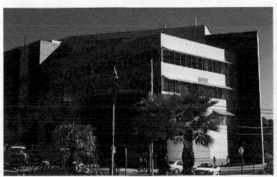
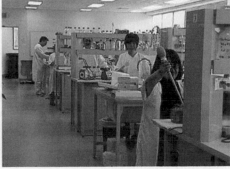

Fig. 3. Research laboratory at St George Hospital, University of New South Wales, Sydney. Research and Education Building, and the orthopedic research institute laboratories, where the author's basic research was conducted.

could have reduced staining with antibodies in their skin,[28–30] making this a useful test for situations in which, as in this case, the proband already was dead and had not been tested. The author and colleagues also recognized a unique variant of JEB caused by the granulomatous eyelid lesions, and in conjunction with Irwin McLean's group, were able to show that this patient had a unique mutation in the same exon of LAMA3a that occurs in laryngo-onycho-cutaneous (LOC) syndrome, proving that LOC was a subtype of JEB.[31,32]

SQUAMOUS CELL CARCINOMA

In conjunction with Jack Arbiser, while in New York, expression of angiogenic factor basic FGF was measured in the urine of the author's patients at Rockefeller. There were extremely high levels in 13 patients, particularly the RDEB patients. This was confirmed in further samples collected.[33] Among the author's cohort of DEB patients, it has not been found that positive staining with collagen VII antibodies LH7.2 and FNC1 increases their risk of developing SCC, or that negative staining protects them from SCC.[34] The author and colleagues also have contributed to international collaborative studies in SCC with the Marinkovich group at Stanford, California and the South group in Dundee, Scotland.

QUALITY OF LIFE

The author's group has worked for the last 3 years on the development of a quality of life (QOL) scale specific for EB that would be useful for clinical trials.[35,36] This is being validated by other groups for its applicability internationally.

NOVEL TREATMENTS FOR EB
Cultured Keratinocyte Skin Substitutes

Mark Eisenberg from Sydney had spent years developing this treatment sourced from neonatal foreskins, which were used successfully in Australian RDEB patients after hand surgery. He established a biotech company, Ortec, based in New York.[37] The author was involved in designing clinical trials of this for EB at Rockefeller University. A similar dressing was developed by Organogenesis and found to be useful in wound healing in EB, but a patent dispute and expensiveness of the treatment unfortunately led to the lack of progress for either of these for EB.

Dressings and Wound Care

To obtain approval for funding of expensive silicone-based dressings for EB in Sydney, the author and colleagues performed a small clinical trial in five patients comparing these with the traditional dressings used. This showed that the time taken to do dressings and the comfort improved, but not the time for wound healing.[38] The author and colleagues published a case report of a teenager with non-Herlitz JEB whose urethral meatal stenosis was improved with nonstick silicone-based dressings instead of instrumentation.[39] Recently, the author and colleagues completed a study demonstrating improved wound healing with topical gentian violet in non-Herlitz JEB.[40]

Allogeneic Fibroblast Cell Therapy for RDEB

The author and colleagues are at the end of a trial of allogenic fibroblast cell therapy for wound healing in severe RDEB, compared with transport media alone, in a randomized, double-blind design, recently presented at the European Society for Dermatologic Research (ESDR) 2009.[21]

Flightless Inhibitors

The author and colleagues commenced a collaborative project with Allison Cowin's group from Adelaide, South Australia in 2007 by selecting a randomly arranged and blinded group of samples of frozen skin of EB cases to be tested by a PhD student, Zlatko Kopecki, with different antibodies to the flightless protein system. After image analysis, the author and colleagues unblinded his results. This showed that the expression of flightless inhibitors was increased in all forms of EB, and the author and colleagues arranged further collaborations with Detlef Zillikens in Germany to look at his epidermolysis bullosa acquisita model, and with Leena Bruckner-Tuderman to look at her mouse model of DEB.[41,42]

COLLABORATION WITH DEBRA AUSTRALIA AND NEW ZEALAND

The author's group has benefited enormously from the support of these charities for their research and support for students to present their work at meetings. Together with three of my medical students, we joined the ski and adventure camp run by DebRA New Zealand for teens with EB, including three wheelchair-bound RDEB patients.[43] The author and colleagues recently completed a national survey of pregnancy and childbirth experiences in EB.[44] DebRA Australia has held three national meetings for its members with talks from professionals and the first EB Professionals conference was held at St George Hospital in 2007.

INTERNATIONAL COLLABORATION

This is the most important aspect of improving the lives of patients with a rare disease, such as EB. The author and colleagues have participated in the latest EB consensus[45] and in the most recent invitation-only research meetings for EB, in 2006 and 2009. They have collaborative projects with their colleagues across not only Australia and New Zealand, but the United States,[46] the United Kingdom,[34] Germany, France, Japan[20,21,47] Austria,[19] Switzerland, Canada,[48] Italy, the Netherlands,[30] Israel, and Ireland. The author and colleagues have set up links and trained dermatologists in EB from Indonesia,[15] India, the Philippines,[20,21] and China.[8,9] The future success for patients and these diseases lies in collaboration, not merely scientific competition.

REFERENCES

1. Yiasemides E, Walton J, Marr P, et al. A comparative study of transmission electron microscopy vs immunofluorescence mapping for the diagnosis of epidermolysis bullosa. Am J Dermatopathol 2006;5:387–94.
2. Kho YC, Agero AL, Rhodes LM, et al. Demographic data from the Australasian epidermolysis bullosa registry. Australas J Dermatol 2008;49(Suppl 1):A55.
3. Kho YC, Robertson S, Agero AL, et al. Epidemiology of epidermolysis bullosa in the Antipodes: the Australasian Epidermolysis Bullosa Registry with a focus on herlitz junctional epidermolysis bullosa. Arch Dermatol 2010, in press.
4. Kho YC, Agero AL, Rhodes LM, et al. Wound data from the Australasian Epidermolysis Bullosa Registry. In: Proceedings of the Seventh National Conference of the Australian Wound Management Association. Western Australia: Australasian Wound Management Association (AWMA), Cambridge Media; 2008. p. 42.
5. Murrell DF. Genotype-phenotype correlations in epidermolysis bullosa. In: Proceedings of Sixty-third Annual American Academy of Dermatology. American Academy of Dermatology. St Louis (MO): Mosby; 2005.
6. Murrell DF. Desmosome gene disorders. Forum on genetic disorders of skin integrity. In: Proceedings of the Sixty-fifth Annual American Academy of Dermatology. St Louis (MO): Mosby; 2007.
7. Murrell DF. What's new in the diagnosis and pathogenesis of EB; what's new in management of EB? Hurwitz Lectureship, Society for Pediatric Dermatology Annual Meeting held in Philadelphia, 2009. Society for Pediatric Dermatology Annual Meeting Program. Indianapolis (IN): Wiley-Blackwell; 2009.
8. Dang NN, Klingberg S, Marr P, et al. Review of collagen VII sequence variants found in Australasian patients with dystrophic epidermolysis bullosa reveals 9 novel COL7A1 variants. J Dermatol Sci 2007;46(3):169–78.
9. Dang NN, Murrell DF. Mutation analysis and characterization of COL7A1 mutations with dystrophic epidermolysis bullosa. Exp Dermatol 2008;17: 553–68.
10. Klingberg S, Mortimore R, Parkes J, et al. Prenatal diagnosis of dominant dystrophic epidermolysis bullosa by collagen VII molecular analysis. Prenat Diagn 2000;20(8):618–622.
11. Kemp MK. Studies in epidermolysis bullosa [PhD thesis]. DF Murrell, supervisor. University of New South Wales, Sydney (Australia); 2005.
12. Premaratne C, Klingberg S, Glass IA, et al. Epidermolysis bullosa simplex Dowling-Meara due to an Arg-Cys substitution in exon 1 of keratin 14. Australas J Dermatol 2002;43:24–7.
13. Cummins RE, Klingberg S, Wesley J, et al. Keratin 14 point mutations at codon 119 of helix 1A resulting in different epidermolysis bullosa simplex phenotypes. J Invest Dermatol 2001;117:1103–7.
14. Kemp MW, Klingberg S, Lloyd L, et al. A novel deletion mutation in keratin 5 causing the removal of 5 amino acids and elevated mutant mRNA levels in Dowling-Meara epidermolysis bullosa simplex. J Invest Dermatol 2005;124:1083–5.
15. Trisnowati N, Klingberg S, Lloyd L, et al. Combined mutations in keratin 5 and keratin 14 genes causing epidermolysis bullosa simplex-Dowling Meara. J Invest Dermatol 2003;121:A1278.
16. Trisnowati N. Mutation detection in EB simplex [MSc thesis]. UNSW, 2004
17. Yan WF, Klingberg S, Lloyd L, et al. Novel and recurrent mutations in KRT5 and KRT14 in epidermolysis bullosa simplex in Australasia. Australas J Dermatol 2007;48(Suppl 1):A64.
18. Yiasemides E, Trisnowati N, Su J, et al. Clinical heterogeneity in recessive epidermolysis bullosa due to mutations in the keratin 14 gene, KRT14. Clin Exp Dermatol 2008;33(6):689–97.
19. Klausseger A, Wadell L, Liu E, et al. Gradual expression of plectin deficiency in a patient with epidermolysis bullosa simplex and adult-onset muscular dystrophy. ESDR Budapest 2009. J Invest Dermatol 2009;129:S51.
20. Yan WF, Halim I, King–Ismael D, et al. A novel keratin 5 splice site mutation in a Filipino family resulting in epidermolysis bullosa simplex associated with ankyloblepharon. ESDR Budapest 2009. J Invest Dermatol 2009;129:S47.
21. Yan WF, Venugopal SS, Frew JW, et al. Investigation of cell therapy for generalized severe recessive dystrophic epidermolysis bullosa by intradermal allogeneic fibroblasts randomized against placebo injections. Clinical oral session, ESDR Budapest 2009 #166. J Invest Dermatol 2009;129:S28.

22. Nakano A, Pulkkinen L, Murrell D, et al. Epidermolysis bullosa with congenital pyloric atresia: novel mutations in the B4 integrin gene (ITGB4) and genotype/phenotype correlations. Pediatr Res 2001;49:618–26.

23. Nakano A, Chao SC, Pulkkinen L, et al. Laminin 5 mutations in junctional epidermolysis bullosa: molecular basis of Herlitz vs non-Herlitz phenotypes. Hum Genet 2002;110(1):41–51.

24. Murrell D. Prenatal diagnosis of EB in Australia. Clinical management of children and adults with epidermolysis bullosa. In: Mellerio J, editor. Proceedings of a Multidisciplinary International Symposium. UK: Debra (UK); 2003. p. 30.

25. Murrell DF, Turner A, Moran K, et al. Prenatal diagnosis of epidermolysis bullosa in Australia. Australas J Dermatol 2004;45:A15–6.

26. Murrell DF, Klingberg S, Dang NN, et al. Herlitz and non-Herlitz junctional epidermolysis bullosa resulting from different types of mutation in the LAMC2 gene. Australas J Dermatol 2006;47(Suppl 1):A23.

27. Dang NN, Klingberg S, Rubin AI, et al. Differential expression of pyloric atresia in junctional epidermolysis bullosa with novel ITGB4 mutations. Acta Derm Venereol 2008;88(5):438–48.

28. Pasmooij AM, Jonkman MF, Pas HH, et al. Dental abnormalities in heterozygous carriers of the COL17A1 823 del A mutation in a family with non-Herlitz junctional EB. J Eur Acad Dermatol Venereol 2005;19(Suppl 2):12.

29. Pasmooij AM, Jonkman MF, Pas HH, et al. Homozygosity for an intragenic deletion in the gene encoding collagen XVII, COL17A1: 823delA results in lethality in a family with non-Herlitz junctional epidermolysis bullosa. J Invest Dermatol 2006;126:S38.

30. Murrell DF, Pasmooij AM, Pas HH, et al. Retrospective diagnosis of fatal BP180-deficient non-Herlitz Junctional epidermolysis bullosa suggested by immunofluorescence (IF) antigen-mapping of parental carriers bearing enamel defects. J Invest Dermatol 2007;127(7):1772–5.

31. Figueira EC, Crotty A, Challinor CJ, et al. Granulation tissue in the eyelid margin and conjunctiva in junctional epidermolysis bullosa with features of laryngo-onycho-cutaneous syndrome. Clin Experiment Ophthalmol 2007;35(2):163–6.

32. Cohn HI, Murrell DF. Laryngo-onycho-cutaneous syndrome. Derm Clin N Am 2010;28(1):89–92.

33. Arbiser JL, Fine JD, Murrell DF, et al. Fibroblast growth factor: a missing link between collagen type VII, increased collagenase, and squamous cell carcinoma in recessive dystrophic epidermolysis bullosa. Mol Med 1998;4:191–5.

34. Yan WF, Kho Y, Frew JW, et al. Reactivity of LH7-2 and FNC1 antibodies against collagen VII does not predict the development of squamous cell carcinoma in recessive dystrophic epidermolysis bullosa [abstract]. J Invest Dermatol 2008;128(Suppl 1):S27.

35. Frew JW, Martin LK, Nijsten T, et al. Development of a quality of life index for epidermolysis bullosa (EB) through the development of the QOLEB questionnaire, an EB-specific quality of life instrument. Br J Dermatol 2009;161(6):1323–30.

36. Frew JW, Murrell DF. Quality of life in epidermolysis bullosa: tools for clinical research and patient care. Derm Clin N Am 2010;28(1):185–90.

37. Eisenberg M, Llewelyn D. Surgical management of hands in children with RDEB: use of allogeneic composite cultured skin grafts. Br J Plast Surg 1998;51:608–13.

38. Martin L, Hrepka P, Murrell DF. An observational study of mepilex dressings in epidermolysis bullosa. Australas J Dermatol 2006;47(Suppl 1):A46.

39. Rubin AI, Moran K, Fine JD, et al. Urethral meatal stenosis in junctional epidermolysis bullosa: a rare complication effectively treated with a novel, and simple modality. Int J Dermatol 2007;46:1076–7.

40. Venugopal SS, Intong LR, Cohn HI, et al. An intra-patient, prospective study of topical gentian violet for the treatment of chronic ulcers in non-Herlitz junctional epidermolysis bullosa. Australas J Dermatol 2009;50(Suppl 2):A55.

41. Kopecki Z, Murrell DF, Cowin AJ. Raising the roof on epidermolysis bullosa: a focus on new therapies. Wound Pract Res 2009;17(2):72–80.

42. Kopecki Z, Arkell R, Ludwig R, et al. Cytoskeletal protein flightless I affects cellular adhesion and blister formation in epidermolysis bullosa. J Invest Dermatol 2009;129:S79 [abstract].

43. Nading MA, Lahmar JJ, Frew JW, et al. A ski and adventure camp for young patients with severe forms of epidermolysis bullosa. J Am Acad Dermatol 2009;61(3):508–11.

44. Intong LRA, Choi SD, Shipman AR, et al. The mother with epidermolysis bullosa—what are the problems? In: Proceedings of the European Academy of Dermatovenereology. 2009. Published on CDROM by documediaS GmbH Hannover A-156-0011-00508 (abstract number).

45. Fine JD, Eady RA, Bauer EA, et al. Revised consensus for definitions of epidermolysis bullosa. J Am Acad Dermatol 2008;58:931–50.

46. Robbins PB, Lin Q, Goodnough JB, et al. In vivo restoration of laminin 5 B3 expression and function in junctional epidermolysis bullosa. Proc Natl Acad Sci U S A 2001;88:5193–8.

47. Lim SW, Su J, Orchard D, et al. Transient dermolysis of the newborn—2 novel amino acid substitutions in COL7A1. Australas J Dermatol 2008;49(Suppl 1):A4.

48. Lara-Corrales I, Mellerio J, Lucky AW, et al. Dilated cardiomyopathy in epidermolysis bullosa, a retrospective, multicenter study. Pediatr Dermatol 2010, in press.

Erratum to "Plectin Gene Defects Lead to Various Forms of Epidermolysis Bullosa Simplex" [Dermatol Clin 28 (2010) 33–41]

In the January 2010 issue of *Dermatologic Clinics* (Volume 28, Issue 1), an error appears in the article "Plectin Gene Defects Lead to Various Forms of Epidermolysis Bullosa Simplex" by Günther A. Rezniczek, Gernot Walko, and Gerhard Wiche. On pages 36 and 37, an unconventional mutation numbering scheme is used in **Table 1** and in the text. The authors have prepared a revised version of the table where mutations are named according to the current guidelines for mutation nomenclature (http://www.hgvs.org/mutnomen/). The new table lists the known plectin mutations, giving their designations on both the cDNA and protein levels. It contains several mutations previously not listed (corresponding references have been added). Additionally, please note that the mutations 1537ins36, 2674del9, and 13480ins16 mentioned in the text (page 36, subsection "Plectin gene mutations and epidermolysis bullosa simplex") should read as 1530_1531ins36, 2677_2685del, and 13459_13474dup, respectively.

ADDITIONAL REFERENCES

84. den Dunnen JT, Antonarakis SE. Mutation nomenclature extensions and suggestions to describe complex mutations: a discussion. Hum Mutat 2000;15:7–12.
85. Sawamura D, Goto M, Sakai K, et al. Possible involvement of exon 31 alternative splicing in phenotype and severity of epidermolysis bullosa caused by mutations in PLEC1. J Invest Dermatol 2007;127:11537–40.
86. Natasuga K, Nishie W, Akiyama M, et al. Plectin expression patterns determine two distinct subtypes of epidermolysis bullosa simplex. Hum Mutat 2010;30:1–9.
87. Koss-Harnes D, Hoyheim B, Jonkman MF, et al. Life-long course and molecular characterization of the original Dutch family with epidermolysis bullosa simplex with muscular dystrophy due to a homozygous novel plectin point mutation. Acta Derm Venerol 2004;84:124–31.

Refers to: Plectin Gene Defects Lead to Various Forms of Epidermolysis Bullosa Simplex, Dermatol Clin, Volume 28, Issue 1, January 2010, Pages 33–41, Günther A. Rezniczek, Gernot Walko, Gerhard Wiche.

Dermatol Clin 28 (2010) 439–441
doi:10.1016/j.det.2010.02.024

Table 1
(Revised) Plectin mutations reported in the literature

Mutation (cDNA Level)[a]	Mutation (Protein Level)[a]	Other Designations Used in Some Publications[c]	Exon[d]	Genotype[e]	References
EBS-MD					
954_956dupGCT	L319dup	956ins3, 1008ins3, 1287ins3	9	c.het. (Q1408X)	73
1530_1531ins36	A510_I511ins12	1530ins36, 1537ins36, 1541ins36	14	c.het. (2677_2685del9)	59,74
2677_2685del	Q893_A895del	2668del9, 2674del9, 2677del9, 2719del9	21	hom.	56
2694-9_2705del	?[b]	2694-9del21, 2745-9del21	22	c.het. (5032delG)	75
3157C>T	Q1053X	Q1053X	24	c.het. (Q1936X)	76
4222C>T	Q1408X	Q1518X	31	c.het. (L319dup)	73
4294_4306dup	V1436GfsX40	430ins13, 4359ins13	31	c.het. (4365delC)	77
4348C>T	Q1450X		31	hom.	85
4365delC	S1456RfsX93	4416delC	31	c.het. (4294_4306dup13)	77
4643_4667dup	K1558GfsX89	R1556fs	31	c.het. (7120C>T)	86
4840G>T	E1614X		31	hom.	59
5018_5036del	L1673RfsX64	5018del19, 5069del19	31	hom.	78
5032delG	V1678WfsX65	5083delG	31	c.het. (2694-9_2505del21)	75
5105_5112del	R1702QfsX14	5105del8, 5148del8	31	hom.	19
5137C>T	Q1713X	5188C>T	31	c.het. (R2351X)	79
5257dupG	E1753GfsX17	5257insG, 5309insG, 5588insG	31	hom.	59, 80
5410G>T	E1804X	E1914X	31	hom.	87
5728C>T	Q1910X		31	hom.	54
5806C>T	Q1936X		31	c.het. (Q1053X)	76
5815delC	L1939WfsX6	5866delC	31	hom.	56
5849_5856dup	E1953WfsX8	5855ins8, 5907ins8	31	hom.	81
5854_5855del	E1952GfsX60	5854del2, 5905del2	31	hom.	78
6013G>T	E2005X		31	c.het. (K4460X)	75
6549_6582del	L2184RfsX21	A2183fs	31	c.het. (13040dupG)	86
6955C>T	R2319X		31	hom.	82

Mutation[a]	Protein[a]	Designation in the literature[c]	Exon[d]	Genotype[e]	Ref.
7051C>T	R2351X		31	c.het. (Q1713X)	79
7120C>T	Q2374X	7102C>T	31	c.het. (4643_4667dup)	86
7261C>T	R2421X		31	c.het. (12578_12581dup)	76
7393C>T	R2465X		31	hom.	83
12578_12581dup	Y4195DfsX41	12581ins4, 12633ins_4	32	c.het. (R2421)	76
13040dupG	I4348HfsX8	G4347fs	32	c.het. (6549_6582del)	86
13378A>T	K4460X		32	c.het. (E2005X)	75
13459_13474dup	E4492GfsX48	13473ins16, 13480ins16, 13803ins16	32	hom.	58
EBS-PA					
913C>T	Q305X		9	hom.; c.het. (1344G>A)	60,67
1344G>A	?[b]		12	c.het. (Q305X)	67
1563_1567del	G522WfsX11	1563del4, 1567del4	14	hom.	60
2680_2693del	E894AfsX84	2680del14, 2727del14	21	hom.	66
2769_2788del[f]	W923CfsX53	2769del21	22	hom.	60
3565C>T	R1189X		27	hom., c.het. (Q2538X)	67
7396C>T	Q2466X		32	c.het. (Q2545X)	85
7612C>T	Q2538X		32	c.het. (R1189)	67
7633C>T	Q2545X		32	c.het. (Q2466X)	85
9085C>T	R3029X		32	hom.	60
EBS-Ogna					
5998C>T	R2000W	R2110W	31	het. (dominant)	62

[a] Mutations are ordered by phenotype (EBS-MD, EBS-PA, and EBS-Ogna) and position within the plectin gene. Numbers correspond to the plectin isoform 1c sequence (also referred to as variant 1; GenBank accession no. NM_000445). Mutations are named following the latest guidelines[84] (see http://www.hgvs.org/mutnomen/), but for brevity, the one-letter amino acid code has been maintained.

[b] Splice sites are affected and the outcome on the transcript/protein level is unknown.

[c] Designations of the mutations in the existing literature that differ from the ones used in this table, for example, due to being based on a different reference sequence.

[d] Exon harboring the mutation.

[e] Genotype of the patient, which is homozygous (hom.), heterozygous (het.), or compound heterozygous (c.het.). Mutation on the other allele is given in parentheses in case of compound heterozygosity.

[f] This mutation was originally described as a 21-bp-deletion (in-frame deletion of 7 amino acids). However, the sequencing data shown by Pfendner and Uitto[60] in Fig. 2 rather correspond to a 20-bp-deletion, resulting in a frameshift and premature termination. This was verified by the authors (J. Uitto, personal communication).

Erratum to "Nail Involvement in Epidermolysis Bullosa" [Dermatol Clin 28 (2010) 153–157]

In the January 2010 issue of *Dermatologic Clinics* (Volume 28, Issue 1), an error appears in the article "Involvement in Epidermolysis Bullosa" by Antonella Tosti, Débora Cadore de Farias, and Dédée F. Murrell. On page 157, the legends for Figs. 4 and 5 should read:

Fig. 4: Periungual blisters and nail atrophy in a patient with Non-Herlitz JEB.

Fig. 5: Herlitz JEB: nail erosions with periungual granulation tissue.

Refers to: Nail Involvement in Epidermolysis Bullosa, Dermatol Clin, Volume 28, Issue 1, January 2010, Pages 153–7, Antonella Tosti, Débora Cadore de Farias, Dédée F. Murrell.

Dermatol Clin 28 (2010) 443
doi:10.1016/j.det.2010.02.025
0733-8635/10/$ – see front matter

Erratum to "Nail involvement in Epidermolysis Bullosa," [Dermatol Clin 28 (2010) 153–157]

In the January 2010 issue of Dermatologic Clinics (Volume 28, Issue 1), an error appears in the article "Nail involvement in Epidermolysis Bullosa," by Amophilip Tosti, Debora Cadore de Farias, and Bertha R. Murrell. On page 157, the legends for Figs. 4 and 5 should read:

Fig. 4. Periungual blisters and nail atrophy in a patient with Hbn-Hedtz JEB.

Fig. 5. Hertiz JEB nail erosions with periungual granulation tissue.

Refers to "Nail Involvement in Epidermolysis Bullosa" and "Nail Clin Volume 28 Issue 1, January 2010, Pages 153–157, Amophilip Tosti, Debora Cadore de Farias, Bertha R. Murrell

Dermatol Clin 28 (2010) 443
doi:10.1016/j.det.2010.02.020

Index

Note: Page numbers of article titles are in **boldface** type.

A

Analgesia
    and epidermolysis bullosa, 319–324
Anesthesia and epidermolysis bullosa, 307, **319–324**, 336–337
    and airway management, 322
    and care of the skin and mucous membranes, 319–320
    complications associated with, 321
    and management of procedural pain, 324
    and medical history, 320–321
    and postoperative recovery, 323–324
    and premedication, 321
    and preoperative assessment, 320

B

Bathing for individuals with epidermolysis bullosa, **265, 266**
    and pool salt, 266
Bone health
    and epidermolysis bullosa, 353–355
    and hormonal factors, 354
    and impaired nutrition, 354
    and inflammation, 354
    and reduced mobility, 353–354
Bone marrow stem cell therapy for recessive dystrophic epidermolysis bullosa, **371–382**
    clinical trials for, 377–379
    and enrichment for optimal donor cell populations, 379
    and homing to the skin, 372–375, 379
    and reprogramming into skin cells, 372–376
    and role of the microenvironment, 373–376
    and tumorigenesis, 379
Bone marrow transplantation
    and recessive dystrophic epidermolysis bullosa, 376–377
Bowen disease
    and epidermolysis bullosa, 284

C

Care of epidermolysis bullosa in Ireland, **397–399**
Caries prevention
    and adjuvant therapies, 305
    and diet, 305
    and epidermolysis bullosa, 304–306
    and fissure sealants, 305
    and oral hygiene, 304–305
Carnitine
    and epidermolysis bullosa, 299, 348–349
Children
    and nutrition in epidermolysis bullosa, 289–300
    and wound management in epidermolysis bullosa, 257–263
Chorionic villus sampling
    and epidermolysis bullosa, 233
Conformation sensitive gel electrophoresis
    and epidermolysis bullosa, 225–226
CSGE. See *Conformation sensitive gel electrophoresis.*
CVS. See *Chorionic villus sampling.*

D

DC. See *Dilated cardiomyopathy.*
DEB. See *Dystrophic epidermolysis bullosa.*
Denaturing gradient gel electrophoresis
    and epidermolysis bullosa, 225–226
Denaturing high-performance liquid chromatography
    and epidermolysis bullosa, 225–227
Dental management
    and epidermolysis bullosa, 305–306
Dental treatment
    and dystrophic epidermolysis bullosa, 304
    and epidermolysis bullosa simplex, 304
    and junctional epidermolysis bullosa, 304
    and Kindler syndrome, 304
DGGE. See *Denaturing gradient gel electrophoresis.*
DHPLC. See *Denaturing high-performance liquid chromatography.*
Dilated cardiomyopathy in epidermolysis bullosa, **347–351**
    and anemia and iron overload, 349
    and carnitine deficiency, 348–349
    genetic predisposition to, 349
    management of, 349–350
    prognosis of, 350
    and selenium deficiency, 348
    virally mediated, 349
DNA sequencing
    and epidermolysis bullosa, 223–228
Dystrophic epidermolysis bullosa
    and dental treatment, 304
    dressing management for, 258, 261–263
    mild recessive and dominant, 261
    severe generalized, 261–263

Dermatol Clin 28 (2010) 445–451
doi:10.1016/S0733-8635(10)00074-4

Index

Moving?

Make sure your subscription moves with you!

To notify us of your new address, find your **Clinics Account Number** (located on your mailing label above your name), and contact customer service at:

Email: journalscustomerservice-usa@elsevier.com

800-654-2452 (subscribers in the U.S. & Canada)
314-447-8871 (subscribers outside of the U.S. & Canada)

Fax number: 314-447-8029

Elsevier Health Sciences Division
Subscription Customer Service
3251 Riverport Lane
Maryland Heights, MO 63043

*To ensure uninterrupted delivery of your subscription, please notify us at least 4 weeks in advance of move.